Cardiovascular Imaging for Clinical Practice

Edited by

Stephen J. Nicholls, MBBS, PhD, FRACP, FACC
*Assistant Professor of Molecular Medicine, Cleveland Clinic Lerner College of
Medicine of Case Western Reserve University
Cardiovascular Director, Cleveland Clinic Coordinated Center for Clinical Research
Director, Atherosclerotic Imaging Core Laboratories, Cleveland Clinic
Cleveland, OH*

Stephen G. Worthley, MBBS, PhD, FRACP
*Helpman Chair of Cardiovascular Medicine
University of Adelaide
Director, Cardiac Catheterisation and Cardiovascular Magnetic Resonance
Cardiovascular Investigation Unit
Royal Adelaide Hospital
Adelaide, Australia*

JONES AND BARTLETT PUBLISHERS
Sudbury, Massachusetts
BOSTON   TORONTO   LONDON   SINGAPORE

World Headquarters

Jones and Bartlett Publishers
40 Tall Pine Drive
Sudbury, MA 01776
978-443-5000
info@jbpub.com
www.jbpub.com

Jones and Bartlett Publishers
Canada
6339 Ormindale Way
Mississauga, Ontario L5V 1J2
Canada

Jones and Bartlett Publishers
International
Barb House, Barb Mews
London W6 7PA
United Kingdom

Jones and Bartlett's books and products are available through most bookstores and online booksellers. To contact Jones and Bartlett Publishers directly, call 800-832-0034, fax 978-443-8000, or visit our website, www.jbpub.com.

Substantial discounts on bulk quantities of Jones and Bartlett's publications are available to corporations, professional associations, and other qualified organizations. For details and specific discount information, contact the special sales department at Jones and Bartlett via the above contact information or send an email to specialsales@jbpub.com.

The authors, editor, and publisher have made every effort to provide accurate information. However, they are not responsible for errors, omissions, or for any outcomes related to the use of the contents of this book and take no responsibility for the use of the products and procedures described. Treatments and side effects described in this book may not be applicable to all people; likewise, some people may require a dose or experience a side effect that is not described herein. Drugs and medical devices are discussed that may have limited availability controlled by the Food and Drug Administration (FDA) for use only in a research study or clinical trial. Research, clinical practice, and government regulations often change the accepted standard in this field. When consideration is being given to use of any drug in the clinical setting, the healthcare provider or reader is responsible for determining FDA status of the drug, reading the package insert, and reviewing prescribing information for the most up-to-date recommendations on dose, precautions, and contraindications, and determining the appropriate usage for the product. This is especially important in the case of drugs that are new or seldom used.

Production Credits
Executive Publisher: Christopher Davis
Senior Acquisitions Editor: Alison Hankey
Editorial Assistant: Sara Cameron
Production Director: Amy Rose
Associate Production Editor: Jessica deMartin
Senior Marketing Manager: Barb Bartoszek
V.P., Manufacturing and Inventory Control: Therese Connell
Composition: Paw Print Media
Cover Design: Kristin E. Parker
Printing and Binding: Malloy, Inc.
Cover Printing: Malloy, Inc.
Cover Image: Main image: © Vesna Njagulj/Dreamstime.com. Thumbnails: © beerkoff/ShutterStock, Inc.; © John Sternig/Dreamstime.com; © Zsolt Nyulaszi/ShutterStock, Inc.; © Vesna Njagulj/Dreamstime.com

Library of Congress Cataloging-in-Publication Data
Cardiovascular imaging for clinical practice / [edited by] Stephen J. Nicholls, Stephen Worthley.
    p. ; cm.
  Includes bibliographical references and index.
  ISBN-13: 978-0-7637-5622-2
  ISBN-10: 0-7637-5622-9
  1. Cardiovascular system—Diseases—Diagnosis. 2. Diagnostic imaging. I. Nicholls, Stephen J. II. Worthley, Stephen.
    [DNLM: 1. Cardiovascular Diseases—diagnosis. 2. Diagnostic Imaging—methods. 3. Diagnostic Techniques, Cardiovascular. WG 141 C2695 2011]
  RC670.C365 2011
  616.1'075—dc22

                              2009041726

6048

Printed in the United States of America
14 13 12 11 10   10 9 8 7 6 5 4 3 2 1

DEDICATION

To Kathy, Emily, Oliver, and Angus
&
Kirsten, Will, Phoebe, and Harry

Contents

PART I: BIOLOGY OF CARDIOVASCULAR DISEASE

PART II: IMAGING TECHNOLOGIES IN
CARDIOVASCULAR DISEASE

PART III: IMAGING AND CARDIOVASCULAR RESEARCH

PART IV: IMAGING IN CLINICAL MANAGEMENT

Preface

Cardiovascular disease is the leading cause of morbidity and mortality in the Western world. Technological advances in imaging modalities enable high-resolution visualization of the cardiovascular system. This book provides the opportunity to employ cardiovascular imaging in order to enhance risk-prediction algorithms, guide invasive interventions, and monitor the response to various therapies.

This textbook presents a state-of-the-art update on the evolution of cardiovascular imaging. Part I provides a review of the biological aspects of cardiovascular disease that are important in terms of developing relevant imaging modalities. The major cardiovascular imaging modalities are described in Part II. Part III reviews imaging data from clinical research that have provided important insights into atherosclerosis progression, myocardial function, and electrical conduction within the heart. In Part IV, a practical approach to integration of cardiovascular imaging modalities into the assessment of common clinical scenarios is presented.

We are in debt to our mentors, colleagues, fellows, and patients who all strive to cure heart disease.

Stephen J. Nicholls
Stephen G. Worthley

Editors and Contributing Authors

EDITORS

Stephen J. Nicholls, MBBS, PhD, FRACP, FACC
Assistant Professor of Molecular Medicine, Cleveland Clinic Lerner College of Medicine of Case Western Reserve University
Cardiovascular Director, Cleveland Clinic Coordinated Center for Clinical Research
Director, Atherosclerotic Imaging Core Laboratories, Cleveland Clinic
Cleveland, OH

Stephen G. Worthley, MBBS, PhD, FRACP
Helpman Chair of Cardiovascular Medicine, University of Adelaide
Director, Cardiac Catheterisation and Cardiovascular Magnetic Resonance
Cardiovascular Investigation Unit, Royal Adelaide Hospital
Adelaide, Australia

CONTRIBUTING AUTHORS

Ashish Aneja, MD
Department of Cardiovascular Medicine, Heart and Vascular Institute, Cleveland Clinic
Cleveland, OH

Peter Barlis, MBBS, MPH, FRACP
Thoraxcenter, Erasmus MC,
Rotterdam, The Netherlands

Christoph R. Becker, MD
Department of Clinical Radiology, Ludwig-Maximillians-University
Munich, Germany

Juan J. Badimon, PhD, FAHA, FACC
Atherothrombosis Research Unit, Cardiovascular Institute, Mount Sinai School of Medicine
New York, NY

Antonio De Miguel, MD
Atherothrombosis Research Unit, Cardiovascular Institute, Mount Sinai School of Medicine
New York, NY
Cardiology Department, Hospital de León
León, Spain.

Hany Dimitri, MBBS, FRACP
Cardiovascular Research Centre, Department of Cardiology, Royal Adelaide Hospital and the Disciplines of Medicine and Physiology, University of Adelaide
Adelaide, Australia

Patrick J.S. Disney, MBBS, FRACP
Cardiovascular Investigation Unit, Royal Adelaide Hospital
Adelaide, Australia

Ben K. Dundon, MBBS
Cardiovascular Investigation Unit,
Royal Adelaide Hospital
Adelaide, Australia

Zahi A. Fayad, PhD, FACC, FAHA
Translational and Molecular Imaging
 Institute, Mount Sinai School of
 Medicine
New York, NY

Hector M. Garcia-Garcia, MD, MSc
Thoraxcenter, Erasmus MC
Rotterdam, The Netherlands

Nieves Gonzalo, MD
Thoraxcenter, Erasmus MC
Rotterdam, The Netherlands

Li-Fern Hsu, MBBS
Department of Cardiology,
 National Heart Centre
Singapore

Borja Ibanez, MD
Atherothrombosis Research Unit,
 Cardiovascular Institute, Mount Sinai
 School of Medicine
New York, NY
Interventional Cardiology Laboratory,
 Cardiology department, Fundación
 Jiménez Díaz-Capio
Madrid, Spain

**Jonathan M. Kalman, MBBS, PhD,
 FRACP**
Department of Cardiology,
 Royal Melbourne Hospital
Department of Medicine,
 University of Melbourne
Victoria, Australia

Theodore D. Karamitsos, MD, PhD
Center for Clinical Magnetic
 Resonance Research, Department
 of Cardiovascular Medicine, John
 Radcliffe Hospital
Oxford, United Kingdom

Philip J. Kilner, MBBS
Royal Brompton Hospital
National Heart and Lung Institute
London, United Kingdom

Pia Lundman, MD, PhD, FESC
Division of Cardiovascular Medicine,
 Department of Clinical Sciences,
 Karolinska Institutet, Danderyd
 Hospital
Stockholm, Sweden

Thomas H. Marwick, MBBS, PhD
University of Queensland
Brisbane, Australia

Vijay Nambi, MD
Section of Atherosclerosis and Vascular
 Medicine, Department of Medicine,
 Baylor College of Medicine
Center for Cardiovascular Disease
 Prevention, Methodist DeBakey
 Heart Center
Houston, TX

Tammy J. Pegg, MRCP
Department of Cardiovascular Surgery,
 University of Oxford
Oxford, United Kingdom

Kurt C. Roberts-Thomson, MBBS, PhD, FRACP
The Department of Cardiology, Brigham
  and Women's Hospital and Harvard
  Medical School
Boston, MA

Prashanthan Sanders, MBBS, PhD, FRACP
Cardiovascular Research Centre,
  Department of Cardiology, Royal
  Adelaide Hospital and the Disciplines
  of Medicine and Physiology,
  University of Adelaide
Adelaide, Australia

Christophe Scavee, MD
Université de Louvain, Cliniques
  Saint-Luc
Brussels, Belgium

Joseph B. Selvanayagam, MBBS (Hons), FRACP, DPhil
Department of Cardiology, Flinders
  Medical Centre
Adelaide, Australia

Patrick W. Serruys, MD, PhD
Thoraxcenter, Erasmus MC
Rotterdam, The Netherlands

William G. Stevenson, MD
The Department of Cardiology, Brigham
  and Women's Hospital and Harvard
  Medical School
Boston, MA

W. H. Wilson Tang, MD
Department of Cardiovascular Medicine,
  Heart and Vascular Medicine,
  Cleveland Clinic
Cleveland, OH

Karen S.L. Teo MBBS, PhD, FRACP
Cardiovascular Investigation Unit,
  Royal Adelaide Hospital
Adelaide, Australia

Louise Thomson, MBChB, FRACP
University of California, Los Angeles
Cedars-Sinai Medical Center, S. Mark
  Taper Foundation Imaging Center
Los Angeles, CA

Stuart Turner, MBBS, PhD, FRACP
Department of Cardiovascular Medicine,
  John Hunter Hospital
Newcastle, Australia

Matthew I. Worthley, MBBS, PhD, FRACP
Cardiovascular Investigation Unit, Royal
  Adelaide Hospital
Adelaide, Australia

Part I

Biology of Cardiovascular Disease

CHAPTER 1

Coronary Artery Disease, Atherobiology, and Thrombosis

Juan J. Badimon, PhD, FAHA, FACC
Borja Ibanez, MD
Antonio De Miguel, MD

INTRODUCTION

Atherothrombosis is the major cause of mortality and morbidity in Western countries, and it is predicted that coronary artery disease will be the dominant cause of mortality worldwide by 2020. The major reasons for the increase are aging of the population, increase in certain risk factors (obesity and diabetes), especially among the youth, and the adoption of an unhealthy lifestyle by developing countries. From the clinical point of view, atherosclerosis is seen as a single diffuse pathologic entity (affecting almost all vascular territories) that progresses silently but with focal clinical manifestations. This chapter is focused on the formation and progression of atherosclerotic lesions leading to high-risk/vulnerable plaques, the triggers for plaque disruption and thrombus formation, as well as potential therapies and strategies for plaque regression.

ATHEROSCLEROTIC PLAQUE HOMEOSTASIS

Atherosclerosis is a systemic disease involving the intima of large and medium-sized arteries (including the aorta, carotids, coronaries, and peripheral arteries) characterized by intimal thickening due to the accumulation of cells and lipids.[1] The deposition of these materials and the subsequent thickening of the wall may significantly compromise the residual lumen leading to ischemic events distal to the arterial stenosis.[2] Rupture or erosion of advanced lesions in coronary arteries initiates platelet activation and aggregation on the surface of the plaque and coagulation cascade activation. This results in acute thrombus formation and subsequent clinical manifestations: unstable angina, non-ST segment elevation acute coronary syndrome, ST elevation myocardial infarction, and sudden cardiac death. These thrombotic episodes largely occur in response to atherosclerotic lesions that have progressed to a high-risk inflammatory/prothrombotic stage. Thus, atherothrombosis is a complex, multifactorial process that involves the two major components (atherosclerosis plus thrombosis) from the pathogenesis of cardiovascular diseases; although distinct from one another, appear to be closely interrelated (Figure 1.1).

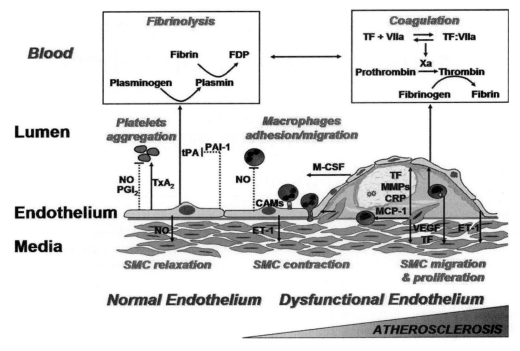

Figure 1.1

Diagram of dysfunctional endothelium and subsequent atherosclerotic lesion development. NO, nitric oxide; ET-1, endothelin; MMP, matrix metalloproteinase; PAI-1, plasminogen activator inhibitor type 1; TF, tissue factor; tPA, tissue plasminogen activator; TXA2, thromboxane A2; CAM: Cell adhesion molecule; CRP: C-reactive protein; MCP: Monocyte chemotactic protein; M-CSF: Monocyte colony stimulating factor; PGI2: Prostacyclin; SMC: Smooth muscle cell; VEGF: Vascular endothelial growth factor.

Corti R, Farkouh ME, Badimon JJ., The vulnerable plaque and acute coronary syndromes, *Am J Med*, 2002 Dec 1;113(8):668–80.

The main components of atherothrombotic plaques are: (1) connective tissue extracellular matrix, including collagen, proteoglycans, and fibronectin elastic fibers; (2) crystalline cholesterol, cholesterol esters, and phospholipids; (3) cells such as monocyte-derived macrophages, T-lymphocytes, and smooth-muscle cells; and (4) thrombotic material with platelets and fibrin deposition. Varying proportions of these components occur in different plaques, thus giving rise to a heterogeneity or spectrum of lesions.

Until recently, atherosclerosis development was seen as a constant progressive process irreversibly associated to aging. However, new evidence indicates that atherosclerotic plaque homeostasis is not necessarily a constant progressing process, and atherosclerotic plaque formation can be slowed, stopped, or even reversed[3] (Figure 1.1).

Endothelial Dysfunction

The initial pathological manifestation of atherosclerosis is a dysfunctional endothelium. Under healthy circumstances, the normally functional endothelium is a dynamic autocrine and paracrine organ that creates an antiatherogenic environment protecting against atherogenesis, since endothelial cells constantly secrete substances into the vascular lumen. This is not only to maintain vascular tone and to avoid abnormal platelet adhesion/activation and clot formation, but with anti-inflammatory and mitogenic regulation activities.[4] This protection is achieved by releasing a series of antithrombotic and vasoactive substances. It is widely accepted that metabolic endothelial dysfunction (even without any mechanical damage) is enough to trigger the pathologic processes leading to plaque formation.

Endothelial dysfunction is often the result of a disturbance in the physiological pattern of blood flow (flow reversal or oscillating shear stress) at bending points and near bifurcations.[5, 6] Therefore, there are areas of endothelium more prone to suffer lesion development, leading to the hypothesis that endothelial activity is regulated by different rheologic conditions in vascular bed. Shear stress and local hemodynamics modulate not only the clinical manifestations of the disease (thrombotic complications), but also the progression of the atherosclerotic plaques. Other than biomechanical shear stress forces (enhanced by hypertension), the coexistence of other cardiovascular risk factors is strongly correlated with the development of endothelial dysfunction.

Endothelial dysfunction is characterized by a change in the pattern of synthesis and secretion of different substances, mainly nitric oxide and prostaglandin (PG) I_2. They unleash not only the internalization and oxidation of circulating lipids into the intimal layer, but also the recruitment of inflammatory cells into the vessel wall, smooth muscle cells proliferation, extracellular matrix deposition and vasoconstriction. This is in addition to a prothrombotic state within the vessel lumen initiating the atherosclerotic process[7, 8] (Figure 1.2). As a result, there are consequences at the systemic level (promoting the activation, adhesion, and aggregation of platelets to the dysfunctional area) and vascular level (endothelial synthesis and exposure of cell adhesive proteins from the selectin superfamily [E- and P-selectins]). These proteins facilitate the homing and internalization of the circulating monocytes into the subendothelial space, where they become macrophages.

Until recently, it was believed that endothelial repair after an injury was carried out only by neighboring cells. However, recent data suggest that the endothelium can be repopulated and repaired by circulating endothelial progenitor cells. The number of these endothelial repairing cells is believed to be a marker of arterial injury in vascular disease,[9] an area of intensive ongoing research.

Cholesterol Accumulation

Lipid accumulation results from an imbalance between the mechanisms responsible for the influx and efflux of lipids into the arterial wall. Cholesterol accumulation plays a

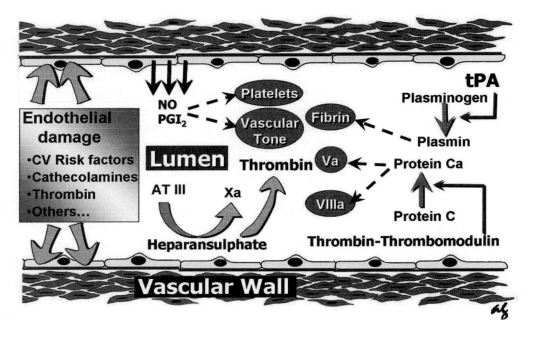

Figure 1.2

Endothelial dysfunction as hallmark of atherothrombotic disease. Simplified diagram of the role of endothelium and the physiologic anticoagulation system. CV: cardiovascular; NO: nitric oxide; tPA: tissue plasminogen activator; PGI2: prostaglandin I2.

From Badimon et al. In Fuster et al. *Hurst's the Heart.*

central role in the atherogenesis process. Low-density lipoprotein cholesterol (LDL-C) infiltrates through the arterial endothelium into the intima and binds to different matrix proteins of the subendothelial space, where it undergoes an oxidative process. This binding seems to be related to an ionic interaction of apolipoprotein (apo) B with matrix proteins, including proteoglycans, collagen, and fibronectin.[10] Secondary changes may occur in the underlying media and adventitia, particularly in advanced disease stages.

LDL is a heterogeneous group of particles that vary in their core content of cholesterol. LDL-C does not reflect the atherogenicity of all of the apo B-containing lipoproteins nor does it necessarily represent the total number of low-density lipoprotein particles (LDL-P) or the distribution of size within those particles. A greater amount of cholesterol in LDL creates larger, more buoyant particles (sometimes referred to as LDL subclass A). A smaller amount of cholesterol in LDL generates smaller, denser particles (sometimes referred to as LDL subclass B). Small dense particles of LDL-C are the ones that participate in cholesterol accumulation in atherosclerotic plaque. In two patients with the same

LDL-C level, the one with a preponderance of small dense LDL-P will have a greater number LDL-P and, more importantly, a significantly greater risk of cardiovascular disease.

There is one molecule of apo B for each LDL-C molecule. Apo B level reflects the total number of atherogenic apo B-containing lipoproteins; however, 90% of total plasma apo B is contained within the LDL-C particles.[11] Thus, for a given LDL-C level, a higher apo-B level indicates higher content of LDL-P. In addition, apo B also appears to be a better predictor of subsequent CAD events in patients on treatment with statins.[12, 13]

Oxidized cholesterol is highly toxic and, as part of a mechanism of defense, it is phagocytosed by the vessel wall macrophages. The presence of the oxidized lipids triggers a series of proinflammatory reactions via different mediators, perpetuating the activation and recruitment of monocytes-macrophages and inflammatory cells. Macrophages, by engulfing the lipid material, become foam cells. Failure of macrophages to remove cholesterol from the vessel wall promotes its apoptotic death, releasing cholesterol to the vessel wall and, more importantly, inflammatory substances like tissue factor (TF)[14] and metalloproteinases (enzymes able to digest the matrix scaffold), making atherosclerotic lesions more prone to rupture (the vulnerable plaque).[15]

Inflammation and Atherothrombosis

Inflammation is another important process playing a dual role on affecting plaque progression, vulnerability, and subsequent thrombus formation, both at the vascular and at the circulating level. It could be considered the link between atherosclerosis and thrombosis. In fact, the relation of inflammation and atherothrombosis could represent different faces of the same disease.

Development of atherosclerosis is influenced by innate and adaptive immune responses. In the first line of innate immunity, scavenger receptors (SR)-A and CD-36 are responsible for the uptake of oxidized LDL, transforming the macrophage into a foam cell,[16] which produces cytokines that activate neighboring smooth muscle cells, resulting in extracellular matrix formation and fibrosis. In the second line of innate immunity, toll-like receptors have a significant role and are involved not only in the initiation but also in the progression and expansive remodeling of atherothrombosis (fibroblast and macrophages location in the intima and adventitia, neointimal formation, intimal lesion.).[17] Adaptive immunity is much more specific than innate immunity and involves an organized immune response leading to generation of T- and B-cell receptors and immunoglobulins.

Different inflammatory markers stand out in the link between atherosclerosis and inflammation. C-reactive protein (CRP), CD40 Ligand (CD40L), interleukin (IL)-6, IL-1, and tumor necrosis factor (TNF). CRP play a proinflammatory role in activating monocyte chemotactic protein-1. CRP levels are high in patients with acute coronary syndrome and can be used to predict outcome in those patients.[18, 19] CD40L is implicated in the various stages of atherogenesis, including the initiation and progression of atherosclerotic lesions, as well as acute complications. Increased levels of soluble CD40L has been observed in unstable angina[20] and hypercholesterolemia,[21] and circulating levels have strong independent prognostic value among apparently healthy individuals.[22]

Advanced Atherosclerosis and High-Risk/Vulnerable Plaque

Continuous exposure to the systemic, proatherogenic environment increases chemotaxis of monocytes leading to lipid accumulation, necrotic core, and fibrous cap formation, evolving into advanced atherosclerosis. Vulnerability to rupture depends on several factors: (1) circumferential wall stress or cap fatigue; (2) location, size, and consistency of the atheromatous core; (3) and blood flow characteristics, particularly the impact of flow on the proximal aspect of the plaque (i.e., configuration and angulation of the plaque). Another important fact is that not all ruptured plaques lead to occlusive thrombus.[15] This observation guided the concept of vulnerable blood in addition to high-risk plaque as a modulator of the clinical manifestations of the disease.[23]

Structural and functional features characterizing these lesions also include eccentric plaque growth with compensatory enlargement of the vessel wall (known as vascular remodeling), vasa vasorum neovascularization leading to lipid core expansion and intraplaque hemorrhage. In addition, inflammation and metalloproteinase expression leads to plaque rupture, often found at the shoulder of large lipid-rich plaques.[15]

Atherosclerotic plaques undergoing remodeling are characterized by a larger lipid core, fewer smooth muscle cells, and increased macrophage infiltration.[24] As the plaque grows eccentrically within the vessel wall, remodeling triggers crucial changes within the tunica media and the adventitia (the increased activity of metalloproteinases-2 and -9 digests the internal elastic lamina, modulating the process of remodeling).

Neovascularization and blood extravasation are involved in plaque destabilization and plaque growth.[25-27] Leaky vasa vasorum with the subsequent red blood cell extravasation has been postulated as a major source for intraplaque cholesterol deposition. This change in composition, characterized by increased extracellular cholesterol within the lipid core and excessive macrophage infiltration, increases the vulnerability of the atherosclerotic lesions. In fact, there is a strong correlation between macrophage infiltration and increased vasa vasorum in human atherosclerotic lesions. Preexisting vasa vasorum in the adventitia are thought to spread into the intima, prompting intimal neovascularization,[26] but intimal disease is considered a prerequisite for vessel wall and plaque neovascularization. This is because neovessels from adventitial vasa vasorum proliferate in response to vessel wall thickness growth derived from atherosclerosis. It is well known that intraplaque hemorrhage is an event leading to plaque rupture and thrombosis. In addition, stable (fibrocalcific) plaques show reduced microvessels compared with lipid-rich and ruptured plaques.

It is important to note that lipid-rich lesions leading to acute coronary syndromes are often mildly stenotic because of significant positive remodeling and, therefore, are not detectable by contrast angiography.[28] This is very important in understanding that early

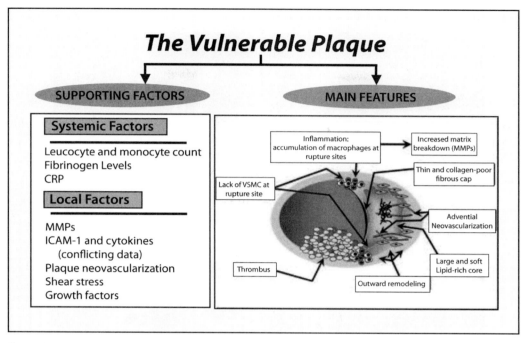

Figure 1.3

The vulnerable plaque. Features and factors associated with plaque vulnerability. MMPs: Matrix metalloproteinases; ICAM: Intercellular cell adhesion molecule; CRP: C reactive protein; VSMC: vascular smooth muscle cells.

Int J Atheroscler, 2006;1(2):143–148

detection of atherosclerosis implies the use of novel imaging modalities that can visualize not only the vessel lumen, but also the entire arterial wall.

On the other hand, the risk of suffering a thrombotic complication depends more on the biochemical and cell composition of the lesions rather than their stenotic severity. At the histological level, these lesions are mildly stenotic. They have a significant lipid-rich necrotic core, separated from the circulating blood by a thin fibrotic cap. At the cellular level, the high-risk lesions show a higher content of macrophages and inflammatory cells. The core is acellular, without the mechanical support of the collagen fibers and delimited by macrophages and cholesterol-loaded cells. The disposition of two zones with different density (fibrotic cap and lipid-rich core) makes these plaques highly unstable and prone to rupture.[15] In addition, in disrupted lesions, the inflammatory cells seem to selectively concentrate in the ruptured areas. Macrophages and mast cells, through phagocytosis and proteolytic enzymes secretion such as plasminogen activators and matrix metalloproteinases (i.e., collagenases, elastases, and gelatinases), degrade the components of extracellular matrix, contributing significantly to plaque rupture.

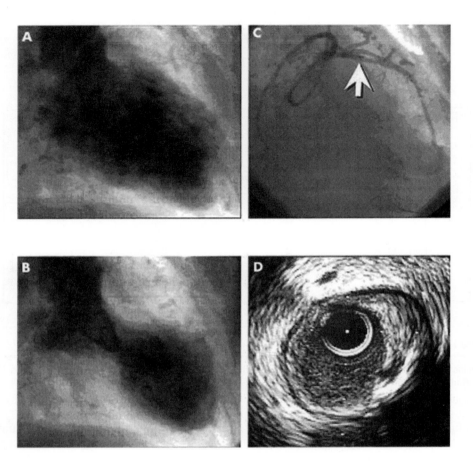

Figure 1.4

Disruption of a nonstenotic plaque leading to acute coronary syndrome. Intravascular ultrasound (IVUS) in the left anterior descending coronary artery of a patient with acute coronary syndrome. Note that contrast angiography reveals no luminal stenosis, while the IVUS clearly depicts a disrupted atherosclerotic plaque.

B Ibanez, M Cordoba, J Farre. Left main coronary artery occlusion in a patient with solitary coronary ostium in the right aortic sinus. *Heart* 2004;90:946 with permission from BMJ Publishing Group, Ltd.

THROMBOSIS FORMATION:
CELLULAR AND MOLECULAR MECHANISMS

Rupture of a high-risk vulnerable plaque changes plaque geometry and triggers coronary thrombosis, resulting in acute occlusion or subocclusion with the subsequent clinical manifestations of unstable angina, acute coronary syndrome, and sudden cardiac death. However, it is known that endothelial denudation/disruption is not an absolute prerequisite for platelet activation and attachment to the arterial wall [29] even under high shear rate conditions.[30]

Thrombus organization mediated by repaired collagen heals the rupture site, but increases plaque volume, contributing to the progression of atherothrombosis. More specifically, different factors (plaque-dependent thrombogenic substrate, rheology, and systemic procoagulant activity) may influence the magnitude and stability of the resulting thrombus and thus, the severity of the acute coronary syndrome.

Platelet Activation and Aggregation Processes

Platelets are the first blood cell to arrive at the scene of vascular damage and they can adhere directly to the dysfunctional endothelial monolayer (even in the absence of endothelial disruption), exposed collagen, and/or macrophages. Accordingly, platelets can also be activated in early stages of the atherosclerotic process. It has been postulated that platelet activation may be attributed to: (a) reduction in the mechanisms implicated in maintaining endothelial antithrombotic properties; (b) reactive oxygen species generated by atherosclerotic risk factors (in fact, the presence of hypertension, hypercholesterolemia, cigarette smoking, and diabetes correlates with a higher number of circulating activated platelets); and (c) an increase in prothrombotic and proinflammatory mediators in the circulation or immobilized on the endothelium.[31] Adhered platelets, in concert with dysfunctional endothelial cells, secrete chemotactic and growth factors, which in turn stimulates migration, accumulation and proliferation of smooth muscle cells and leukocytes in the intima layer.

The initial recognition of damaged vessel wall by platelets involves: (a) adhesion, activation, and adherence to recognition sites on the thromboactive substrate (extracellular matrix proteins such as von Willebrand Factor [vWF], collagen, fibronectin, vitronectin, laminin); (b) spreading of the platelet on the surface; and (c) aggregation of platelets to form a platelet plug or white thrombus.[32] The efficiency of platelet recruitment will depend on the underlying substrate and local geometry (local factors). A final step involving the recruitment of other blood cells also occurs. Erythrocytes, neutrophils, and, occasionally, monocytes are found on evolving mixed thrombus. Plaque rupture facilitates the interaction of inner plaque components with the circulating blood; among these components, TF exhibits a potent activating effect on platelets and coagulation.

Platelet function depends on the adhesive interaction of several compounds. Most of the glycoproteins in the platelet membrane surface are receptors for adhesive proteins or mediate cellular interactions. At the site of vascular lesions, circulating vWF binds to the exposed collagen which subsequently binds to the glycoprotein (GP) Ib/IX receptor on the platelet membrane.[33-35] Under pathological conditions and in response to changes in shear stress, vWF can be secreted from the storage organelles in platelets or endothelial cells, reinforcing the activation process. Although GPIb/IX-vWF interaction is enough to promote binding of platelets to subendothelium, it is highly transient, resulting in rapid dislocation of platelet to the site of injury. GPVI binding to matrix collagen has slower binding kinetics, but once initiated promotes a firm adhesion of platelet to the vessel surface.[36] Finally, both GPIb/IX and GPVI also regulate

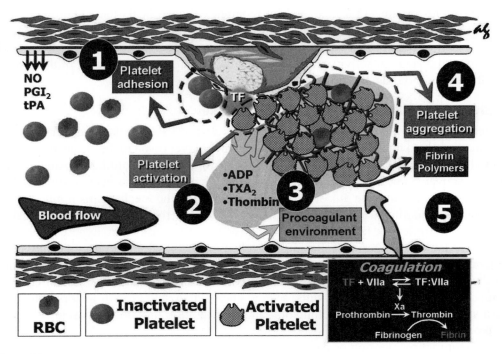

Figure 1.5

Mechanism involved in thrombus formation. Healthy endothelium (left) presents antithrombotic properties since it is able to release vascular protective substances such as nitric oxide (NO), prostacyclin (PGI2), tissue plasminogen activator (tPA), and tissue factor pathway inhibitor (TFPi). On the contrary, dysfunctional endothelium (right) not only favors platelet adhesion, activation, and aggregation, but also promotes vascular lipid deposition, macrophage migration, and tissue factor (TF) expression (activation of the coagulation cascade). Following platelet adhesion, activation is characterized by platelet shape change. Activated platelets secrete different agonists prompting activation of circulating platelets, and a procoagulant environment. This pro-thrombotic milieu will favor thrombus formation and the subsequent clinical manifestations. ADP: adenosine diphosphate; TXA2: thromboxane A2; RBC: red blood cell.

Ibanez et al. *European Heart Journal Supplements* 8(2006): G3 (Under permission of the copyright holder: Oxford University Press).

platelet-leukocyte adhesion and, thereby, are implicated in other vascular processes, such as inflammation and atherosclerosis.[37-39] Perfusion studies conducted at high shear rates have shown that vWF binds to platelet membrane glycoproteins both in adhesion (platelet-substrate interaction) and aggregation (platelet-platelet interaction), leading to thrombus formation.[40-42]

Circulating agents such as epinephrine, thrombin, serotonin, thromboxane A_2 (TXA_2), and adenosine diphosphate (ADP) are powerful platelet agonists and can also activate platelets via specific platelet surface receptors. These agonists stimulate different membrane receptors promoting subsequent platelet free-ionic Ca^{2+} release of platelet granule components in a process called platelet degranulation (discharge of platelet granule contents from the platelet dense granules). Once activated, platelets suffer a considerable shape change and ensuing calcium translocation within the platelet.

ADP plays a key role in platelet function because it amplifies the platelet response induced by other platelet agonists.[43] This ADP release from platelet granules has an autocrine effect promoting stable platelet aggregation by interacting with specific ADP receptors in the membrane (P2Y$_1$ and P2Y$_{12}$). It also promotes a paracrine effect by binding to ADP-receptors of neighboring platelets and amplifying the activation process, which are intracellular signaling events that result in activation of the GP IIb/IIIa receptor, dense granule release, amplification of platelet aggregation, platelet shape change and stabilization of the platelet aggregate. Although not activated by ADP, platelets possess a third purinergic receptor (P2X1), which is a fast adenosine triphosphate (ATP)-gated calcium channel receptor mainly involved in platelet shape change.

On the other hand, platelet activation also induces phospholipase-A$_2$ activation that triggers arachidonic acid metabolism. Platelet cyclooxygenase (COX)-1 catalyzes the conversion of arachidonic acid to PG G$_2$/H$_2$, and the latter is converted to TXA$_2$, which is released to the circulation, where it binds to thromboxane receptors thus enhancing platelet activation and vasoconstriction. Therefore, platelet activation triggers intracellular signaling and expression of platelet membrane receptors for adhesion and initiation of cell contractile processes that induce shape change and secretion of the granular contents.

On activated platelets, the expression of the integrin IIb/IIIa (αIIbβ_3) receptors for adhesive glycoprotein ligands (mainly fibrinogen and vWF) in the circulation initiates platelet-to-platelet interaction. The process is perpetuated by the arrival of platelets from the circulation. The initial binding of fibrinogen to IIb/IIIa receptor is a reversible process that is followed seconds to minutes later by an irreversible stabilization of the fibrinogen linkage to the IIb/IIIa complex. This not only results in the binding of fibrinogen but, once fibrinogen is bound inside out, signalling also occurs causing amplification of the initial signal and further platelet activation. This leads to further aggregation of platelets and accumulation at the site of vessel injury resulting in thrombus formation.

Coagulation Cascade Activation

During plaque rupture, in addition to platelet deposition in the injured area, the clotting mechanism is activated by the exposure of the plaque contents. The activation of coagulation leads to the generation of thrombin, which is a powerful platelet agonist, in addition to being an enzyme that catalyzes the formation and polymerization of fibrin. Fibrin is essential in the stabilization of the platelet thrombus and its ability to withstand removal forces by flow, shear, and high intravascular pressure. The efficacy of fibrinolytic agents demonstrates the importance of fibrin in thrombosis associated with myocardial infarction.

The blood coagulation system involves a sequence of reactions integrating zymogens (proteins susceptible to activation into enzymes via limited proteolysis) and cofactors

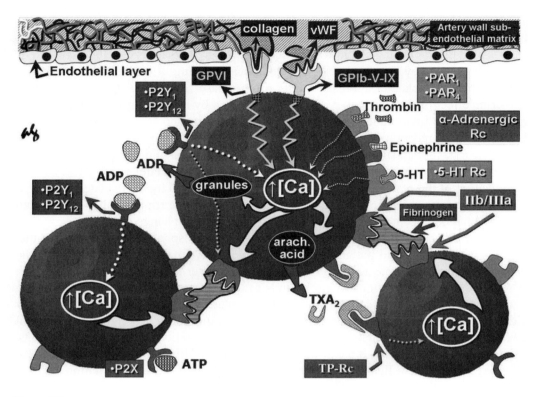

Figure 1.6

Mechanisms and agonists involved in platelet adhesion, activation, and aggregation. PAR: protease-activated receptor; GP: glycoprotein; vWF: Von Willebrand factor; TP: thromboxane receptor; TXA: thromboxane.

Ibanez et al. *European Heart Journal Supplements* 8(2006): G3 (Under permission of the copyright holder: Oxford University Press).

(nonproteolytic enzyme activators) in three groups: (1) contact activation (generation of factor XIa via the Hageman factor) and TF-dependent activation pathways; (2) the conversion of factor X to factor Xa in a complex reaction requiring the participation of factors IX and VIII; and (3) the conversion of prothrombin to thrombin and fibrin formation.[44] Platelets may provide the membrane requirements for the activation of factor X, although the participation of cells of the vessel wall (in exposed injured vessels) has not been excluded.[45]

Activated factor XI induces the activation of factor IX in the presence of Ca^{++}. Factor IXa forms a catalytic complex with factor VIII on a membrane surface and efficiently activates factor X in the presence of Ca^{++} (factors II, VII, and IX are vitamin K–dependent enzymes). Factor VIII forms a noncovalent complex with vWF in plasma, and its function in coagulation is the acceleration of the effects of IXa on the activation of X to Xa.

The TF pathway, previously known as the extrinsic coagulation pathway, through the TF-factor VIIa complex in the presence of Ca^{++}, induces the formation of Xa. A second TF-dependent reaction catalyzes the transformation of IX into IXa. TF is an integral membrane protein that serves to initiate the activation of factors IX and X and to localize the reaction to cells on which TF is expressed. Other cofactors include factor VIIIa, which binds to platelets and forms the binding site for IXa, thereby forming the machinery for the activation of X; and factor Va, which binds to platelets and provides a binding site for Xa.

Activated platelets provide a procoagulant surface for the assembly and expression of both intrinsic Xase and prothrombinase enzymatic complexes. These complexes respectively catalyze the activation of factor X to factor Xa and prothrombin to thrombin. The expression of activity is associated with the binding of both of the proteases, factor IXa and factor Xa, and the cofactors, VIIIa and Va, to procoagulant surfaces. The binding of IXa and Xa is promoted by VIIIa and Va, respectively, such that Va, and likely VIIIa, provide the equivalent of receptors for the proteolytic enzymes. The surface of the platelet expresses the procoagulant phospholipids that bind coagulation factors and contribute to the procoagulant activity of the cell.[46]

Activated Xa converts prothrombin into thrombin. The complex that catalyzes the formation of thrombin consists of factors Xa and Va in a 1:1 complex. The interaction of the four components of the prothrombinase complex (Xa, Va, phospholipid, and Ca^{++}) enhances the efficiency of the reaction.[46] Thrombin acts on multiple substrates, including fibrinogen, factor XIII, factors V and VIII, and protein C, in addition to its effects on platelets. It plays a central role in hemostasis and thrombosis. The catalytic transformation of fibrinogen into fibrin is essential in the formation of the hemostatic plug and in the formation of arterial thrombi. Thrombin binds to the fibrinogen central domain and cleaves fibrinopeptides A and B, resulting in the formation of fibrin monomer and polymer formation.[47] The fibrin mesh holds the platelets together and contributes to the attachment of the thrombus to the vessel wall.

Role of Local Factors in the Regulation of Coronary Thrombosis

The cellular and molecular mechanisms of platelet deposition and thrombus formation following vascular damage are modulated by the type of injury, the local geometry at the site damage (degree of stenosis), and local hemodynamic conditions.[48-51] Similarly, three major factors also determine the vulnerability of the fibrous cap: (1) circumferential wall stress, or cap fatigue; (2) lesion characteristics (location, size, and consistency); and (3) blood-flow.[52]

Effects Derived from the Severity of Vessel Wall Damage

Exposure of de-endothelialized vessel wall, native fibrillar collagen type I bundles with a rough surface, or atherosclerotic plaque components at similar blood shear rate conditions

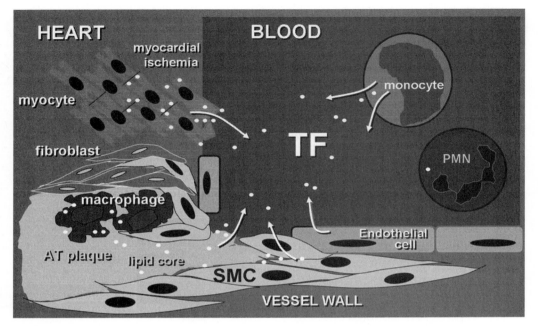

Figure 1.7

Suggested sources of circulating Tissue Factor (TF). PMN: polymorphonuclear leukocytes; AT: atherosclerotic; SMC: smooth muscle cell.

From Badimon et al. In Fuster et al. *Hurst's the Heart.*

leads to increasing degrees of platelet deposition.[48] Thromboplastin or TF, readily available in the atherosclerotic intimal space exposed by endothelial loss, contributes to the high thrombogenicity of atherosclerotic plaques.[53] Overall, it is likely that when injury to the vessel wall is mild, the thrombogenic stimulus is relatively limited and the resulting thrombotic occlusion is transient, as occurs in unstable angina. On the other hand, deep vessel injury secondary to plaque rupture or ulceration results in exposure of collagen, TF, and other elements of the vessel matrix, leading to relatively persistent thrombotic occlusion and subsequent acute myocardial infarction. The analysis of the relative contribution of different components of human atherosclerotic plaques show that atheromatous core is up to six times more active than the other substrates in triggering thrombosis.[54] Other common features directly related to higher plaque thrombogenicity are high density of activated inflammatory (monocytes/macrophages) and T-cells, downregulation expression of lysil-oxidase in vascular wall cells due to LDL, cell apoptosis and microparticles with procoagulant activity and postulated apoptotic origin, and matrix metalloproteinases secretion.

Effects Derived from Geometry

The degree of stenosis caused by the ruptured plaque and the overlying mural thrombi are also key factors for determining thrombogenicity at the local arterial site. Acute platelet deposition after plaque rupture is highly modulated by the degree of narrowing after rupture. Thus, changes in geometry may increase platelet deposition, whereas sudden growth of thrombus at the injury site may create further stenosis and thrombotic occlusion.[50, 55]

Spontaneous lysis of thrombus does occur, but the presence of a residual mural thrombus creates a predisposition to recurrent thrombotic vessel occlusion. Two main contributing factors for the development of rethrombosis have been identified: (1) platelet deposition increases with increasing degrees of vessel stenosis; and (2) fragmented thrombus appears to present one of the most powerful thrombogenic surfaces. The fact that a clear predilection exists for lesion formation at arterial branch points strongly indicates the important influence of local hemodynamics and rheologic conditions on atherosclerosis.

Role of Systemic Factors in the Regulation of Coronary Thrombosis

The severity of coronary thrombosis and associated acute coronary syndrome is modulated by the magnitude and/or stability of the formed thrombus. Once a plaque ruptures, in addition to the local factors, there are circulating systemic factors that modulate, predispose, or lead to acute coronary syndrome. This knowledge leads to the concept of vulnerable patient as a composite of vulnerable plaque plus vulnerable blood.[56, 57] Two major pathways are deeply involved in systemic procoagulant activity: coronary risk factors and circulating tissue factor (hyper-thrombotic state triggered by systemic factors).

Systemic factors, including elevated LDL, decreased high-density lipoprotein cholesterol (HDL-C), cigarette smoking, diabetes, and disregulated hemostasis, are associated with increased thrombotic complications.[57-60]

TF, a major local player in the vulnerability and thrombogenicity of atherosclerotic plaques, is highly expressed in atherosclerotic plaques, and its content has been related to plaque thrombogenicity.[61] Increased levels of circulating TF activity seems to be associated with cardiovascular risk factors. Improvement in glycemic control showed a reduction in circulating TF, suggesting that circulating TF may be the mechanism of action responsible for the increased thrombotic complications associated with the presence of these cardiovascular risk factors.[62]

Thrombogenic systemic factors can be modulated by controlling the cardiovascular risk factors and by dietary and pharmacologic strategies. Currently, it is well known that inflammatory circulating markers correlate with cardiovascular events and severity of the disease. Therefore, atherosclerosis and inflammation could represent different faces of the same disease. Several inflammatory markers are being postulated as having a significant prognostic value for recurrent cardiovascular events.[63] However, it is clear that the best weapon for treating inflammation in cardiovascular disease is an aggressive management of all the cardiovascular risk factors (i.e., statins, angiotensin converting enzyme-inhibitor, hypoglycemic agents, and antiplatelet agents). Interestingly, the use of these therapeutic interventions have been demonstrated to not only offer significant benefits, but to reduce the systemic levels of proinflammatory markers.[63]

PLAQUE REGRESSION: EMERGING THERAPIES LEADING TO PLAQUE REGRESSION

Atherosclerosis is initiated by the deposition, retention, and oxidative modification of apo-B-containing lipoproteins, notably LDL, within the subendothelial space in the vessel wall. This triggers the recruitment of inflammatory cells, a defensive mechanism that by self-perpetuation becomes injurious and leads to the development and progression of atherosclerotic lesions. The accumulation of lipid material is the result of an imbalance between the influx and efflux of cholesterol within the arterial wall. The mechanism responsible for the influx of cholesterol is mostly driven by the plasma levels of low-density lipoprotein LDL-C, while apo A-I/HDL-C seems to be responsible for its efflux.[3, 64, 65]

Reverse Cholesterol Transport

The discovery that intravascular deposition of cholesterol is not an irreversible process led to the concept of reverse cholesterol transport (RCT). RCT is the transfer of excess cholesterol from lipid-laden macrophages (foam cells) present in peripheral tissues to the liver via HDL particles, with subsequent catabolism of cholesterol or excretion into bile. Therefore, atherosclerosis can regress and regression is often accompanied by changes in plaque composition favoring stability and decreased likelihood of rupture (Figure 1.8).

In the vessel wall, cholesterol ester stored in macrophages can be converted to free cholesterol by cholesterol ester hydrolase, whereas acyl-cholesterol acyltransferase can esterify cholesterol within macrophages to form atherogenic foam cells. The liver and intestine synthesize lipid-poor apo A-I, which can interact with the adenosine triphosphate–binding cassette transporter A1 (ABCA1), located on the arterial macrophages, transporting free cholesterol to the extracellular lipid-poor HDL. Lipidation of the HDL particles generates nascent (pre-α) HDL. Subsequently, lecithin-cholesterol acyltransferase (LCAT) esterifies free cholesterol within nascent HDL to produce mature α-HDL particles (i.e., HDL3 [smaller, more dense particles] and HDL2 [larger, less dense particles]). These mature α-HDL particles can further take up free cholesterol via the macrophage adenosine triphosphate–binding cassette transporter G1 (ABCG1). Interconversion of mature α-HDL subspecies (HDL3 and HDL2) can occur in the arterial wall and in plasma mediated by hepatic lipase, endothelial lipase, and LCAT. Mature HDL has at least two metabolic fates: (1) in the direct pathway of hepatic cholesterol uptake, cholesteryl esters contained within HDL can undergo selective uptake by hepatocytes and steroid hormone–producing cells via the SR-B1 following catabolism and subsequent excre-

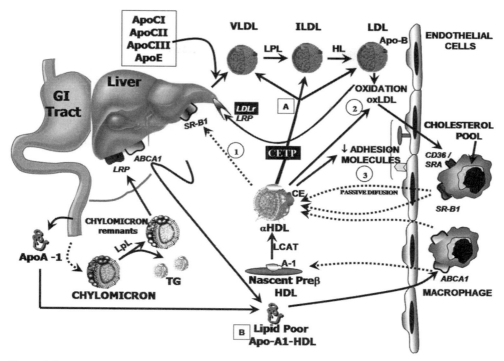

Figure 1.8

Schematic view of cholesterol metabolism and reverse cholesterol transport. CATP: cholesterol ester transfer protein; LRP: lipoprotein receptor protein; LCAT: lecithin-cholesterol acyltransferase; OXLDL: oxydized low-density lipoprotein; HDL: high-density lipoprotein; VLDL: very low-density lipoprotein; ILDL: intermediate low-density lipoprotein; ABC A1: ATP-binding cassette A1; SR-B1: scavenger receptor B1; LPL: lipoprotein lipase; TG: triglyceride; GI: gastrointenstinal; APO: apolipoprotein.

Choi BG, Vilahur G, Yadegar D, Viles-Gonzalez JF, Badimon JJ. The role of high-density lipoprotein cholesterol in the prevention and possible treatment of cardiovascular diseases. *Curr Mol Med* 2006 Aug;6(5):571–87.

tion into the bile; (2) in the indirect pathway, cholesteryl esters within HDL particles can be moved to apolipoprotein B–rich particles (LDL and very low-density lipoprotein [VLDL] particles) through the action of cholesteryl ester transfer protein (CETP). The VLDL- and LDL-C can be taken up by LDL receptors in the liver or be transported back to the vessel wall, releasing cholesterol inside the vessel wall. The understanding of this process led to the development of therapies aiming to increase HDL with the purpose of increasing RCT.[66]

In addition to its major role in RCT, HDL has other biologic activities that may contribute to its protective effects against atherosclerosis. These include antithrombotic/profibrinolytic effects, antioxidant effects, anti-inflammatory effects, and vasoprotective effects.[66]

HDL particles can vary substantially in size, density, composition, and functional properties, potentially affecting their relationship to atherosclerosis. Furthermore, levels of plasma HDL do not predict its functionality. Particle size is an important predictor of HDL function. Some analyses suggest that small particles are anti-inflammatory, while others indicate that small particles may not be protective in settings of increased oxidative stress.[67-70] The apolipoproteins within HDL are significant determinants of its function.[71] The major HDL apolipoprotein, apo A-I, helps to stimulate the activity of ABCA1 and lecithin-cholesterol acyltransferase and is a ligand for scavenger receptor type B1.[72] On the other hand, apo A-II, another component of HDL, has been shown to be proatherogenic in animal models[72] Thus, therapeutic strategies that selectively increase apo A-I levels may be more atheroprotective than those that increase levels of both apo A-I and apo A-II.

In humans, LDL-C can be lowered effectively with statins therapy, and successive guidelines have advocated progressively lower LDL-C targets. Currently, 70 mg/dl (1.8 mmol/l) has been suggested for secondary prevention in the patients with highest risk. Despite the effect on LDL-C seen at 6 weeks with intensive statin treatment atherosclerotic plaque regression needs longer (1 or 2 years), showing that long treatments with statins are needed in order to induce lesion regression.[73] In isolation, even with optimal LDL-C lowering, LDL-C reduction with statins prevents only a minority of vascular events. There remains a relatively high risk of atherothrombotic events, and from epidemiological observations, HDL-C is considered a stronger predictor of risk than LDL-C. Increased cardiovascular risk associated with low HDL-C persists at all levels of LDL-C and there also seems to be synergy such that the effects of HDL-C are much more pronounced where non-HDL-C is low. This suggests that a clinical strategy of simultaneously lowering LDL-C to reduce cholesterol deposition in the vessel wall, and raising HDL-C to promote reverse cholesterol transport, might produce considerable plaque regression. Emerging strategies for additional atherosclerosis treatment include increasing HDL-C to promote reverse cholesterol transport and direct targeting of plaque inflammation and macrophage lipid metabolism.

Potentially beneficial effects of HDL increase include reverse cholesterol transport HDL-C and anti-inflammatory and antioxidant actions in vitro.[74, 75] One mechanism of benefit from HDL increase could be improvement in endothelial function observed after infusion of reconstituted HDL.[76] Currently available lipid-modifying agents that can raise HDL-C include statins, fibrates and nicotinic acid. Emerging HDL related strategies include the APO-AI mimetics and the inhibition of CETP. Above all, appropriate strategies to increase HDL-C include aggressive overall lifestyle modification: regular aerobic exercise, tobacco cessation, moderate intake of alcohol (30–40g per day), weight loss, and diets in rich polyunsaturated fats.

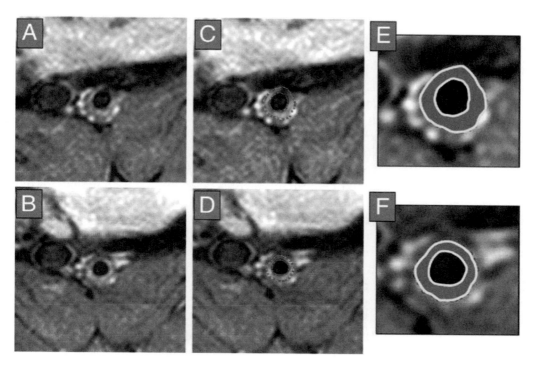

Figure 1.9

Atherosclerotic Plaque Regression in an Animal Receiving Recombinant apoA-IMilano. Magnetic resonance images before (A) and after (B) treatment at the same level of the abdominal aorta. (C and D) The same images as panels A and B but highlighting the autotracing of luminal and total vessel area contours. (E and F) Magnification of panels A and B drawing the plaque area. Plaque size in this segment regressed by 20.5% after 2 doses of apoA-IMilano. Apo: apolipoprotein.

Ibanez B et al. Rapid change in plaque size, composition, and molecular footprint after recombinant apolipoprotein A-1$_{Milano}$ (ETC-216) administration. *J Am Coll Cardiol* 2008; 51:1104–1109.

Emerging Therapies Raising HDL-C Levels

Epidemiological evidence has associated high levels of HDL cholesterol/apo A-I with protection against atherosclerotic disease.[3, 65 77] Recently, research efforts have been focused in ApoA-I$_{Milano}$, a naturally occurring mutation of apoA-I with potent antiatherogenic properties. Benefits associated with the administration of the recombinant form of apoA-I$_{Milano}$ (rApoA-I$_M$) have been described in experimental models of atherosclerosis[78-80] and even in humans.[81] Acute administration of rApoA-I$_M$ induces a rapid regression of advanced atherosclerotic lesions in a rabbit model of atherosclerosis, and the rapid plaque regression observed was associated with molecular changes suggesting a transition to a more stable plaque phenotype[82] (Figure 1.9). A limitation of current apoA-I mimetics, though, is that they must be administered parenterally because gastrointestinal proteases prevent effective oral use. Novel apoA-I oral peptides are currently under active investigation.

Another potential intervention to raise HDL-C is the inhibition of CETP. Torcetrapib, a CETP inhibitor, was tested in several clinical trials.[83, 84] Despite significant increases in HDL-C levels, the trial was stopped because torcetrapib therapy resulted in an increased risk of mortality and morbidity of unknown mechanism.[85] Whether this deleterious effect was related to a class effect should be further tested. Preliminary observations have shown that a different CETP inhibitor (RO4607381) has some differences in side effects (i.e., this novel compound does not increase blood pressure as torcetrapib[83]). While it is well known that lipid-poor Apo A-I-HDL binds avidly to macrophages removing their cholesterol, there is no information on the fate of the spherical, and perhaps dysfunctional, big HDL-C particles generated by CETP inhibition. Following this observation, it could be argued that the quality of HDL, rather than the quantity, is the major determinant of the beneficial effect on cardiovascular events prevention. This is because accumulation of cholesteryl ester in large HDL particles may increase the measured level of HDL-C but does not necessarily indicate increased functionality in respect of reverse cholesterol transport.

Targeting Atherogenesis at the Plaque Level

Modifications of LDL-C and HDL-C previously described may have indirect effects on plaque biology, but there is also increasing interest in developing direct plaque interventions. Targets include inflammation and thrombogenicity, and pathways of cholesterol uptake and efflux from macrophages. Many genes involved in macrophage lipid homeostasis and the inflammatory process are collectively under the control of certain transcriptional regulators (notably peroxisome proliferator activated receptors [PPARs] and liver X receptors [LXRs]). Fibrate and thiazolidinedione (glitazone) drugs are agonists of PPARα and PPARγ, respectively. One attractive strategy is to increase evacuation of foam cell cholesterol by upregulating expression of the ABCA-1 membrane transporters that mediate cholesterol transfer from cells to HDL that are under the transcriptional control of the PPAR and LXR families.

Despite initial enthusiasm because of reduced progression of atherosclerosis with rosiglitazone therapy,[86] successive data have shown serious adverse cardiovascular effects of treatment with rosiglitazone. Rosiglitazone was associated with a significant increase in the risk of myocardial infarction and with an increase in the risk of death from cardiovascular causes.[87] More research is required before there is widespread adoption of the glitazones as antiatherosclerotic treatments. For instance, rosiglitazone and pioglitazone differ markedly in their effects on lipids, in particular on triglycerides and LDL-C.[88] Further PPAR agonists are under development, including combined agonists of PPARα and PPARα.

LXR agonists are also under development, but one problem might be lack of specificity. Current LXR agonists under investigation seem able to activate expression of ATP-binding cassette proteins, and have provided encouraging preliminary effects in mouse atherosclerosis.[89] However, direct translation to human use will require the development of more specific LXR agonists because currently available drugs have been associated with the development of hepatic steatosis.

The enzyme acyl-cholesterol acyltransferasa (ACAT) esterifies cholesterol within macrophages to form atherogenic foam cells. Enzymes with ACAT activity are present in multiple tissues including the liver and intestine (in the context of atherosclerosis, the ACAT-1 subtype is present in macrophages). In human patients with coronary atherosclerosis, addition of the ACAT inhibitor avasimibe to standard treatment, including statins, had no beneficial effect on plaque size assessed by intravascular ultrasound.[90]

◇◇◇◇◇◇◇◇◇◇◇◇

REFERENCES

1. Corti R, Badimon JJ. Biologic aspects of vulnerable plaque. *Curr Opin Cardiol.* Nov 2002;17(6):616-625.
2. Fuster V, Fayad ZA, Moreno PR, Poon M, Corti R, Badimon JJ. Atherothrombosis and high-risk plaque: Part II: approaches by noninvasive computed tomographic/magnetic resonance imaging. *J Am Coll Cardiol.* Oct 4 2005;46(7):1209-1218.
3. Badimon JJ, Badimon L, Galvez A, Dische R, Fuster V. High density lipoprotein plasma fractions inhibit aortic fatty streaks in cholesterol-fed rabbits. *Lab Invest.* Mar 1989;60(3):455-461.
4. Bonetti PO, Lerman LO, Lerman A. Endothelial dysfunction: a marker of atherosclerotic risk. *Arterioscler Thromb Vasc Biol.* Feb 1 2003;23(2):168-175.
5. Ravensbergen J, Ravensbergen JW, Krijger JK, Hillen B, Hoogstraten HW. Localizing role of hemodynamics in atherosclerosis in several human vertebrobasilar junction geometries. *Arterioscler Thromb Vasc Biol.* May 1998;18(5):708-716.
6. Nerem RM. Vascular fluid mechanics, the arterial wall, and atherosclerosis. *Journal of biomechanical engineering.* Aug 1992;114(3):274-282.
7. Ignarro LJ, Napoli C. Novel features of nitric oxide, endothelial nitric oxide synthase, and atherosclerosis. *Curr Atheroscler Rep.* Jul 2004;6(4):281-287.
8. Voetsch B, Jin RC, Loscalzo J. Nitric oxide insufficiency and atherothrombosis. *Histochemistry and Cell Biology.* Oct 2004;122(4):353-367.
9. Hill JM, Zalos G, Halcox JP, Schenke WH, Waclawiw MA, Quyyumi AA, Finkel T. Circulating endothelial progenitor cells, vascular function, and cardiovascular risk. *N Engl J Med.* Feb 13 2003;348(7):593-600.
10. Khalil MF, Wagner WD, Goldberg IJ. Molecular interactions leading to lipoprotein retention and the initiation of atherosclerosis. *Arterioscler Thromb Vasc Biol.* Dec 2004;24(12):2211-2218.
11. Sniderman AD. How, when, and why to use apolipoprotein B in clinical practice. *Am J Cardiol.* Oct 17 2002;90(8A):48i-54i.
12. Barter PJ, Ballantyne CM, Carmena R, Castro Cabezas M, Chapman MJ, Couture P, de Graaf J, Durrington PN, Faergeman O, Frohlich J, Furberg CD, Gagne C, Haffner SM, Humphries SE, Jungner I, Krauss RM, Kwiterovich P, Marcovina S, Packard CJ, Pearson TA, Reddy KS, Rosenson R, Sarrafzadegan N, Sniderman AD, Stalenhoef AF, Stein E, Talmud PJ, Tonkin AM, Walldius G, Williams KM. Apo B versus cholesterol in estimating cardiovascular risk and in guiding therapy: report of the thirty-person/ten-country panel. *J Intern Med.* Mar 2006;259(3):247-258.

13. Gotto AM, Jr., Whitney E, Stein EA, Shapiro DR, Clearfield M, Weis S, Jou JY, Langendorfer A, Beere PA, Watson DJ, Downs JR, de Cani JS. Relation between baseline and on-treatment lipid parameters and first acute major coronary events in the Air Force/Texas Coronary Atherosclerosis Prevention Study (AFCAPS/TexCAPS). *Circulation.* Feb 8 2000;101(5):477-484.

14. Hutter R, Valdiviezo C, Sauter BV, Savontaus M, Chereshnev I, Carrick FE, Bauriedel G, Luderitz B, Fallon JT, Fuster V, Badimon JJ. Caspase-3 and tissue factor expression in lipid-rich plaque macrophages: evidence for apoptosis as link between inflammation and atherothrombosis. *Circulation.* Apr 27 2004;109(16):2001-2008.

15. Vilahur G, Ibanez B, Badimon J. Characteristic Features of Atherosclerotic Plaques that are Vulnerable to Rupture. Brief Review. *Int J Atheroscler.* 2006;1(2):143-148.

16. Hansson GK. Immune mechanisms in atherosclerosis. *Arterioscler Thromb Vasc Biol.* Dec 2001;21(12):1876-1890.

17. Hollestelle SC, De Vries MR, Van Keulen JK, Schoneveld AH, Vink A, Strijder CF, Van Middelaar BJ, Pasterkamp G, Quax PH, De Kleijn DP. Toll-like receptor 4 is involved in outward arterial remodeling. *Circulation.* Jan 27 2004;109(3):393-398.

18. Liuzzo G, Biasucci LM, Gallimore JR, Grillo RL, Rebuzzi AG, Pepys MB, Maseri A. The prognostic value of C-reactive protein and serum amyloid a protein in severe unstable angina. *N Engl J Med.* Aug 18 1994;331(7):417-424.

19. Ridker PM, Cushman M, Stampfer MJ, Tracy RP, Hennekens CH. Inflammation, aspirin, and the risk of cardiovascular disease in apparently healthy men. *N Engl J Med.* Apr 3 1997;336(14):973-979.

20. Aukrust P, Muller F, Ueland T, Berget T, Aaser E, Brunsvig A, Solum NO, Forfang K, Froland SS, Gullestad L. Enhanced levels of soluble and membrane-bound CD40 ligand in patients with unstable angina. Possible reflection of T lymphocyte and platelet involvement in the pathogenesis of acute coronary syndromes. *Circulation.* Aug 10 1999;100(6):614-620.

21. Cipollone F, Mezzetti A, Porreca E, Di Febbo C, Nutini M, Fazia M, Falco A, Cuccurullo F, Davi G. Association between enhanced soluble CD40L and prothrombotic state in hypercholesterolemia: effects of statin therapy. *Circulation.* Jul 23 2002;106(4):399-402.

22. Schonbeck U, Varo N, Libby P, Buring J, Ridker PM. Soluble CD40L and cardiovascular risk in women. *Circulation.* Nov 6 2001;104(19):2266-2268.

23. Naghavi M, Falk E, Hecht HS, Jamieson MJ, Kaul S, Berman D, Fayad Z, Budoff MJ, Rumberger J, Naqvi TZ, Shaw LJ, Faergeman O, Cohn J, Bahr R, Koenig W, Demirovic J, Arking D, Herrera VL, Badimon J, Goldstein JA, Rudy Y, Airaksinen J, Schwartz RS, Riley WA, Mendes RA, Douglas P, Shah PK. From vulnerable plaque to vulnerable patient--Part III: Executive summary of the Screening for Heart Attack Prevention and Education (SHAPE) Task Force report. *Am J Cardiol.* Jul 17 2006;98(2A):2H-15H.

24. Ward MR, Pasterkamp G, Yeung AC, Borst C. Arterial remodeling. Mechanisms and clinical implications. *Circulation.* Sep 5 2000;102(10):1186-1191.

25. Moreno PR, Purushothaman KR, Fuster V, Echeverri D, Truszczynska H, Sharma SK, Badimon JJ, O'Connor WN. Plaque neovascularization is increased in ruptured atherosclerotic lesions of human aorta: implications for plaque vulnerability. *Circulation.* Oct 5 2004;110(14):2032-2038.

26. Virmani R, Kolodgie FD, Burke AP, Finn AV, Gold HK, Tulenko TN, Wrenn SP, Narula J. Atherosclerotic plaque progression and vulnerability to rupture: angiogenesis as a source of intraplaque hemorrhage. *Arterioscler Thromb Vasc Biol.* Oct 2005;25(10):2054-2061.

27. Fuster V, Moreno PR, Fayad ZA, Corti R, Badimon JJ. Atherothrombosis and high-risk plaque: part I: evolving concepts. *J Am Coll Cardiol.* Sep 20 2005;46(6):937-954.

28. Ibanez B, Navarro F, Cordoba M, Marcos-Alberca P, Farre J. Tako-tsubo transient left ventricular apical ballooning: is intravascular ultrasound the key to resolve the enigma? *Heart.* Jan 2005;91(1):102-104.

29. Massberg S, Brand K, Gruner S, Page S, Muller E, Muller I, Bergmeier W, Richter T, Lorenz M, Konrad I, Nieswandt B, Gawaz M. A critical role of platelet adhesion in the initiation of atherosclerotic lesion formation. *J Exp Med.* Oct 7 2002;196(7):887-896.

30. Massberg S, Gruner S, Konrad I, Garcia Arguinzonis MI, Eigenthaler M, Hemler K, Kersting J, Schulz C, Muller I, Besta F, Nieswandt B, Heinzmann U, Walter U, Gawaz M. Enhanced in vivo platelet adhesion in vasodilator-stimulated phosphoprotein (VASP)-deficient mice. *Blood.* Jan 1 2004;103(1):136-142.

31. Huo Y, Ley KF. Role of platelets in the development of atherosclerosis. *Trends Cardiovasc Med.* Jan 2004;14(1):18-22.

32. Ibanez B, Vilahur G, Badimon J. Pharmacology of thienopyridines: rationale for dual pathway inhibition *Eur Heart J Suppl.* 2006;8:G3-G9.

33. Ruggeri ZM. Mechanisms initiating platelet thrombus formation. *Thromb Haemost.* Jul 1997;78(1):611-616.

34. Ruggeri ZM. Platelets in atherothrombosis. *Nat Med.* Nov 2002;8(11):1227-1234.

35. Alevriadou BR, Moake JL, Turner NA, Ruggeri ZM, Folie BJ, Phillips MD, Schreiber AB, Hrinda ME, McIntire LV. Real-time analysis of shear-dependent thrombus formation and its blockade by inhibitors of von Willebrand factor binding to platelets. *Blood.* Mar 1 1993;81(5):1263-1276.

36. Nieswandt B, Watson SP. Platelet-collagen interaction: is GPVI the central receptor? *Blood.* Jul 15 2003;102(2):449-461.

37. Gawaz M. Role of platelets in coronary thrombosis and reperfusion of ischemic myocardium. *Cardiovasc Res.* Feb 15 2004;61(3):498-511.

38. Andrews RK, Gardiner EE, Shen Y, Berndt MC. Platelet interactions in thrombosis. *IUBMB life.* Jan 2004;56(1):13-18.

39. Weyrich AS, Lindemann S, Zimmerman GA. The evolving role of platelets in inflammation. *J Thromb Haemost.* Sep 2003;1(9):1897-1905.

40. Coughlin SR. Thrombin receptor structure and function. *Thromb Haemost.* Jul 1 1993;70(1):184-187.

41. Sakariassen KS, Bolhuis PA, Sixma JJ. Human blood platelet adhesion to artery subendothelium is mediated by factor VIII-Von Willebrand factor bound to the subendothelium. *Nature.* Jun 14 1979;279(5714):636-638.

42. Badimon L, Badimon JJ, Turitto VT, Fuster V. Role of von Willebrand factor in mediating platelet-vessel wall interaction at low shear rate; the importance of perfusion conditions. *Blood.* Mar 1989;73(4):961-967.

43. Cattaneo M, Gachet C. ADP receptors and clinical bleeding disorders. *Arterioscler Thromb Vasc Biol.* Oct 1999;19(10):2281-2285.

44. Viles-Gonzalez JF, Badimon JJ. Atherothrombosis: the role of tissue factor. *Int J Biochem Cell Biol.* Jan 2004;36(1):25-30.

45. Nemerson Y. *Mechanisms of coagulation.* New York: McGraw-Hill; 1990.

46. Mann KG. *Membrane-bound enzyme complexes in blood coagulation.* New York: Grunne & Stratton; 1984.

47. Comp PC. *Kinetics of plasma coagulation factors.* New York: McGraw-Hill; 1990.

48. Badimon L, Badimon JJ, Turitto VT, Vallabhajosula S, Fuster V. Platelet thrombus formation on collagen type I. A model of deep vessel injury. Influence of blood rheology, von Willebrand factor, and blood coagulation. *Circulation.* Dec 1988;78(6):1431-1442.

49. Badimon L, Badimon JJ, Galvez A, Chesebro JH, Fuster V. Influence of arterial damage and wall shear rate on platelet deposition. Ex vivo study in a swine model. *Arteriosclerosis.* May-Jun 1986;6(3):312-320.

50. Badimon L, Badimon JJ. Mechanisms of arterial thrombosis in nonparallel streamlines: platelet thrombi grow on the apex of stenotic severely injured vessel wall. Experimental study in the pig model. *J Clin Invest.* Oct 1989;84(4):1134-1144.

51. Lassila R, Badimon JJ, Vallabhajosula S, Badimon L. Dynamic monitoring of platelet deposition on severely damaged vessel wall in flowing blood. Effects of different stenoses on thrombus growth. *Arteriosclerosis.* Mar-Apr 1990;10(2):306-315.

52. Fuster V, Badimon L, Badimon JJ, Chesebro JH. The pathogenesis of coronary artery disease and the acute coronary syndromes (1). *N Engl J Med.* Jan 23 1992;326(4):242-250.

53. Mackman N. Role of tissue factor in hemostasis, thrombosis, and vascular development. *Arterioscler Thromb Vasc Biol.* Jun 2004;24(6):1015-1022.

54. Fernandez-Ortiz A, Badimon JJ, Falk E, Fuster V, Meyer B, Mailhac A, Weng D, Shah PK, Badimon L. Characterization of the relative thrombogenicity of atherosclerotic plaque components: implications for consequences of plaque rupture. *J Am Coll Cardiol.* Jun 1994;23(7):1562-1569.

55. Frojmovic M, Nash G, Diamond SL. Definitions in biorheology: cell aggregation and cell adhesion in flow. Recommendation of the Scientific Subcommittee on Biorheology of the Scientific and Standardisation Committee of the International Society on Thrombosis and Haemostasis. *Thromb Haemost.* Apr 2002;87(4):771.

56. Naghavi M, Libby P, Falk E, Casscells SW, Litovsky S, Rumberger J, Badimon JJ, Stefanadis C, Moreno P, Pasterkamp G, Fayad Z, Stone PH, Waxman S, Raggi P, Madjid M, Zarrabi A, Burke A, Yuan C, Fitzgerald PJ, Siscovick DS, de Korte CL, Aikawa M, Juhani Airaksinen KE, Assmann G, Becker CR, Chesebro JH, Farb A, Galis ZS, Jackson C, Jang IK, Koenig W, Lodder RA, March K, Demirovic J, Navab M, Priori SG, Rekhter MD, Bahr R, Grundy SM, Mehran R, Colombo A, Boerwinkle E, Ballantyne C, Insull W, Jr., Schwartz RS, Vogel R, Serruys PW, Hansson GK, Faxon DP, Kaul S, Drexler H, Greenland P, Muller JE, Virmani R, Ridker PM, Zipes DP, Shah PK, Willerson JT. From vulnerable plaque to vulnerable patient: a call for new definitions and risk assessment strategies: Part I. *Circulation.* Oct 7 2003;108(14):1664-1672.

57. Naghavi M, Libby P, Falk E, Casscells SW, Litovsky S, Rumberger J, Badimon JJ, Stefanadis C, Moreno P, Pasterkamp G, Fayad Z, Stone PH, Waxman S,

Raggi P, Madjid M, Zarrabi A, Burke A, Yuan C, Fitzgerald PJ, Siscovick DS, de Korte CL, Aikawa M, Airaksinen KE, Assmann G, Becker CR, Chesebro JH, Farb A, Galis ZS, Jackson C, Jang IK, Koenig W, Lodder RA, March K, Demirovic J, Navab M, Priori SG, Rekhter MD, Bahr R, Grundy SM, Mehran R, Colombo A, Boerwinkle E, Ballantyne C, Insull W, Jr., Schwartz RS, Vogel R, Serruys PW, Hansson GK, Faxon DP, Kaul S, Drexler H, Greenland P, Muller JE, Virmani R, Ridker PM, Zipes DP, Shah PK, Willerson JT. From vulnerable plaque to vulnerable patient: a call for new definitions and risk assessment strategies: Part II. *Circulation.* Oct 14 2003;108(15):1772-1778.

58. Shah PK. Thrombogenic risk factors for atherothrombosis. *Rev Cardiovasc Med.* Winter 2006;7(1):10-16.

59. Markovitz JH, Tolbert L, Winders SE. Increased serotonin receptor density and platelet GPIIb/IIIa activation among smokers. *Arterioscler Thromb Vasc Biol.* Mar 1999;19(3):762-766.

60. Badimon JJ, Badimon L, Turitto VT, Fuster V. Platelet deposition at high shear rates is enhanced by high plasma cholesterol levels. In vivo study in the rabbit model. *Arterioscler Thromb.* Mar-Apr 1991;11(2):395-402.

61. Badimon JJ, Lettino M, Toschi V, Fuster V, Berrozpe M, Chesebro JH, Badimon L. Local inhibition of tissue factor reduces the thrombogenicity of disrupted human atherosclerotic plaques: effects of tissue factor pathway inhibitor on plaque thrombogenicity under flow conditions. *Circulation.* Apr 13 1999;99(14):1780-1787.

62. Sambola A, Osende J, Hathcock J, Degen M, Nemerson Y, Fuster V, Crandall J, Badimon JJ. Role of risk factors in the modulation of tissue factor activity and blood thrombogenicity. *Circulation.* Feb 25 2003;107(7):973-977.

63. Jaffe AS, Babuin L, Apple FS. Biomarkers in acute cardiac disease: the present and the future. *J Am Coll Cardiol.* Jul 4 2006;48(1):1-11.

64. Viles-Gonzalez JF, Fuster V, Corti R, Badimon JJ. Emerging importance of HDL cholesterol in developing high-risk coronary plaques in acute coronary syndromes. *Curr Opin Cardiol.* Jul 2003;18(4):286-294.

65. Badimon JJ, Badimon L, Fuster V. Regression of atherosclerotic lesions by high density lipoprotein plasma fraction in the cholesterol-fed rabbit. *J Clin Invest.* Apr 1990;85(4):1234-1241.

66. Singh IM, Shishehbor MH, Ansell BJ. High-density lipoprotein as a therapeutic target: a systematic review. *Jama.* Aug 15 2007;298(7):786-798.

67. Navab M, Ananthramaiah GM, Reddy ST, Van Lenten BJ, Ansell BJ, Fonarow GC, Vahabzadeh K, Hama S, Hough G, Kamranpour N, Berliner JA, Lusis AJ, Fogelman AM. The oxidation hypothesis of atherogenesis: the role of oxidized phospholipids and HDL. *J Lipid Res.* Jun 2004;45(6):993-1007.

68. Ansell BJ, Fonarow GC, Fogelman AM. High-density lipoprotein: is it always atheroprotective? *Curr Atheroscler Rep.* Sep 2006;8(5):405-411.

69. Zheng L, Nukuna B, Brennan ML, Sun M, Goormastic M, Settle M, Schmitt D, Fu X, Thomson L, Fox PL, Ischiropoulos H, Smith JD, Kinter M, Hazen SL. Apolipoprotein A-I is a selective target for myeloperoxidase-catalyzed oxidation and functional impairment in subjects with cardiovascular disease. *J Clin Invest.* Aug 2004;114(4):529-541.

70. Ansell BJ, Navab M, Hama S, Kamranpour N, Fonarow G, Hough G, Rahmani S, Mottahedeh R, Dave R, Reddy ST, Fogelman AM. Inflammatory/antiinflammatory properties of high-density lipoprotein distinguish patients from control subjects better than high-density lipoprotein cholesterol levels and are favorably affected by simvastatin treatment. *Circulation.* Dec 2 2003;108(22):2751-2756.

71. Shah PK, Kaul S, Nilsson J, Cercek B. Exploiting the vascular protective effects of high-density lipoprotein and its apolipoproteins: an idea whose time for testing is coming, part I. *Circulation.* Nov 6 2001;104(19):2376-2383.

72. Meyers CD, Kashyap ML. Pharmacologic elevation of high-density lipoproteins: recent insights on mechanism of action and atherosclerosis protection. *Curr Opin Cardiol.* Jul 2004;19(4):366-373.

73. Corti R, Fuster V, Fayad ZA, Worthley SG, Helft G, Smith D, Weinberger J, Wentzel J, Mizsei G, Mercuri M, Badimon JJ. Lipid lowering by simvastatin induces regression of human atherosclerotic lesions: two years' follow-up by high-resolution noninvasive magnetic resonance imaging. *Circulation.* Dec 3 2002;106(23):2884-2887.

74. Cockerill GW, Rye KA, Gamble JR, Vadas MA, Barter PJ. High-density lipoproteins inhibit cytokine-induced expression of endothelial cell adhesion molecules. *Arterioscler Thromb Vasc Biol.* Nov 1995;15(11):1987-1994.

75. Watson AD, Berliner JA, Hama SY, La Du BN, Faull KF, Fogelman AM, Navab M. Protective effect of high density lipoprotein associated paraoxonase. Inhibition of the biological activity of minimally oxidized low density lipoprotein. *J Clin Invest.* Dec 1995;96(6):2882-2891.

76. Spieker LE, Sudano I, Hurlimann D, Lerch PG, Lang MG, Binggeli C, Corti R, Ruschitzka F, Luscher TF, Noll G. High-density lipoprotein restores endothelial function in hypercholesterolemic men. *Circulation.* Mar 26 2002;105(12):1399-1402.

77. Franceschini G, Sirtori CR, Capurso A, 2nd, Weisgraber KH, Mahley RW. A-IMilano apoprotein. Decreased high density lipoprotein cholesterol levels with significant lipoprotein modifications and without clinical atherosclerosis in an Italian family. *J Clin Invest.* Nov 1980;66(5):892-900.

78. Ameli S, Hultgardh-Nilsson A, Cercek B, Shah PK, Forrester JS, Ageland H, Nilsson J. Recombinant apolipoprotein A-I Milano reduces intimal thickening after balloon injury in hypercholesterolemic rabbits. *Circulation.* Oct 1994;90(4):1935-1941.

79. Shah PK, Nilsson J, Kaul S, Fishbein MC, Ageland H, Hamsten A, Johansson J, Karpe F, Cercek B. Effects of recombinant apolipoprotein A-I(Milano) on aortic atherosclerosis in apolipoprotein E-deficient mice. *Circulation.* Mar 3 1998;97(8):780-785.

80. Kaul S, Coin B, Hedayiti A, Yano J, Cercek B, Chyu KY, Shah PK. Rapid reversal of endothelial dysfunction in hypercholesterolemic apolipoprotein E-null mice by recombinant apolipoprotein A-I(Milano)-phospholipid complex. *J Am Coll Cardiol.* Sep 15 2004;44(6):1311-1319.

81. Nissen SE, Tsunoda T, Tuzcu EM, Schoenhagen P, Cooper CJ, Yasin M, Eaton GM, Lauer MA, Sheldon WS, Grines CL, Halpern S, Crowe T, Blankenship JC, Kerensky R. Effect of recombinant ApoA-I Milano on coronary atherosclerosis in patients with acute coronary syndromes: a randomized controlled trial. *Jama.* Nov 5 2003;290(17):2292-2300.

82. Ibanez B, Vilahur G, Cimmino G, Speidl W, Pinero A, Choi BG, Zafar MU, Santos-Gallego CG, Krause B, Badimon L, Fuster V, Badimon J. Rapid Change in Plaque Size, Composition and Molecular Footprint Following Recombinant ApoA-I$_{Milano}$ (ETC-216) Administration. *Magnetic Resonance Imaging Study in an Experimental Model of Atherosclerosis. J Am Coll Cardiol.* 2008;51(11):1104-1109.

83. Nissen SE, Tardif JC, Nicholls SJ, Revkin JH, Shear CL, Duggan WT, Ruzyllo W, Bachinsky WB, Lasala GP, Tuzcu EM. Effect of torcetrapib on the progression of coronary atherosclerosis. *N Engl J Med.* Mar 29 2007;356(13):1304-1316.

84. Barter PJ, Caulfield M, Eriksson M, Grundy SM, Kastelein JJ, Komajda M, Lopez-Sendon J, Mosca L, Tardif JC, Waters DD, Shear CL, Revkin JH, Buhr KA, Fisher MR, Tall AR, Brewer B. Effects of torcetrapib in patients at high risk for coronary events. *N Engl J Med.* Nov 22 2007;357(21):2109-2122.

85. Tall AR, Yvan-Charvet L, Wang N. The failure of torcetrapib: was it the molecule or the mechanism? *Arterioscler Thromb Vasc Biol.* Feb 2007;27(2):257-260.

86. Sidhu JS, Kaposzta Z, Markus HS, Kaski JC. Effect of rosiglitazone on common carotid intima-media thickness progression in coronary artery disease patients without diabetes mellitus. *Arterioscler Thromb Vasc Biol.* May 2004;24(5):930-934.

87. Nissen SE, Wolski K. Effect of rosiglitazone on the risk of myocardial infarction and death from cardiovascular causes. *N Engl J Med.* Jun 14 2007;356(24):2457-2471.

88. Goldberg RB, Kendall DM, Deeg MA, Buse JB, Zagar AJ, Pinaire JA, Tan MH, Khan MA, Perez AT, Jacober SJ. A comparison of lipid and glycemic effects of pioglitazone and rosiglitazone in patients with type 2 diabetes and dyslipidemia. *Diabetes Care.* Jul 2005;28(7):1547-1554.

89. Tangirala RK, Bischoff ED, Joseph SB, Wagner BL, Walczak R, Laffitte BA, Daige CL, Thomas D, Heyman RA, Mangelsdorf DJ, Wang X, Lusis AJ, Tontonoz P, Schulman IG. Identification of macrophage liver X receptors as inhibitors of atherosclerosis. *Proc Natl Acad Sci U S A.* Sep 3 2002;99(18):11896-11901.

90. Tardif JC, Gregoire J, L'Allier PL, Anderson TJ, Bertrand O, Reeves F, Title LM, Alfonso F, Schampaert E, Hassan A, McLain R, Pressler ML, Ibrahim R, Lesperance J, Blue J, Heinonen T, Rodes-Cabau J. Effects of the acyl coenzyme A:cholesterol acyltransferase inhibitor avasimibe on human atherosclerotic lesions. *Circulation.* Nov 23 2004;110(21):3372-3377.

CHAPTER 2

Heart Failure:
Role of Cardiac Imaging

Ashish Aneja, MD
W. H. Wilson Tang, MD

INTRODUCTION

Definition and Epidemiology

Heart failure is defined as a complex clinical syndrome that can result from any structural or functional cardiac disorder that impairs the ability of the ventricle to fill or eject blood.[1] It manifests with shortness of breath, easy fatigability, or fluid retention, either alone or in combination. The clinical syndrome can result from disorders of the pericardium, myocardium, endocardium, or the great vessels; but the majority of cases result from myocardial dysfunction. In the United States, approximately 5 million people have heart failure, and about 550,000 new patients are diagnosed with heart failure every year. It accounts for 12 to 15 million office visits, approximately 1 million hospitalizations (where heart failure is the primary diagnosis), and more than 50,000 deaths annually in the United States.[2, 3] The lifetime risk of developing heart failure has been estimated at 20% for the U.S. population. Heart failure is also the single largest expense for any diagnosis-related group for Medicare, with an approximate annual cost of $33 billion.[1] In the Western world, the most common causative factors for heart failure include myocardial ischemia, hypertension, or rhythm disturbances. Valvular heart disease is also a common cause of heart failure, particularly in the developing world because of the high prevalence of rheumatic heart disease. In many cases, the precise cause of heart failure may remain undetermined even with existing diagnostic modalities.

According to the American College of Cardiology and American Heart Association (ACC/AHA) guideline, chronic heart failure is classified into four stages. Stage A identifies patients at risk for heart failure without the symptoms or structural abnormalities. Stage B consists of patients with structural heart disease without symptoms or signs of heart failure. Stage C constitutes the presence of structural heart disease with prior or current symptoms of heart failure and Stage D stands for heart failure refractory to standard therapy. This staging system lends itself well to interpretation from the imaging perspective because it represents a structural and clinical continuum. Determination of altered cardiac structure and performance by different imaging techniques has provided valuable insights into the pathophysiology and causation of heart failure. However, it is important to emphasize that the clinical syndrome of heart failure is not synonymous with the presence of ventricular dysfunction. In patients presenting the symptoms and signs of heart failure, standard transthoracic echocardiography is most commonly used. It can often display a spectrum of abnormalities ranging from a normal sized left ventricle (LV) and preserved ejection fraction (EF) to a dilated and poorly functioning LV with impaired EF. Irrespective of the EF, abnormalities in both systolic and diastolic function commonly coexist. Nevertheless, a completely normal echocardiographic study with normal filling patterns and chamber characteristics may argue against such diagnosis in an otherwise symptomatic patient.

Systolic Versus Diastolic Heart Failure

Approximately half of heart failure patients have evidence of LV systolic dysfunction (so-called systolic heart failure) and distinguishing between patients with and without LV systolic dysfunction on clinical grounds is generally difficult. Therefore, at present, the information presented in a well-executed imaging study is essential for the management and long-term follow up of patients with symptomatic heart failure. The ACC/AHA Clinical Guideline recommends an echocardiographic study (or alternative imaging means) when heart failure is suspected, when a change in the clinical condition is noted, and when a new treatment with potential for cardiotoxicity is instituted (e.g., in recipients of doxorubicin, sunitinib, trastuzumab, or mitoxantrone).

The other half consists of patients with "diastolic heart failure" or "heart failure with preserved ejection fraction" (HFpEF, also referred to as "heart failure with normal ejection fraction"). The diagnosis of HFpEF can be complex and controversial and is evident from elevated LV end-diastolic pressure and altered stiffness (e.g., hemodynamic measurements like *tau*) measured by specialized catheters during cardiac catheterization. Patients with HFpEF often present with reduced exercise capacity and propensity for acute pulmonary edema.[4] The main causes of HFpEF are listed in Table 2.1. This syndrome manifests most commonly in the elderly with comorbidities such as hypertension, coronary artery disease, diabetes mellitus, and renal dysfunction. Patients with HFpEF frequently have left ventricular hypertrophy and myocardial fibrosis, which can result in increased diastolic stiffness.[5]

Mechanistic studies in humans with HFpEF have not demonstrated any characteristic abnormalities in end-diastolic pressure volume relations (EDPVRs).[6,7] These studies suggest that EDPVR curves in patients with HFpEF can be variable, and can shift to lower, similar, or higher volumes than control subjects. Patients with HFpEF can have heart failure caused by diastolic dysfunction and/or reduced stroke volume resulting from small ventricular volumes (as seen in patients with hypertrophic cardiomyopathy) or can have mildly dilated hearts with subtle or no abnormalities in pressure volume relationships (as seen in patients with hypertension and HFpEF).[4,8] Direct measurements of EDPVR during

Table 2.1 Major Causes of Heart Failure with Preserved Ejection Fraction

Hypertension	Severe valvular stenosis
Restrictive cardiomyopathy	Severe valvular regurgitation
Infiltrative cardiomyopathy	Pericardial disease
Hypertrophic cardiomyopathy	Cardiac tamponade
Noncompaction cardiomyopathy	Constrictive pericarditis
Right heart failure	Intracardiac mass
Severe pulmonary hypertension	Atrial myxoma
Right ventricular infarct	Apical eosinophilic thrombus
Arrhythmogenic right ventricular dysplasia	Pulmonary vein stenosis
Atrial septal defect	Congenital heart diseases
Valvular heart diseases	

exercise in patients with HFpEF have further demonstrated the ability of the ventricle to accommodate an increased diastolic volume with little impact on EDPVRs, challenging the traditional construct of a necessary link between HFpEF and diastolic dysfunction.

In contrast, the natural history of chronic systolic heart failure is thought to be preceded by a prolonged period of myocardial dysfunction, during which cardiac systolic function and output is maintained at normal or near normal by compensatory hypertrophy and dilatation. In the early stages, the symptoms of heart failure do not manifest at rest because of compensatory structural changes. With exercise, the cardiac output may not rise or fall, eventually declining even at rest. In addition, systemic vascular resistance, which normally declines with exercise, fails to do so in overt heart failure, further contributing to ventricular hypertrophy and dilatation.

Cardiac Remodeling

Cardiac remodeling has been defined as genome expression, molecular, cellular, and interstitial changes that are manifested clinically as changes in size, shape, and function of the heart after cardiac injury.[9] Cardiac remodeling occurs to accommodate the abnormal heart physiology and is pivotal in the development and progression of heart failure. Therefore, early recognition and management of the presence and extent of remodeling with imaging can have considerable therapeutic and prognostic impact in overall disease management.

In the majority of patients, remodeling and heart failure are the result of myocardial failure or external work overload. Common examples of the former include myocardial infarction, valvular disease, and cardiomyopathy (e.g., caused by hypertension). Less common mechanisms include sustained tachycardia, pericardial abnormalities, inflammation, toxins, and congenital malformations. These processes may vary, are often interdependent, and can occur as primary phenomena and epiphenomena. For example, patients with a primary idiopathic dilated cardiomyopathy often develop mitral valve regurgitation because of altered chamber size and symmetry, which in turn may further link to deterioration of myocardial function. Distinguishing between the primary and the secondary processes remains to be challenging despite advances in imaging technology.

Remodeling following myocardial infarction starts rapidly (can be within hours), and can lead to further progression over weeks and months, depending upon the extent of injury, degree of neurohormonal activation, and immediacy/type of treatment instituted. The initial process of remodeling is considered beneficial because it may involve repair of the damaged myocardium with scar tissue, which can help maintain pump function. With myocardial stretch, local neurohormonal mechanisms including adrenergic, endothelin, and angiotensin mechanisms are activated, leading to hypertrophy, fibrosis, and apoptosis. In addition, activation of inflammatory processes, expressed by elevated tumor necrosis factor levels, accompanies remodeling and contributes to myocardial necrosis. Whereas the primary target of remodeling is the myocyte, other areas of the heart including the interstitium also undergo changes (include fibroblast activation and proliferation). Fibrin and collagen deposition often accompanies and contributes to interstitial remodeling. These changes are dynamic, and can influence the contractile and relaxant properties of surrounding myocytes.

In terms of mechanical changes at the cellular level, ventricular dilation results from an increase in myocyte length, limited by a maximum sarcomere length of approximately 2.2μm. If these forces are maintained chronically, sarcomeres are added longitudinally, resulting in more permanent dilatation. With systolic pressure overload, sarcomeres are added in parallel within the myocytes, leading to progressive ventricular hypertrophy. Both mechanisms may help to reduce the resting myocardial tension but eventually contribute to maladaptive changes leading to progression of heart failure.

The structural effects of remodeling are grossly manifest by transformation of the normally ellipsoid LV into a somewhat spherical structure. Changes in ventricular volumes and mass contribute to the process. Primary imaging measures of cardiac remodeling include cardiac size, shape, mass, ejection fraction, end-diastolic and end-systolic volumes, and contractile force. The ability of such changes allows preservation of stroke volume in the setting of reduced myocardial contractility. These measurements are ascertained most commonly by echocardiography but, more accurately by magnetic resonance imaging (MRI) as described in the following sections. In patients with a recent myocardial infarction, even small increases in chamber volume within days can be associated with an independent increase in mortality. Assessment of disordered regional ventricular contraction (known as dysynergy) can also be measured reliably with echocardiography and MRI techniques.

IMAGING MODALITIES IN HEART FAILURE

Echocardiography

Estimation of Myocardial Structure and Performance

Figure 2.1 demonstrates standard echocardiographic views for assessment of cardiac function. Because of its two-dimensional views, echocardiographic measurements of LVEF have traditionally been limited by acquisition errors and overall lack of precision and reproducibility in interpretation. Although there is poor correlation between symptoms and LVEF, the estimation of LVEF remains to be one of the most important measurements in echocardiography because of its independent correlation with long-term prognosis. In addition, LVEF measurements are an essential guide in assessing treatment efficacy and management decisions. This is largely historical, as clinical trials have utilized a reduced LVEF as a necessary confirmation of underlying systolic dysfunction as primary cause of heart failure. The American Society of Echocardiography recommends the biplane method for estimations of EF in patients with a well-defined endocardial border and discourages the use of visual assessment.[9] The cut off for an abnormal LVEF is < 55%; < 45% constitutes moderate dysfunction, and < 30% is severe LV dysfunction. Normal values for LV dimensions are based on the body surface area. Dimensions of 2.4–3.2cm/m^2 are considered normal,[10] with values of 3.5cm/m^2 and 3.9cm/m^2 representative of moderate to severe ventricular dilation.

Other clinically useful assessments of chamber characteristics include right ventricular systolic function and right atrial enlargement for right-sided dysfunction, and left atrial enlargement (especially indexed to body size) for underlying LV diastolic dysfunction. These measurements can also be challenging because of the irregular shape and configuration of these chambers. While we recognize the interdependence between the left and right heart chambers as they share the septal wall, few reliable echocardiographic parameters can quantify such interactions.

Several integrated parameters have also been developed for potential clinical applications. The myocardial performance index (MPI, also known at "the Tei index") is a Doppler-based assay of both myocardial systolic and diastolic function. It is important in patients with heart failure because of the almost invariable coexistence of the two forms of ventricular dysfunction. It is defined as the sum of isovolumetric contraction time (IVCT) and isovolumetric relaxation time (IVRT), divided by ejection time (ET) (IVCT + IVRT/ET).[11] This index is independent of heart rate and blood pressure and independent of any geometrical assumptions, has been validated in studies, and shows good correlation with outcomes in patients with dilated and infiltrative cardiomyopathies. In patients with dilated cardiomyopathy, MPI > 0.77 has been shown to be prognostically superior to EF.[12] Despite the fact that MPI changes with age, it has been successful in predicting future heart failure in elderly patients with no evidence of baseline ventricular dysfunction,[13] and may help to predict a lack of overall response to treatment for heart failure.[14]

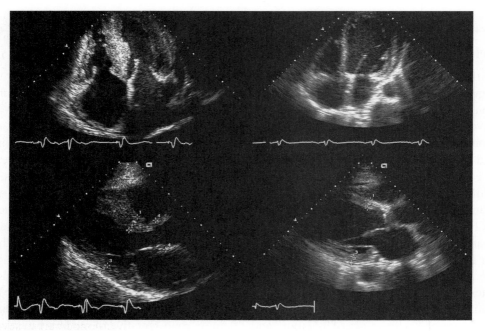

Figure 2.1

Standard Echocardiographic Views for Cardiac Evaluation. (Left panel) Hypertrophic cardiomyopathy; (Right panel)
Dilated cardiomyopathy.

Reproduced from Francis GS, Tang WH. *Clinical Evaluation of Heart Failure. Heart Failure: A Companion to Braunwald's Heart Disease*, Mann D ed.,
W.B. Saunders, 2003.

Assessment of Hemodynamics

Over the decades, there has been an ongoing search for a noninvasive substitute for
invasive techniques to measure hemodynamics. Echocardiography can provide reliable
estimates of cardiac output by pulse wave Doppler recordings of the ventricular outflow
tract. It can also help estimate right-sided atrial and ventricular systolic pressures and
pulmonary artery pressures (systolic, diastolic, and mean), thus providing valuable information about the etiology and prognosis of heart failure. However, such measurements
are limited by their measurement techniques, as their values are dependent on Doppler
cursor alignment with blood flow. Care must be exercised in the interpretation of these
findings because even small degrees of valvular regurgitation can result in overestimation
of cardiac measurements. Similarly, estimation of pulmonary artery pressures is dependent on reliable estimations of the degree of tricuspid regurgitation, pulmonary valve
regurgitation, and right atrial pressure. Furthermore, Doppler signals can be influenced
by a wide range of factors including loading conditions, patient positioning and stability,
as well as underlying heart rate and rhythm.

Assessing Diastolic Dysfunction

Echocardiography has also proven valuable in estimating diastolic function, as well as left atrial and left ventricular end-diastolic pressures. Diastolic dysfunction (which represents impaired ventricular relaxation and contributes significantly to the pathogenesis of HFpEF) has been classified by echocardiography into three broad categories based on measurements of early diastolic flow velocity (E-wave) and atrial contraction (A-wave). Mild dysfunction is expressed as a reversal of the normal E/A ratio from > 1 to < 1. Moderate dysfunction is characterized by a return of the E/A to a normal appearing pattern (also known as pseudonormalization), which is explained by the progressive increase in the early flow velocity (E) to near-normal levels in the face of increased atrial filling pressures (A) with an E/A ratio ranging from 1.0–1.5. Severe dysfunction (also known as the restrictive filling pattern) consists of a significant increase in the rate of early filling and equalization of left atrial and ventricular pressures, resulting an E/A ratio > 2. However, such measures of diastolic dysfunction are dependent on the heart rate and loading conditions. The Valsalva maneuver, which reduces early filling, can change the pseudonormalized pattern to the early dysfunction pattern (E/A < 1) and the restrictive pattern to a pseudonormalized one. Overall, patients with heart failure with a persistently restrictive pattern despite the Valsalva maneuver or with optimal treatment have a poor prognosis, although most validation studies have been conducted in patients with less severe LV systolic dysfunction.[15]

Doppler echocardiography is also commonly utilized in measurement of additional parameters of diastolic function. Figure 2.2 demonstrates transmitral Doppler inflow patterns, color M-mode, and tissue Doppler indices. Many of these echocardiographic criteria are less dependent on loading conditions and heart rate and correlate well with ventricular filling pressures. Pulmonary vein (PV) Doppler parameters including an abnormal ratio of pulmonary venous systolic and diastolic pulmonary vein velocities (S/D < 1), a pulmonary venous forward flow (SF) systolic fraction of < 40%, and an early LV filling flow propagation slope (Vp) of < 45cm/s have shown excellent prognostic value in patients with diastolic dysfunction and heart failure. This is especially true in those with underlying systolic dysfunction.

Several newer derived measurements have been evaluated and adopted as reliable measurements of diastolic dysfunction. The tissue Doppler-derived measure of the ratio between peak early mitral flow velocity (E) to peak early diastolic mitral velocity (Ea) has been widely examined. A E/Ea ratio of ≤ 8 predicts a left ventricular end diastolic pressure (LVEDP) of < 15mmHg, and a E/Vp ratio of ≥ 1.5 predicts an LVEDP > 15mmHg.[16, 17, 18] In addition, a left atrial volume index > 32ml/m^2 is predictive of increased morbidity.[19] Table 2.2 summarizes the prognostic significance of the various Doppler measures in the assessment of diastolic dysfunction in single component studies and Table 2.3 assesses it in composite studies. Figure 2.3 summarizes the Doppler criteria for classifying diastolic dysfunction and Figure 2.4 summarizes the diagnostic criteria for diastolic heart failure.

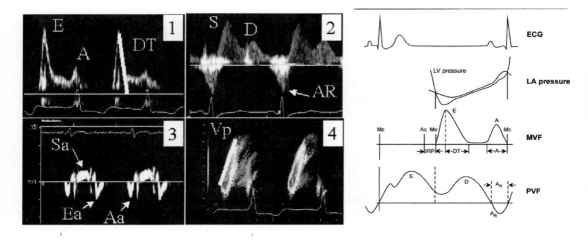

Figure 2.2

Transmitral Doppler inflow patterns, color M-mode, and tissue Doppler indices.

Reprinted from Plasma B-type natriuretic peptide levels in systolic heart failure: importance of left ventricular diastolic function and right ventricular systolic function, Troughton et al., *J Am Coll Cardiol* 2004; 43:(3), with permission from Elsevier.

Assessment of Left Ventricular Mass

Left ventricular mass is an independent risk factor for poor prognosis in patients with heart failure and it increases in patients with remodeled failing hearts, hypertensive heart disease, renal failure, diabetes mellitus, and various other causes of cardiomyopathy. An echocardiographic substudy of the Studies of Left Ventricular Dysfunction (SOLVD) trial has suggested that LV hypertrophy is independently associated with a higher mortality in patients with chronic heart failure.[20] Reversal of LV hypertrophy has also been associated with better long-term prognosis in hypertensive patients with largely preserved LV function.

Left ventricular mass calculations from echocardiography are based on geometric assumptions, whether linear (with the LV assumed to be an ellipse) or two-dimensional (2D) methods are employed. In heart failure patients with heavily remodeled ventricles, these estimations can be inaccurate. Left ventricular mass measurements are gender-dependent, and women have smaller reference values (67–162g by linear and 66–150g by two-dimensional methods). Corresponding numbers for men are 88–224g and 96–200g, respectively. However, the degree of LV hypertrophy is generally described qualitatively (especially with description of interventricular septal or posterior wall thicknesses) based on direct visualization, and may not be as apparent if concomitant ventricular dilatation is present.

Table 2.2   Prognostic Significance of Echocardiographic Diastolic Dysfunction Measures: Single Component Studies

MODALITY	PATIENT POPULATION	CUTOFF VALUES	OUTCOME
	**Mitral inflow Doppler**		
E/A	2,671 elderly patients, no CVD	<0.7 or >1.5	Incident heart failure
E/A	1,839 hypertensive patients	Age- and heart rate-adjusted ratio below median	Cardiovascular events
E/A	3,008 Native Americans	<0.6 or >1.5	Death or cardiac death
DT	110 patients, EF <50%, no CAD	<115 ms, persisting after 3 months' heart failure treatment	Death or transplant at 4 yrs
Peak E	2,671 elderly, no CVD	Continuous	Incident heart failure
DT	571 patients post-AMI	<130 ms	Death at 4 yrs
DT	79 heart failure patients, no CAD	<115 ms	Death or transplant
M-mode IVRT	185 elderly heart failure patients	≤30 ms	Death
	**Pulmonary vein Doppler**		
PV AR dur – MV A dur	145 LV dysfunction patients	≥30 ms	Cardiac death or hospital stay
S/D	115 patients, EF <45%	<1	heart failure hospital readmission or heart failure death at 1 yr
	**Tissue Doppler**		
E/E'	250 patients post-AMI	>15	Death
E/E'	45 patients, NYHA functional class III or IV heart failure	Continuous	Predictor of NYHA functional class, heart failure hospital stay, cardiac death
E/E'	130 chronic heart failure patients	>12.5	Composite: cardiac death, heart failure hospital stay, urgent transplant
E/E'	110 patients hospitalized with heart failure	≥15	Cardiac death or hospital readmission for heart failure
E', E/E'	518 patients referred for echocardiography	E' <3 or 3–5 cm/s, E/E' >20	Cardiac death
Systolic mitral	185 patients, EF <45%	Continuous	Death or transplant annular velocity
LA volume	1,375 elderly patients with preserved EF	≥ 32 ml/m^2	Incident heart failure

Table 2.2   Prognostic Significance of Echocardiographic Diastolic Dysfunction Measures: Single Component Studies (continued)

Modality	Patient Population	Cutoff Values	Outcome
		Flow propagation	
E/Vp	67 post-MI patients	E/Vp ≥1.5	Death and heart failure readmission
Vp	125 post-MI patients	Vp <45 cm/s	Cardiac death

A = atrial filling velocity; AMI = acute myocardial infarction; CAD = coronary artery disease; CVD = cardiovascular disease; D = diastolic pulmonary vein wave; DT = deceleration time of E-wave; E = early diastolic filling velocity; E' = tissue Doppler early filling velocity; EF = ejection fraction; IVRT = interventricular relaxation time; LA = left atrium; LV = left ventricle; MV A dur = mitral valve atrial wave duration; NYHA = New York Heart Association; PV AR dur = pulmonary vein atrial reversal duration; S = systolic pulmonary vein wave; Vp = flow propagation velocity slope.

*New onset event = myocardial infarction, sudden cardiac death, unstable angina, revascularization, stroke/transient ischemic attack, hospital stay for heart failure (heart failure), symptomatic aorto-iliac disease, end-stage renal disease.

Table 2.3   Prognostic Significance of Echocardiographic Diastolic Dysfunction Measures: Composite Studies

Composite Study	Patient Population	Components	Outcome	Degree of Predictive Significance
Mild diastolic dysfunction vs. normal	2,042 patients >45 yrs	E/A <0.75, E/A Valsalva <0.5, E/E' <10, S >D, PV ARdur >MV Adur	Death	HR 8.31
Moderate or severe diastolic dysfunction vs. normal	2,042 patients >45 yrs	E/A 0.75–1.5, DT >140 ms, E/A Valsalva ≥0.5, E/E' ≥10, S <D, PV AR dur – MV A dur >30 ms E/A >1.5, DT <140 ms, E/A Valsalva <0.5, E/E' ≥10, S <D, PV AR dur – MV A dur >30 ms	Death	HR 10.17
Restrictive vs. nonrestrictive	311 heart failure patients evaluated for transplant	E/A >2 or DT ≤140 ms	Death or transplant	RR 2.4
Restrictive vs. nonrestrictive	98 chronic heart failure patients	E/A >1 and DT ≤130 ms	Cardiac death or transplant	NA
Restrictive vs. nonrestrictive	100 patients, EF <40%	E/A ≥2 or 1–2 plus DT <140 ms	Cardiac death at 2 yrs	RR 8.6

Table 2.3 Prognostic Significance of Echocardiographic Diastolic Dysfunction Measures: Composite Studies (continued)

Composite Study	Patient Population	Components	Outcome	Degree of Predictive Significance
Restrictive vs. nonrestrictive	193 heart failure patients, EF <45%	E/A >2, DT <150 ms, E'<8 cm/s	Cardiac death or early transplant	RR 6.62
Restrictive vs. nonrestrictive	63 patients with amyloid cardiomyopathy	E/A >1 and DT <150 ms	Cardiac death at 1 yr	RR 4.87
AR vs. PN vs. RFP	115 patients admitted with heart failure	E/A <1 or >2, DT <140 or >230 ms, PV AR dur/MV A dur >1.2		

Assessment of Contractile Reserve, Ischemia, and Viability

Even though stress echocardiography plays an important role in viability assessment, it has a low predictive value compared to MRI or positron emission tomography (PET) based determinations. Common approaches to determine the presence of underlying infarcted regions utilize grading of wall motions of different myocardial segments to generate a composite score. In akinetic areas with end-diastolic wall thickness ≥ 6mm, additional testing can reveal nonviable myocardium in 40% of these regions.[21] Wall thickness measurements can provide additional clues in viability assessment by echocardiography. It is generally believed that akinetic regions with an end-diastolic thickness < 6mm are unlikely to be viable and respond to revascularization.[21]

Stress echocardiographic responses vary according to the myocardial substrate. A normal response is characterized by normal segmental motion at rest and normal or hyperkinetic response with stress. With stress, ischemic myocardium manifests a dyskinetic response (from normokinesis at rest). Necrotic myocardium remains akinetic both at rest and stress. Viable myocardium responds to stress by an improvement in resting dysfunction.

"Contractile reserve" is defined as the difference between values of an index of LV contractility during peak stress and baseline values. Echocardiography with exercise or pharmacologic stress is one of the most commonly used techniques for identifying contractile reserve and estimating the amount of viable hibernating myocardium. The presence of contractile reserve can predict favorable response to drug or device interventions (such as beta-adrenergic blockers or resynchronization therapy).

With pharmacologic testing, viable myocardium can respond in a biphasic fashion improvement at low dose and a dyskinetic response at high dose. The sensitivity

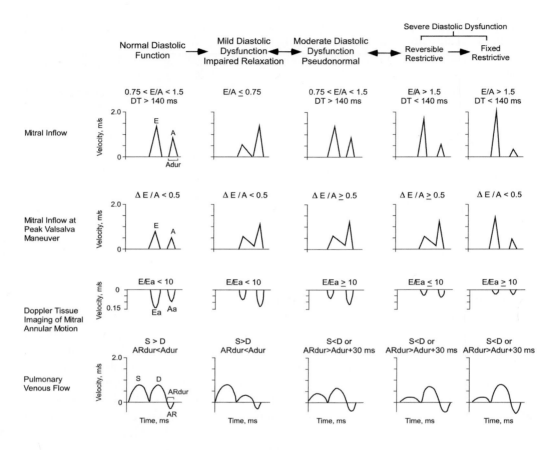

Figure 2.3

Doppler Criteria for Classification of Diastolic Function (Abbreviations: E, peak early filling velocity; A, velocity at atrial contraction; DT, deceleration time; Adur, A duration; ARdur, AR duration; S, systolic forward flow; D, diastolic forward flow; AR, pulmonary venous atrial reversal flow; e', velocity of mitral annulus early diastolic motion; a', velocity of mitral annulus motion with atrial systole; DT, mitral E velocity deceleration time.)

and specificity of dobutamine stress echocardiography (DSE) for predicting recovery of regional function following revascularization is approximately 80%. The sensitivity of DSE can be limited by resting tachycardia, which may result in ischemia at rest and worsened by dobutamine or by critical reductions in myocardial perfusion that do not permit any improvement in contractility. On the other hand, the specificity of DSE can be adversely impacted by a tethering effect of injured subendocardial myocardium.[22] How-

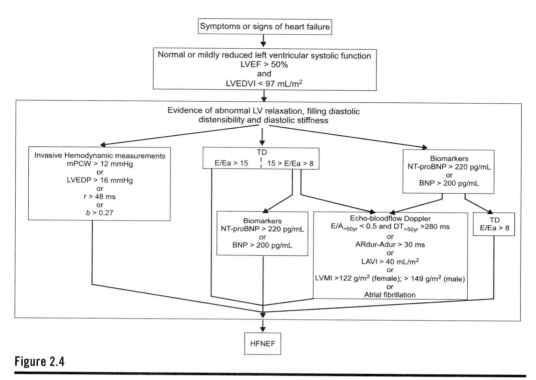

Figure 2.4

Diagnostic criteria for diastolic heart failure (2007 European Society of Cardiology Consensus Statement).

From Paulus et al. *Eur Heart J* 2007.

ever, improvements in global myocardial function and symptoms following revascularization are generally not demonstrable unless a significant proportion of the myocardium is jeopardized. Generally speaking, improved contractility with stress or dobutamine in ≥ 4 viable segments (about 20% of the LV) predicts postrevascularization global improvements in EF. However, these improvements in function may not occur consistently despite the presence of these discriminating criteria.[23]

Stress-induced improvement in LVEF in patients with significantly depressed LV function generally portends a good prognosis, and a lack of improvement is indicative of poor outcomes, even in patients with idiopathic dilated cardiomyopathy.[24, 25] Even though the primary goal of stress echocardiography in this case is to demonstrate underlying contractile reserve, it is equally important to point out that ischemia, obstruction at the LV outflow track, or worsening mitral regurgitation can also be provoked and can be part of the differential diagnosis. Assessment of underlying pulmonary hypertension, right ventricular function, and diastolic function are also incremental.

Assessment of Mechanical Dyssynchrony

Apart from its important role in the assessment of hemodynamics and diastolic function, tissues Doppler imaging (TDI) plays an important role in the assessment of dyssynchrony. Assessment of ventricular dyssynchrony is pivotal to the use of cardiac resynchronization therapy (CRT), which has emerged an important therapeutic modality for patients with heart failure. Generally speaking, CRT is indicated for patients with ischemic and dilated cardiomyopathy with EF < 35% and a QRS duration > 120–150ms. A prolonged QRS duration is currently considered the best predictor of response to CRT but assessment of mechanical dyssynchrony by TDI is considered important for management of patients before and after CRT and is likely to play an even greater role in the future. Mechanical dyssynchrony in the heart can occur at many levels and includes atrioventricular (AV) dyssynchrony. AV can occur either when AV conduction is delayed (delayed LV contraction) or with delayed interatrial conduction (delayed left atrial contraction). AV dyssynchrony can result in erratic mitral valve function with late diastolic mitral regurgitation, simultaneous early and active phases (E and A) of ventricular filling, and a reduced filling period. Tissue Doppler imaging can also help quantify interventricular dyssynchrony, which is characterized by a significant delay in the activation of the LV following the RV (> 40ms). Intraventricular dyssynchrony, which can be reliably estimated by TDI, refers to an abnormal sequence of contraction of different LV walls during systole. Several echocardiographic techniques can be used to assess intraventricular dyssynchrony and include M-mode imaging, tissue velocity imaging, tissue tracking, strain and strain rate imaging, and tissue synchronization imaging. However, the routine use of TDI requires considerable technical expertise and the presence of sinus rhythm for reliable estimates.

Mechanical dyssynchrony, especially intraventricular dyssynchrony, is considered a poor prognostic sign in patients with heart failure. Studies have suggested that the prognostic effect of mechanical dyssynchrony is independent of QRS duration and EF[26] and may indeed be one of the most important predictors of clinical and echocardiographic response to CRT.[27, 28] Tissue Doppler imaging can also help with wall selection for lead placement in patients undergoing CRT by its ability to determine the sequence of LV wall activation. It is also useful in assessing response to CRT, optimization of pacemaker parameters and periodic echocardiographic follow-up of patients who have received CRT.

Three-Dimensional Echocardiography

Three-dimensional (3D) echocardiography can help overcome some other limitations of two-dimensional (2D) echocardiography, including foreshortening and errors associated with geometric assumptions. It can also allow simultaneous assessment of all cardiac segments but, like 2D echocardiography, is limited by imaging quality. Additional expenses for software and probe are usually required for real-time image acquisition, which is a significant advance in the field. Studies suggest that volumetric data are more accurate with 3D echocardiography.[29, 30] Estimations of EF and LV size with 3D echocardiography have compared well with MRI in some studies and are superior to conventional imaging techniques.[31] Despite the advantages, 3D echocardiography has not achieved widespread clinical use but holds promise for accurately assessing chamber volumes, EF, and segmental wall motion for diagnosis, prognosis and follow-up of heart failure patients. Recent availability of real-time analysis utilized 3D technologies with transesophageal echocardiography may also contribute to more broad applications.

Limitations of Echocardiography

Two-dimensional echocardiographic measurements of LVEF are based upon the geometric assumption of the LV as an ellipsoid, and can be hampered by foreshortening. The LV shape in heart failure is frequently nonellipsoidal because of remodeling and segmental motion abnormalities, which can result in inaccuracies. Another major limitation of echocardiography is poor acoustic windows that usually result from body habitus, chest wall deformities, or lung disease. Using tissue harmonic imaging can overcome some of the limitations of conventional methods.[32] Other limitations of echocardiography include high dependence on technical expertise, great interobserve and intraobserver differences, and subjectivity in interpretation. Major advantages include no risk of ionic radiation, renal failure, universal and around-the-clock availability, low cost, and portability.

MAGNETIC RESONANCE IMAGING

Cardiac MRI is considered the gold standard for the assessment of ventricular mass, size, and function. The biggest advantage of MRI over echocardiography is independence from geometric assumptions, which translates into low interobserver and intraobserver variability. This is advantageous when MRI used as an investigative tool because it reduces the sample size. Current advancements in imaging technology have allowed study completion within 5 minutes with a lesser need for breath-holding. MRI is noninvasive and poses no ionizing radiation risk. The images produced have high temporal and spatial resolution with clear definition of soft tissues, without the need for contrast. It can also acquire images in any imaging plane and is not limited by chest wall deformity or body habitus.

In addition to accuracy, MRI has the best interstudy reproducibility for ventricular mass and volume. Myocardial mass is calculated by multiplying volume by the specific gravity of muscle (1.05g/mL). For perfusion and viability assessment, MRIs with gadolinium-diethylenetriaminepenta-acetic acid (Gd-DTPA) provides excellent images and can be performed in most patients with a low risk of dermal toxicity. MRI is particularly useful in determining the etiology and prognosis of various cardiomyopathies because of characteristic images. In patients with atrial fibrillation and other arrhythmias, MRI images quality may get compromised, but real-time imaging can usually provide images of adequate quality. MRI is also being evaluated in measurement of diastolic dysfunction with velocity mapping, tagging and ventricular torsion. However, echocardiography is preferred because MRI currently lacks in temporal resolution.

In evaluation of inducible myocardial ischemia, MRI has also facilitated complete evaluation of all ventricular segments, which is often limited with echocardiography. MRI can also be used with dobutamine (low- and high-dose) for assessment of viability and ischemia respectively and, when used in conjunction with tagging and Gd-DTPA contrast, an accurate assessment of viability can be obtained. Myocardial tagging is a technique commonly utilized with MRI that works by intersecting the myocardium into grids that undergo distortion with myocardial motion during contraction and relaxation. A computer-based analysis of the motion of the points on the grids permits an accurate assessment of myocardial motion in various axes and myocardial layers (sub-epicardium and endocardium). Figure 2.5 demonstrates an MRI images that utilizes the technique of myocardial tagging.

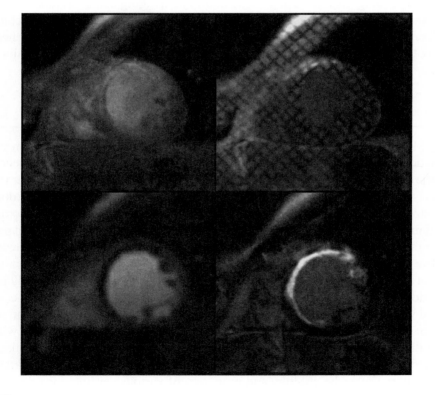

Figure 2.5

Magnetic resonance imaging for evaluation of cardiomyopathy, including myocardial tagging and delay-enhanced gadolinium.

From Francis GS, Tang WH. Clinical Evaluation of Heart Failure. *Heart Failure: A Companion to Braunwald's Heart Disease*, Mann D ed. W.B. Saunders, 2003.

An accurate assessment of myocardial viability using MRI has been made possible with Gd-DTPA contrast because of its propensity to localize to the interstitium after leaving the intravascular space and its inability to enter intact cells. Therefore, areas with myocardial edema and fibrosis preferentially take up Gd-DTPA, giving rise to the characteristically bright signal and delayed hyperenhancement at sites of myocardial scarring. On the other hand, viable myocardium does not take up the contrast agent, hibernating myocardium shows < 50% transmural hyperenhancement and decreased contractility, while scarred tissue has > 50% hyperenhancement.[33] These findings correlate closely with PET findings, but MRI provides superior spatial resolution. Assessment of myocardial perfusion with MRI also requires the use of Gd-DTPA contrast. At rest, ischemic areas do not demonstrate signal intensity change, in contrast to well-perfused areas. If not present at rest, these defects become evident with agents that provoke ischemia, such as dobutamine and adenosine. Direct visualization of coronary anatomy with MRI is currently not reliable because of cardiac motion and low spatial resolution. Therefore, MRI is generally used for detecting abnormal coronary anatomy and bypass grafts.

In addition to its important role in assessment of myocardial anatomy, viability, and ischemia, MRI can help determine the underlying etiology of nonischemic cardiomyopathy and heart failure. Some of the specific types of cardiomyopathy and the role of MRI are discussed in the following sections.

Idiopathic Dilated Cardiomyopathy (IDC)

IDC is a diagnosis of exclusion and primarily requires differentiation from ischemic dilated cardiomyopathy secondary to coronary heart disease. A small percentage (up to 41%) of patients with IDC manifests myocardial scarring on MRI. The scarring resembles an ischemic pattern in 13% and 28% in a midwall nonischemic pattern.[34] It is typically seen in the midwall, and involves basal or mid-portions of the interventricular septum. By contrast, patients with ischemic cardiomyopathy have consistent evidence of prior myocardial infarction. Therefore, in patients without scarring (if present, only in the midwall section) and with LV dysfunction should be considered to have IDC. The presence of myocardial scarring in IDC patients has prognostic significance and predicts a propensity for ventricular arrhythmia and hospital admission.[35]

Myocarditis

Patients with acute myocarditis, who can present with acute and with severe heart failure, demonstrate myocardial hyperenhancement compared to normal myocardium.[36] The pattern of hyperenhancement is typically most prominent in the subepicardium, spares the endocardium, and frequently involves the lateral and inferolateral walls. The sensitivity in diagnosing chronic myocarditis is lower with hyperenhancement patterns resembling those seen with IDC, leading to the belief that some patients with IDC have progressed from chronic myocarditis.

Hypertrophic Cardiomyopathy

Hypertrophic cardiomyopathy (HCM) is characterized by genetically inherited patterns of myocardial structural abnormalities, often associated with dynamic obstruction to the flow of blood because of asymmetric septal hypertrophy and systolic anterior movement of the mitral valve. MRI is the most accurate diagnostic modality for the diagnosis of HCM and allows a clear visualization of the disordered anatomy, level and degree of dynamic obstruction, and tissue characteristics. For the apical form of HCM, MRI offers superior diagnostic ability over echocardiography, which can miss the diagnosis in a significant proportion. Wall thickness is an important predictor of sudden death in HCM patients and MRI is considerably superior to other imaging methodologies in this regard. MRI can also quantify the degree of scarring in HCM, which appears to progress with time and seems to have prognostic value.

Iron Overload Cardiomyopathy

Iron overload of the myocardium is commonly encountered in patients who are transfusion-dependent, including thalassemia and the myelodysplastic syndromes. Patients with primary hemochromatosis are particularly susceptible but the condition is much less common. In addition, MRI can image the amount of iron deposition in the liver which can prove helpful in diagnosis.

Sarcoidosis

Cardiac involvement in sarcoidosis is much more common than is clinically evident and typically manifests as a restrictive cardiomyopathy. Sarcoid nodules are visualized with good accuracy using MRI and manifests similar to myocarditis with subepicardial hyperenhancement. The diagnosis is important because of the high incidence of sudden death in cardiac sarcoidosis.

Arrhythmogenic Right Ventricular Cardiomyopathy or Dysplasia (ARVC/D)

ARVD is a cardiomyopathy that involves the right ventricle and is characterized by progressive replacement of the right ventricular myocardium with fibro-fatty tissue and by a high risk of malignant arrhythmia and right ventricular failure. It is difficult to diagnose clinically, and MRI is considered the gold standard test because of the outstanding resolution of right ventricular anatomy.

Amyloid Cardiomyopathy (or "Cardiac Amyloidosis")

Systemic amyloidosis commonly involves the myocardium (approximately 50% of patients), and carries a poor prognosis once the diagnosis is established. Since echocardiography lacks sensitivity and specificity in diagnosing amyloid cardiomyopathy, the gold standard for diagnosis is myocardial biopsy, usually multiple biopsies. MRI offers an attractive alternative means of diagnosis and prognosis based on the pattern of hyperenhancement.

In addition to diagnosing common conditions, cardiac MRI can aid in the diagnosis of less common conditions such as restrictive cardiomyopathies, pericardial disease, Fabry's disease, Chagas' cardiomyopathy, endomyocardial fibroelastosis, uremic cardiomyopathy, and myocardial noncompaction. Cardiac MRI can also play a role in monitoring response to treatment in patients with heart failure.

Limitations of Cardiac MRI

The traditional contraindications and limitations of MRI include claustrophobia and safety concerns related to the presence of metallic objects in the body, including pacemakers and implantable cardioverter defibrillators. These devices are commonly implanted in patients with heart failure, somewhat limiting the usefulness of MRI in this population. Newer-generation devices and wires in the future may be MRI-compatible. In addition, it is not as widely accessible as echocardiography, is considerably more expensive, and carries a small risk of a dermopathy in patients with renal failure when Gd-DTPA contrast is used. However, MRI is safe in most patients with prosthetic cardiac valves, with sternal wires and coronary stents.

NUCLEAR IMAGING

Radionuclide ventriculography has traditionally been used for an accurate assessment of EF in patients with cardiovascular disease. At present it is seldom used for this indication, except in the case of serial measurements following cardiotoxic chemotherapy or more precise estimation of LVEF for borderline cases when determining the indications for device implantation (defibrillators or pacemakers). In patients with heart failure, nuclear cardiology technology is commonly used for assessment of myocardial viability with PET scanning (which evaluates glucose uptake with ^{18}F-FDG) and SPECT (which evaluates perfusion, cell membrane integrity, and intactness of mitochondria with ^{201}Tl or ^{99}Tc-labeled agents) for evaluation of ischemia and viability. Viable tissue can display reduced perfusion and normal ^{18}F-FDG uptake suggesting hibernation or normal perfusion and ^{18}F-FDG uptake suggesting stunning. The larger issue of a therapeutic response to revascularization in terms of improved EF or symptoms has been evaluated in some studies. Pooled data from 12 viability studies with ^{18}F-FDG have demonstrated that in patients with evidence of viability, revascularization improves the EF from 37% to 47%, but no improvement is observed in patients without evidence of viability. Similar results were reported with ^{201}Tl studies, albeit with a smaller number of patients.[37] Numerous studies evaluating the functional impact of revascularizing viable myocardium detected by ^{18}F-FDG have demonstrated improvement in symptoms and lower event rates in patients undergoing revascularization.[38]

FUTURE DIRECTIONS

Molecular imaging in patients with heart failure is in its infancy at present but is likely to assume a larger role in the future. The areas of interest for molecular imaging in heart failure patients include assessment of the myocardial renin-angiotensin system with ^{18}F-labeled captopril and lisinopril, which are investigative tools in explaining the role of the angiotensin converting enzyme and angiotensin 1 receptors in the pathogenesis of fibrosis and progression of heart failure. Other studies have demonstrated a role for ^{123}I-MIBG imaging in providing diagnostic and prognostic imaging in heart failure patients. MIBG scans have been shown to evaluate the cardiac sympathetic nervous system redistribution and function. Molecular cardiac imaging is now able to demonstrate the heightened role of apoptosis in heart failure. In animal models, reducing the rate of apoptosis has resulted in a corresponding decrease in the progression to ventricular remodeling and heart failure. In a human study of IDC patients with ^{99m}Tc-labeled Annexin A5, uptake of the isotope (which is avid for regions with apoptosis) signaled progression of LV dysfunction. Patients without an increased uptake maintained stable ventricular function, further demonstrating a role for apoptosis in the pathogenesis of heart failure in humans.[39]

Clinical application of imaging techniques at the point of care is another promising area. Echocardiographic machines have been miniaturized to hand-held sizes and affordable, portable scanning equipment allows everyday application for determining physiologic variations in different clinical settings. Recent data imply the potential for devising algorithms to accurately estimate filling pressures at the bedside using simple algorithms,[40] although more validations are needed to determine the reproducibility and reliability of such measurements.

CONCLUSION

Heart failure is a clinical syndrome which relies heavily upon imaging modalities for confirmation of diagnosis, prognosis, treatment decisions, and monitoring of response to treatments. Echocardiography is the most commonly utilized imaging modality in heart failure because of its broad availability, convenience, tolerability, and low cost. New applications of echocardiography have expanded its conventional role in the traditional diagnostic and therapeutic paradigms. However, MRI scanning also plays an increasingly important role in the detection of specific cardiomyopathies as well as the tissue characterization and morphologic and functional assessment of the failing heart. Nuclear cardiac imaging is still widely used in ischemic and viability assessments, particularly in decisions regarding revascularization in patients with ischemic cardiomyopathy. Molecular imaging in heart failure patients is currently in its infancy but likely to assume a larger future role.

◇◇◇◇◇◇◇◇◇◇◇◇◇

REFERENCES

1. Hunt SA; American College of Cardiology; American Heart Association Task Force on Practice Guidelines (Writing Committee to Update the 2001 Guidelines for the Evaluation and Management of Heart Failure). ACC/AHA 2005 guideline update for the diagnosis and management of chronic heart failure in the adult: a report of the American College of Cardiology/American Heart Association Task Force on Practice Guidelines (Writing Committee to Update the 2001 Guidelines for the Evaluation and Management of Heart Failure). *J Am Coll Cardiol* 2005 Sep 20;46(6):e1-82. Erratum in: *J Am Coll Cardiol* 2006 Apr 7;47(7):1503-1505.

2. American Heart Association, Heart Disease and Stroke Statistics 2005 Update, American Heart Association, Dallas, Tex (2005).

3. Koelling TM, Chen RS, Lubwama RN, L'Italien GJ, Eagle KA. The expanding national burden of heart failure in the United States the influence of heart failure in women, *Am Heart J* 147 (2004), pp. 74-78.

4. Maurer MS, Kronzon I, Burkhoff D. Ventricular pump function in heart failure with normal ejection fraction: insights from pressure-volume measurements. *Prog Cardiovasc Dis* 2006 Nov-Dec;49(3):182-95.

5. Kirkpatrick JN, Vannan MA, Narula J, Lang RM. Echocardiography in heart failure: applications, utility, and new horizons. *J Am Coll Cardiol* 2007 Jul 31;50(5):381-96. Epub 2007 Jul 13.

6. Kawaguchi M, Hay I, Fetics B, et al: Combined ventricular systolic and arterial stiffening in patients with heart failure and preserved ejection fraction: Implications for systolic and diastolic reserve limitations. *Circulation* 107:714-720, 2003.

7. Liu CP, Ting CT, Lawrence W, et al: Diminished contractile response to increased heart rate in intact human left ventricular hypertrophy. Systolic versus diastolic determinants. *Circulation* 88:1893-1906, 1993.

8. Redfield MM: Understanding "diastolic" heart failure. *NEJM* 350: 1930-31, 2004.

9. Cohn JN, Ferrari R, Sharpe N. Cardiac remodeling--concepts and clinical implications: a consensus paper from an international forum on cardiac remodeling. Behalf of an International Forum on Cardiac Remodeling. *J Am Coll Cardiol* 2000 Mar 1;35(3):569-82.

10. Gottdiener J, Bednarz J, Devereux R, et al. American Society of Echocardiography recommendations for use of echocardiography in clinical trials. *J Am Soc Echocardiogr* 2004;17:1086-119.

11. Tei C, Dujardin KS, Hodge DO, Kyle RA, Tajik AJ, Seward JB. Doppler index combining systolic and diastolic myocardial performance: clinical value in cardiac amyloidosis. *J Am Coll Cardiol* 1996; 28: 658-664.

12. Yeo TC, Dujardin KS, Tei C, Mahoney DW, McGoon MD, Seward JB. Value of a Doppler-derived index combining systolic and diastolic time intervals in predicting outcome in primary pulmonary hypertension. *Am J Cardiol* 1998;81:115-7.

13. Arnlov J, Ingelsson E, Riserus U, Andren B, Lind L. Myocardial performance index, a Doppler-derived index of global left ventricular function, predicts congestive heart failure in elderly men. *Eur Heart J* 2004;25:2220-5.

14. Chuang M, Hibberd M, Salton C, Beaudin R, Riley M, Parker R, et al. Importance of imaging method over imaging modality in noninvasive determination of left ventricular volumes and ejection fraction. *J Am Coll Cardiol* 2000;35:477-84.

15. Lang RM, Bierig M, Devereaux RB, et al. Recommendations for chamber quantification. *J Am Soc Echocardiogr* 2005;18:1440-63.

16. Pinamonti B, Zecchin M, Di Lenarda A, Gregori D, Sinagra G, Camerini F. Persistence of restrictive left ventricular filling pattern in dilated cardiomyopathy: an ominous prognostic sign. *J Am Coll Cardiol* 1997;29:604-12.

17. Dini FL, Dell' Anna R, Micheli A, Michelassi C, Rovai D. Impact of blunted pulmonary venous flow on the outcome of patients with left ventricular systolic dysfunction secondary to either ischemic or idiopathic dilated cardiomyopathy. *Am J Cardiol* 2000;85:1455-60.

18. Garcia MJ, Smedira NG, Greenberg NL, et al. Color M-mode Doppler flow propagation velocity is a preload insensitive index of left ventricular relaxation: animal and human validation. *J Am Coll Cardiol* 2000;35:201-8.

19. Garcia MJ, Ares MA, Asher C, Rodriguez L, Vandervoort P, Thomas JD. An index of early left ventricular filling that combined with pulsed Doppler peak E velocity may estimate capillary wedge pressure. *J Am Coll Cardiol* 1997;29:448-54.

20. Nagueh SF, Zoghbi WA. Clinical Assessment of LV Diastolic Filling by Doppler Echocardiography. *ACC Current Journal Review* 2001; July/Aug: 45-49.

21. Quinones MA, Breenberg BH, Kopelen HA, et al., for the SOLVD Investigators. Echocardiogaphic predictors of clinical outcomes in patients with left ventricular dysfunction enrolled in the SOLVD registry and trials: significance of left ventricular hypertrophy. *J Am Coll Cardiol* 2005;35:1237-44.

22. Schinkel AF, Bax JJ, Boersma E, Elhendy A, Vourvouri EC, Roelandt JR, Poldermans D. Assessment of residual myocardial viability in regions with chronic electrocardiographic Q-wave infarction. *Am Heart J* 2002, 144:865-869.

23. Senior R, Lahiri A. Role of dobutamine echocardiography in detection of myocardial viability for predicting outcome after revascularization in ischemic cardiomyopathy. *J Am Soc Echocardiogr* 2001, 14:240-248.

24. Bax JJ, Poldermans D, Elhendy A, Cornel JH, Boersma E, Rambaldi R, Roelandt JR, Fioretti PM. Improvement of left ventricular ejection fraction, heart failure symptoms and prognosis after revascularization in patients with chronic coronary artery disease and viable myocardium detected by dobutamine stress echocardiography. *J Am Coll Cardiol* 1999, 34:163-169.

25. Nagaoka H, Isobe N, Kubota S, Iizuka T, Imai S, Suzuki T, Nagai R: Myocardial contractile reserve as prognostic determinant in patients with idiopathic dilated cardiomyopathy without overt heart failure. *Chest* 1997, 111:344-350.

26. Pratali L, Picano E, Otasevic P, Vigna C, Palinkas A, Cortigiani L, Dodi C, Bojic D, Varga A, Csanady M, Landi P. Prognostic significance of the dobutamine echocardiography test in idiopathic dilated cardiomyopathy. *Am J Cardiol* 2001, 88:1374-1378.

27. Bader H, Garrigue S, Lafitte S, Reuter S, Jais P, Haissaguerre M, et al. Intra-left ventricular electromechanical asynchrony; a new independent predictor of severe cardiac events in heart failure patients. *J Am Coll Cardiol* 2004;43:248-56.

28. Bax JJ, Bleeker GB, Marwick TH, Molhoek SG, Boersma E, Steendijk P, et al. Left ventricular dyssynchrony predicts response and prognosis after cardiac resynchronization therapy. *J Am Coll Cardiol* 2004;44:1834-40.

29. Sogaard P, Egeblad H, Pedersen AK, Kim WY, Kristensen BO, Hansen PS, et al. Sequential versus simultaneous biventricular resynchronization for severe heart failure; evaluation by tissue Doppler imaging. *Circulation* 2002;106:2078-84.

30. Jenkins C, Bricknell K, Hanekom L, Marwick T. Reproducibility and accuracy of echocardiographic measurements of left ventricular parameters using real-time three-dimensional echocardiography. *J Am Coll Cardiol* 2004;44:878-86.

31. Mikkelsen KV, Moller JE, Bie P, Ryde H, Videbaek L, Haghfelt T. Tei index and neurohormonal activation in patients with incident heart failure: serial changes and prognostic value. *Eur J Heart Fail* 2006;8:599-608.

32. Malm S, Frigstad S, Sagberg E, Larsson H, Skjaerpe T. Accurate and reproducible measurement of left ventricular volume and ejection fraction by contrast echocardiography: a comparison with magnetic resonance imaging. *J Am Coll Cardiol* 2004;44:1030-5.

33. Soriano CJ, Ridocci F, Estornell J, et al. Noninvasive diagnosis of coronary artery disease in patients with heart failure and systolic dysfunction of uncertain etiology, using late gadolinium-enhanced cardiovascular magnetic resonance. *J Am Coll Cardiol* 2005;45(5):743-8.

34. McCrohon JA, Moon JC, Prasad SK, et al. Differentiation of heart failure related to dilated cardiomyopathy and coronary artery disease using gadolinium-enhanced cardiovascular magnetic resonance. *Circulation* 2003;108(1):54-9.

35. Assomull RG, Prasad SK, Lyne J, et al. Cardiovascular magnetic resonance, fibrosis, and prognosis in dilated cardiomyopathy. *J Am Coll Cardiol* 2006; 48:1977-85.

36. Friedrich MG, Strohm O, Schulz-Menger J, et al. Contrast media-enhanced magnetic resonance imaging visualizes myocardial changes in the course of viral myocarditis. *Circulation* 1998;97(18):1802-9.

37. Maddahi J, Schelbert H, Brunken R, Di Carli M. Role of thallium-201 and PET imaging in evaluation of myocardial viability and management of patients with coronary artery disease and left ventricular dysfunction. *J Nucl Med* 1994;35: 707-715.

38. Schinkel AF, Poldermans D, Elhendy A, Bax JJ. Assessment of myocardial viability in patients with heart failure. *J Nucl Med* 2007 Jul;48(7):1135-46. Epub 2007 Jun 15.

39. Kietselaer BL, Reutelingsperger CP, Boersma HH, et al. Noninvasive detection of programmed cell loss with 99mTc-labeled annexin A5 in heart failure. *J Nucl Med* 2007; 48 (4):562-7.

40. Nguyen VT, Ho JE, Ho CY, Givertz MM, Stevenson LW. Handheld echocardiography offers rapid assessment of clinical volume status. *Am Heart J* 2008;156(3):537-42.

CHAPTER 3

Atrial Arrythmias

Li-Fern Hsu, MBBS
Christophe Scavee, MD
Prashanthan Sanders, MBBS, PhD, FRACP

INTRODUCTION

The increasing availability of advanced and sophisticated electrophysiologic techniques for the study of cardiac cells and tissues, together with the ability to study arrhythmias in experimental models and in patients, has contributed much to our present knowledge about the mechanisms of arrhythmias. Although much remains to be understood, such knowledge has enabled us to devise strategies, both pharmacologic and nonpharmacologic, to treat these rhythm disorders. This chapter first provides a brief overview of these mechanisms, followed by a more detailed discussion of the pathophysiology of arrhythmias arising from the atrium, and ends with a short review of how such understanding has been translated into curative therapy, specifically catheter ablation.

GENERAL MECHANISMS OF ATRIAL ARRHYTHMIAS

Arrhythmias are caused by disorders of impulse formation, disorders of impulse conduction, or a combination of both.[1, 2] However, it is important to realize that, unlike tissue or experimental models, the mechanisms of some clinically occurring arrhythmias are difficult to determine using present technology. In addition, some tachyarrhythmias can be started by one mechanism and be precipitated by another.

Disorders of Impulse Formation

Atrial arrhythmias caused by disorders of impulse formation can be due to normal or abnormal automaticity, or triggered activity. Anatomically, they can be considered as: (1) inappropriate discharge rate from a normal pacemaker, the sinus node, or (2) discharge from an ectopic pacemaker that takes over control of the atrial rhythm.

Automaticity

Automaticity is the property of a cell to initiate an impulse spontaneously, without the need for prior stimulation. Such cells are called pacemaker cells and are located in the sinus node, as well as in specialized fibers in the atria, atrioventricular (AV) junction, and the His-Purkinje system. Normally, the dominant pacemaker of the heart is the sinus node, which usually discharges at a rate of 60–100 beats per minute in adults. The other tissue-containing pacemaker cells are known as latent pacemakers.

In sinus tachycardia, the sinus node fires at a rate >100 beats per minute, but is still the dominant pacemaker of the heart. This arrhythmia is a result of *normal automaticity*, since the cellular mechanism for depolarization is unchanged from normal sinus rhythm. An ectopic rhythm occurs when the site of the dominant pacemaker shifts to a site other than the sinus node.[3] This can occur when the intrinsic rate of the sinus node decreases, allowing the ectopic pacemaker activity to manifest, or when the intrinsic rate of the ectopic pacemaker site increases, leading to overdrive suppression of the sinus node. These arrhythmias can be due to normal automaticity, if they originate from the latent pacemakers, or abnormal automaticity, from both latent pacemakers and atrial myocardial tissue. *Abnormal automaticity* can occur under certain conditions, often with intrinsic cardiac disease, whereby the cells have reduced maximum diastolic potentials, resulting in spontaneous diastolic (Phase 4) depolarization.[4]

Triggered Activity
This is a form of impulse initiation caused by after-depolarizations, which are depolarizing oscillations in cell membrane voltage induced by a preceding action potential.[5, 6] They may occur during Phases 2 or 3 of the action potential (early after-depolarizations) or following complete membrane repolarization (delayed after-depolarizations).[7] In summary, they constitute pacemaker activity resulting from a preceding impulse or series of impulses (trigger).

Disorders of Impulse Conduction
Conduction delay and block can result in tachyarrhythmias because of reentrant excitation. The conduction block can be anatomic or functional.

Reentry
During a normal cardiac cycle, the impulse from the pacemaker sequentially activates the atria, the AV conduction system, and the ventricles, and dies out after all the fibers have been activated and are completely refractory. The heart must then wait for a new impulse for each subsequent activation. Reentry occurs when the impulse does not die out but continues to propagate and reactivate the heart because the activation wavefront continuously encounters excitable cardiac tissue.[1] Most clinically important tachyarrhythmias are caused by reentry.

For reentry to occur, certain conditions must be fulfilled: (1) there must be a substrate capable of supporting reentry, usually a region of slow conduction, (2) the activation wavefront must encounter unidirectional block, and (3) the activation wavefront must be able to circulate or rotate around a central obstacle, which can be anatomic or functional.[8] The concept of reentry is illustrated in Figure 3.1.

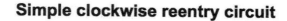

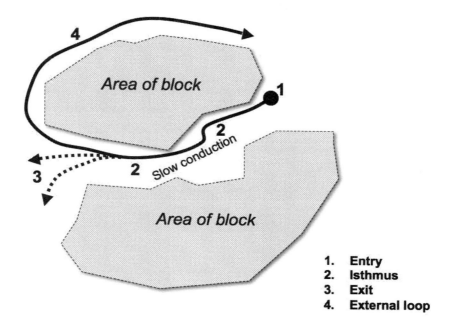

Figure 3.1

Schemetic diagram of reentrant circuit around a central area of conduction block.

The classical form of reentry, *anatomic reentry*, describes a simple circus movement in which the wavefront propagates around an anatomically-defined circuit with a central anatomic obstacle.[9, 10] It is a characterized by a stable circuit, which is relatively fixed in length and location. In *functional reentry*, the circuit is not constrained by anatomical obstacles. Instead, it is defined by the dynamic heterogeneities of the electrophysiologic properties in the involved tissues. It can be fixed and stable, or unstable, changing in size and location.[11, 12]

Clinically, the features suggestive of reentry include: (1) initiation and termination of tachycardia with premature stimuli, (2) initiation of tachycardia dependent on pacing site, (3) initiation requiring a critical degree of conduction slowing, (4) inverse relationship between the coupling interval of the premature stimulus and the interval to the first beat of tachycardia, (5) demonstration of entrainment of the tachycardia, (6) correlation of continuous fragmented electrical activity with the tachycardia, and (7) termination of the tachycardia by interrupting the circuit at a single point.[13]

PATHOPHYSIOLOGY AND FEATURES OF ATRIAL ARRHYTHMIAS

Clinically, atrial arrhythmias were initially classified based on their ECG features, including their regularity and features of the P-waves. However, a greater understanding of their mechanisms has revealed the limitations of such an approach and created the need for a mechanistic classification, with implications for their therapy, especially in the field of catheter ablation.[14]

Sinus Tachyarrhythmias

These arrhythmias occur in the region of the sinus node. Sinus tachycardia occurs in response to an appropriate physiologic stimulus, as well as to inappropriate or excessive stimuli, such as thyrotoxicosis. Inappropriate sinus tachycardia may occur because of the failure of the mechanisms controlling sinus rate. In addition, reentry may also occur within or close to the sinus node, resulting in sinus node reentrant tachycardia.

Sinus Tachycardia

Sinus tachycardia is defined as an increase in the sinus rate to more than 100 beats per minute in keeping with the level of physical, emotional, pharmacologic, or pathologic stress.[15] It is often a physiologic response to various stimuli, although it is sometimes a sign of significant underlying pathologies. It results from physiologic influences on individual pacemaker cells and from an anatomic shift in atrial depolarization site superiorly within the sinus node.[16]

Inappropriate Sinus Tachycardia

Inappropriate sinus tachycardia is defined as a persistent increase in resting heart rate or sinus rate unrelated to, or out of proportion with, the level of physical, emotional, pathologic, or pharmacologic stress.[15] It has been thought to result from either enhanced automaticity of the sinus node,[17] or abnormal autonomic regulation of the sinus node, with excessive sympathetic and reduced parasympathetic tone.[18] It is sometimes considered a form of focal atrial tachycardia originating in the sinus node. However, in general, the site of atrial depolarization/origin shifts inferiorly down along the crista terminalis as function of changes in autonomic tone, whereas the origin remains fixed in focal atrial tachycardia.[14]

It is diagnosed on the basis of the following: (1) the presence of persistent sinus tachycardia with excessive rate increase in response to activity and nocturnal rate normalization, (2) the nonparoxysmal nature of the tachycardia and symptoms, (3) identical P-wave morphology and endocardial activation to sinus rhythm, and (4) exclusion of secondary/systemic causes.[19, 20]

Focal Atrial Tachycardia

Focal atrial tachycardia is characterized by atrial activity starting at a small area, or focus, from where it spreads centrifugally.[21, 22]

Mechanism

Focal activity can be to the result of automaticity, triggered activity or reentry involving very small circuits (microreentry). Clinically, an automatic mechanism is suggested by the following: (1) a progressive increase in rate at the beginning (warm up) and/or a progressive decrease in rate before termination (cool down), (2) initiation with isoprotroterenol, (3) inability of pacing maneuvers to initiate, entrain, or terminate the tachycardia, and (4) transient suppression with overdrive atrial pacing, with subsequent resumption of tachycardia characterized by a gradual increase in atrial rate.[21, 23] Triggered activity is suggested by the following: (1) initiation and termination by atrial premature stimuli, which is dependent on cycle length, (2) absence of entrainment, although overdrive suppression and termination are present, and (3) presence of delayed after-depolarizations on recordings of monophasic action potentials just before the onset of tachy-cardia.[7, 21, 24, 25] Reentry is suggested by the presence of some of the features discussed in the previous section,[21, 26-28] although very small, localized circuits may be very difficult to define, requiring high-density mapping.[29]

Distribution

Anatomically, focal atrial tachycardias are not randomly distributed, but tend to cluster over certain anatomic regions. The majority of right atrial tachycardias originate along the crista terminalis,[30] with lesser involvement of other sites, including the septum, appendage and tricuspid annulus, coronary sinus and superior vena cava.[31, 32, 33] In the left atrium, the foci are often found in the pulmonary veins, septum or mitral annulus.[32-35]

Diagnosis

The ECG typically shows discrete P-waves, with a clearly defined isoelectric baseline between the P-waves in all leads (Figure 3.2). The morphology of the P-waves will vary with the location of the focus, and can be used to approximately localize it before electrophysiologic study and ablation.[32, 36] However, the ECG features can vary widely in the presence of rapid rates, atrial conduction disturbances, the presence of structural heart disease, or cardiac surgery. In such cases, the diagnosis of focal atrial tachycardia can be established for certainty only by an electrophysiology study and endocardial mapping demonstrating a focus with centrifugal activation of the surrounding atrial tissue.

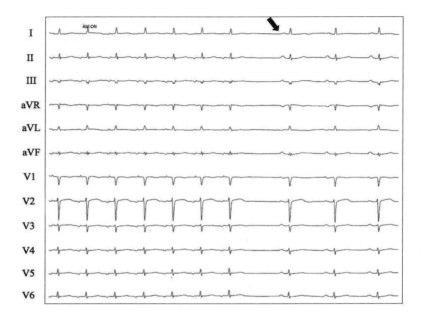

Figure 3.2

An example of focal atrial tachycardia. The ECG shows atrial tachycardia which terminated shortly after commencement of ablation (Abl: ON), resulting in restoration of sinus rhythm (arrow). Note the difference in P-wave morphology.

Multifocal Atrial Tachycardia

Multifocal atrial tachycardia is diagnosed based on the finding of an irregular tachycardia characterized by three or more different P-wave morphologies at different rates.[37] The rhythm is always irregular and is sometimes confused with atrial fibrillation. It is most commonly associated with underlying chronic pulmonary disease, but may also result from metabolic or electrolyte disorders.

Macroreentrant Atrial Tachycardia

This implies reentrant activation around a large central obstacle. Examples of these obstacles are a normal, valve annulus, or abnormal structure, like scar tissue. There is no single point or origin of activation, and the circuit includes large portions of the atria. Activation should be recorded continuously throughout the tachycardia cycle length. Although a reference point may be assigned as the start of activation during an electrophysiological study, it should be understood that this is arbitrary.[38]

The best-characterized macroreentrant atrial tachycardias are right atrial, typical (isthmus-dependent) atrial flutters and postatriotomy (or incisional) atrial tachycardias.

However, our understanding of left atrial flutters has improved dramatically in recent years, and with the increasing popularity of atrial fibrillation ablation and surgery, macroreentrant tachycardias arising after these procedures are increasingly encountered.

Typical Atrial Flutter

This is the most common type of macroreentrant atrial tachycardia. The term *atrial flutter* is an ECG diagnosis characterized by an organized atrial rhythm with a rate typically between 250 and 350 beats/min, with the P-wave producing an undulating appearance on the ECG.

Mechanism

The reentrant circuit is in the right atrium, bound anteriorly by the tricuspid valve, and posteriorly by a combination of anatomical obstacles (the Eustachian ridge and orifices of the superior and inferior vena cava) and functional barriers (crista terminalis).[39-43] The superior part of the circuit commonly involves the right atrial roof between the superior vena cava and tricuspid annulus,[44, 45] although sometimes activation can cross the superior portion of the crista terminalis. Inferiorly, the circuit always involves the cavotricuspid isthmus, between the inferior vena cava and tricuspid annulus,[46, 47] hence the term *isthmus-dependent*. The descending limb of the circuit involves the lateral and anterior right atrium, and the ascending limb involves the septum and part of the posterior wall with the boundaries.[46] This is called counterclockwise reentry as seen from the left anterior oblique perspective.[14] Less commonly, reentry can proceed in the reverse (clockwise) direction over the typical flutter circuit. This is called reverse typical atrial flutter.[48, 49] In both cases, the left atrium is a passive bystander (Figure 3.3).

The Cavotricuspid Isthmus

The cavotricuspid isthmus forms the inferior border of the reentrant circuit. It is bounded anteriorly by the inferior part of the tricuspid orifice and posteriorly by the inferior vena cava and Eustachian ridge. Its structure, width, and thickness are very variable, and the musculature can be very complex, especially near the septal end.[50] The large width of the ascending and descending limbs of the circuit and the size of the roof make the cavotricuspid isthmus the narrowest part of the circuit. Therefore, it is the ideal target for ablation, not because it is an area of slow conduction or disease, but because it is accessible, narrow, safe, and essential for the integrity of the circuit.

Diagnosis

The ECG for typical atrial flutter is very specific, showing a characteristic sawtooth pattern best observed in the inferior leads. The pattern consists of a succession of gently downsloping segments followed by a sharper negative deflection, then a sharp positive upstroke with a slight positive overshoot leading to the next cycle. Lead V1 often shows a positive deflection while V6 is negative. Conversely, reverse typical atrial flutter is characterized by the presence of broad, positive deflections in the inferior leads, wide

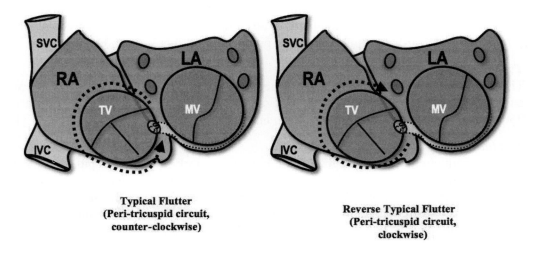

**Typical Flutter
(Peri-tricuspid circuit,
counter-clockwise)**

**Reverse Typical Flutter
(Peri-tricuspid circuit,
clockwise)**

Figure 3.3

Schematic representation of both atria in the left anterior oblique view. The activation patterns of typical and reverse typical flutter are shown by the arrows. The left atrium is activated passively.

negative or biphasic deflections in lead V1 and a positive deflection in V6.[48, 51] Both are illustrated in Figure 3.4.

In most instances, typical atrial flutter can be diagnosed based on the classical ECG findings alone. However, patients may sometimes show unusual ECG patterns, and confirmation of cavotricuspid isthmus involvement can only be made by activation and entrainment studies.[44]

Other Cavotricuspid Isthmus-Dependent Circuits

Isthmus-dependent flutter may also occur as double-wave reentry or lower-loop reentry. Double wave reentry is defined as a circuit in which two wavefronts circulate simultaneously in the usual flutter pathway.[52] This is an unstable rhythm and is usually transient, but at times may deteriorate into atrial fibrillation. Lower loop reentry is defined as a circuit in which the reentrant wavefront circulates around the inferior vena cava due to conduction across the crista terminalis.[53,54] The anterior arm of the circuit is the cavotricuspid isthmus, while the posterior arm is the low posterior right atrial wall.

Noncavotricuspid Isthmus-Dependent Right Atrial Circuits

Atrial flutter caused by macroreentrant circuits that do not use the cavotricuspid isthmus are less common. These circuits are often associated with a fixed anatomical obstacle, usually a scar/lesion, or sometimes a functional barrier in the region of the crista terminalis.

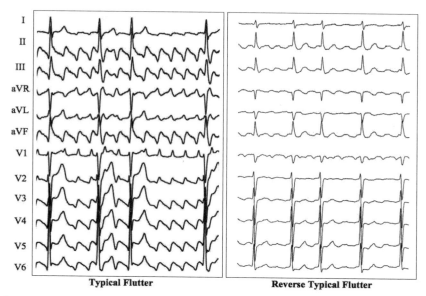

Figure 3.4

The ECG of typical and reverse typical atrial flutter. Typical flutter shows a slowly descending segment preceding a shart negative deflection in the inferior leads, while the flutter wave in V1 is usually positive, with transition to negative waves towards V6. Reverse typical flutter shows a broad positive deflection in the inferior leads, while V1 is negative or biphasic.

Lesion-Related Macroreentrant Atrial Tachycardia

In this macroreentrant circuit, the central obstacle is an atrial lesion, which could be an atriotomy scar (Figure 3.5A), a septal prosthetic patch, a suture line, or a fixed line of conduction block caused by an atrial maze procedure or radiofrequency ablation.[14, 38, 55-58] Atrial mapping can reveal low-voltage electrograms characterizing areas of scar, flat bipolar recordings characterizing a prosthetic patch, or lines of double potentials at linear scar lines.[38] Rarely, in patients who have not had prior cardiac surgery, abnormal areas of low amplitude electrical activity can be detected at the right atrial free wall, consistent with spontaneously occurring scar tissue of uncertain cause (Figure 3.5B).[59, 60]

Sometimes, these incisional/lesion macroreentrant flutters can coexist with a cavotricuspid isthmus-dependent flutter, resulting in multiple circuits. For example, the simultaneous circulation of wavefronts through two loops can create a complex figure-8 reentrant circuit (Figure 3.5C).[55] Very complex and/or multiple reentrant circuits are often seen after surgery for congenital heart disease. For example, after the Mustard, Senning, or Fontan procedures.[56-58]

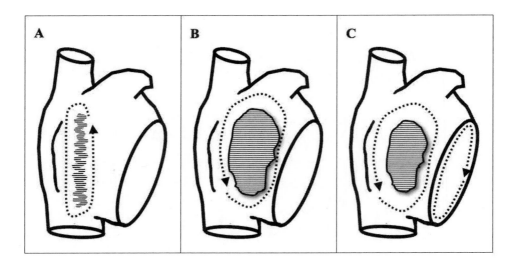

Figure 3.5

Schemetic representation of non-isthmus-dependent atrial flutter. (A) Incisional macroreentry from atriotomy scar. (B) Macroreentry around a spontaneously occurring atrial scar. (C) Complex dual-loop or figure-of-eight macroreentry, with a counterclockwise loop around the scar and a clockwise loop around the tricuspid annulus.

The ECG features of these arrhythmias can be highly variable, sometimes appearing similar to typical atrial flutter or focal atrial tachycardia. In some cases the P-wave can be difficult to identify, possibly because of extensive atrial scarring.[14] Thus definitive diagnosis requires intracardiac mapping.

Other Noncavotricuspid Isthmus-Dependent Right Atrial Tachycardias

Upper loop reentry describes an unusual macroreentrant circuit confined to the right atrial free wall with the central obstacle composed of the superior vena cava (anatomical block) and upper part of the crista terminalis (functional block). The wavefront rotates around this obstacle and a conduction gap in the crista terminalis is essential for maintenance of this circuit.[54,61]

Left Atrial Macroreentrant Tachycardia

Macroreentrant circuits occurring in the left atrium were much less common than right atrial circuits. However, with the increasing application of catheter and surgical ablation for atrial fibrillation, the incidence of left atrial macroreentry has increased significantly.

Spontaneous Left Atrial Macroreentrant Tachycardia

Left atrial macroreentrant circuits can occur spontaneously, although often in the context of structural heart disease.[62] The central obstacles include the mitral annulus, pulmonary veins, areas of low voltage or scarring, and the septum primum.[62-64] Multiple and complex circuits were also observed.[62]

As in other forms of noncavotricuspid isthmus dependent flutters, the ECG features are variable, although a positive F (flutter)-wave in lead V1 is suggestive of left atrial origin.[62] Definitive diagnosis requires detailed intracardiac mapping.

Lesion-Related Left Atrial Macroreentrant Tachycardia

Catheter or surgical treatment of atrial fibrillation involves the creation of lesions, using radiofrequency or cryo-energy (or surgical cut and sew), to isolate the pulmonary veins electrically, and further modify the left atrial substrate.

The incidence of atrial tachycardia after catheter ablation for atrial fibrillation is high, ranging from about 10% to 30%.[65-68] The vast majority are macroreentrant and are related to the presence of gaps, or recovery of conduction, across the ablation lesions.[69-72] Fixed anatomic barriers like the mitral annulus and septum are also important central obstacles, as the most common reentrant circuits in these patients are peri-mitral and septal in location.[70, 71] Complex and multiple circuits are also observed, as are localized circuits confined to the anterior left atrium.[73]

Similarly, left atrial tachycardia has been observed after maze surgery for atrial fibrillation. The mechanisms and locations are similar to those occurring after catheter ablation.[74, 75] Detailed intracardiac mapping is required to characterize these often complex circuits.

Atrial Fibrillation

Atrial fibrillation is characterized by rapid, uncoordinated atrial activation, with consequent deterioration of atrial mechanical function. It is usually associated with an irregular and frequently rapid ventricular response (Figure 3.6), although the ventricular response depends on the conduction properties of the AV node and other factors.[76]

It is the most common arrhythmia, with an estimated prevalence of 0.4 to 1% in the general population, increasing with age.[77, 78] Its incidence increases from less than 0.1% per year in those younger than 40 years old to 1.5% per year in women and 2.0% in men older than 80 years.[79, 80] The lifetime risk for developing this arrhythmia is 1 in 6.[81]

The importance of atrial fibrillation lies in its clinical consequences. It is associated with 5 times more strokes in patients without valvular disease,[80, 82, 83] and 17 times more among those with rheumatic heart disease.[84] It can cause heart failure or potentiate the effects and worsen the prognosis of patients who already have heart failure.[85] It is associated with a doubling of mortality compared to patients in sinus rhythm, even after adjusting for other preexisting heart conditions.[86]

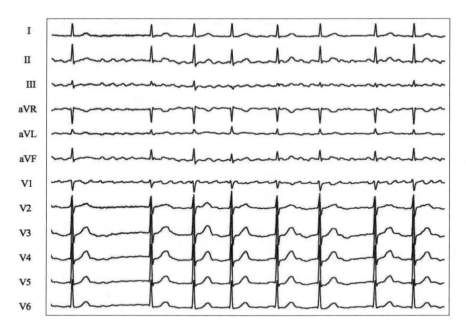

Figure 3.6

Typical ECG of atrial fibrillation, with rapid irregular atrial depolarizations (undulating baseline) and irregular ventricular response.

Causes and Associated Conditions

Atrial fibrillation is often a manifestation of underlying cardiac disease, although approximately 30–45% of paroxysmal and 20–25% of persistent atrial fibrillation are observed in younger patients without demonstrable underlying heart disease (lone atrial fibrillation).[76] Atrial fibrillation can also be associated with other noncardiac disorders, some of which can be reversible. The causes and related conditions are listed in Table 3.1.

Atrial Pathology in Atrial Fibrillation

Atrial Structural Pathology Causing Atrial Fibrillation

The most common findings in patients with atrial fibrillation are atrial fibrosis and atrial dilation. Histologic examination of atrial tissue in these patients revealed patches of fibrous tissue juxtaposed with normal atrial fibers.[87, 88] This may account for heterogeneous conduction and act as the substrate for atrial fibrillation. Atrial fibrosis may be caused by genetic defects, inflammation, and atrial dilation, which can occur in any type of car-

Table 3.1   Causes and Conditions Associated with Atrial Fibrillation

Associated Heart Disease
Valvular heart disease
Ischemic heart disease
Hypertension (especially with left ventricular hypertrophy)
Cardiomyopathies – hypertrophic, dilated, restrictive
Congenital heart disease
Pericardial disease
Heart failure
Other arrhythmias – atrial flutter, Wolff-Parkinson-White syndrome
Medical Conditions
Endocrine disorders – Hyperthyroidism, Phaeochromocytoma
Drugs
Alcohol
Post-Operative
Cardiac surgery
Thoracic surgery / Esophageal surgery
Neurogenic or Autonomic Influences
Increased sympathetic or parasympathetic activity
Subarachnoid hemorrhage
Stroke
Idiopathic (Lone AF)
Familial AF

diac disease.[76] Atrial dilation can be the result of atrial stretch, which activates several molecular pathways, including the renin-angiotensin-aldosterone system. The resultant upregulation of angiotensin II and transforming growth factor-beta1 (TGF-beta1) induces the production of connective tissue growth factor, leading to fibrosis.[76, 89]

In addition, studies of patients with heart failure and atrial septal defect demonstrated that chronic atrial stretch resulted in structural and electrophysiologic changes, such as areas of scarring, reduction of voltage, slow of conduction, and alterations in refractory periods.[90, 91] These changes were similar to those that occur as a consequence of aging.[92]

Atrial Structural Pathology Caused by Atrial Fibrillation
Just as atrial dilation and fibrosis can result in atrial fibrillation, the reverse can also occur. Atrial structural remodeling can be difficult to distinguish from the degenerative changes discussed previously. The initial changes are mainly cellular, with a large proportion of atrial myocytes showing marked changes in their cellular structures, such as loss of

myofibrils, accumulation of glycogen, changes in mitochondrial shape and size, loss of sarcoplasmic reticulum, and dispersion of nuclear chromatin.[93, 94] However, fibrosis can occur later when atrial dilation occurs as a result of loss of contractility and changes in compliance.[95, 96]

These changes have been noted to closely resemble those seen in ventricular myocytes in the hibernating myocardium associated with chronic ischemia.[94, 97] As these changes appear to protect the myocytes against the high metabolic stress associated with rapid rates, it has been speculated that these structural changes occur in response to the relative ischemia associated with the rapid atrial rates.

Mechanisms of Atrial Fibrillation

Automatic Focus Theory of Atrial Fibrillation

A focal origin of atrial fibrillation had been postulated for many years, supported by experimental models.[98] However, this theory received minimal attention until the fairly recent observation that a focal source of atrial fibrillation could be identified in humans, and ablation of this source could eliminate the arrhythmia (Figure 3.7A).[99] Whereas pulmonary veins are the most frequent source of these initiating ectopic beats, nonpulmonary vein sources have also been reported, particularly in the superior vena cava, crista terminalis, coronary sinus and other atrial locations.[100-103]

Due to their primacy as triggers for atrial fibrillation, substantial research has been invested in the anatomic and electrical properties of pulmonary veins. Histologically, atrial myocardium with preserved electrical properties has been observed to extend into the pulmonary veins.[104, 105] These sleeves of myocardium possess a complex and highly variable architecture, possibly with nonhomogeneous anisotropic properties, hence serve as a trigger or substrate for atrial fibrillation.[106] Their electrophysiologic properties are different from other parts of the atria, and from the pulmonary veins of patients without atrial fibrillation, exhibiting shorter refractory periods and decremental conduction.[107]

Although the pulmonary veins were initially considered as triggers, with close-coupled ectopic beats or short rapid salvoes triggering atrial fibrillation (Figure 3.8), it has been recognized that they can serve as substrates or potentiators as well. Sustained pulmonary vein tachycardia can occur because of rapid focal firing, or reentry, and this persistent rapid tachycardia can maintain atrial fibrillation.[108-110]

The use of spectral analysis has increased our knowledge of focal activity in the maintenance of atrial fibrillation. In experimental models, a focal dominant fibrillation frequency has been demonstrated to maintain atrial fibrillation.[111, 112] This has been replicated in humans,[113, 114] and proven by ablation of these sites, with resultant prolongation of atrial fibrillation cycle length and termination of paroxysmal atrial fibrillation.[114] Spectral analysis has demonstrated the importance of pulmonary vein activity in the maintenance of paroxysmal atrial fibrillation but less so for permanent atrial fibrillation, for which atrial substrate is still the more important factor.[115]

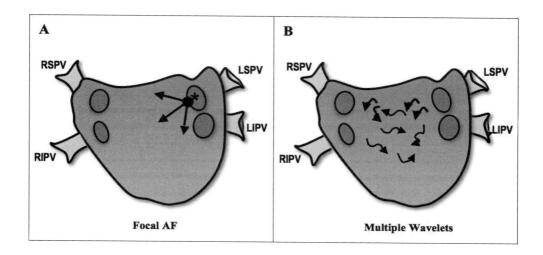

Figure 3.7

The main hypotheses for atrial fibrillation. (A) Automatic focus hypothesis, and (B) multiple wavelet reentry.

Multiple-Wavelet Hypothesis for Atrial Fibrillation

This hypothesis as the mechanism of reentrant atrial fibrillation was first advanced by Moe and colleagues, who proposed that fractionation of wavefronts propagating through the atria results in self-perpetuating daughter wavelets.[116] The initial wavefronts could arise from any of the triggers discussed previously, and these fragment into multiple reentering wavelets if the wavelength is sufficiently short (see Figure 3.7B).[117] This hypothesis is supported in humans by intraoperative electrophysiologic mapping using simultaneous recordings from multiple electrodes.[118]

The presence of an abnormal atrial substrate to maintain atrial fibrillation is important and has been demonstrated in many studies on patients with idiopathic atrial fibrillation. The markers indicating atrial vulnerability include a greater coefficient of dispersion of atrial refractoriness and more easily induced arrhythmia,[119] more widespread distribution of abnormal electrograms,[120] and prolongation of intra-atrial conduction. In patients with preexisting structural heart disease, the associated atrial structural pathology has been discussed previously. However, the extent to which these changes in atrial architecture contribute to the initiation and maintenance of atrial fibrillation is uncertain.

Atrial Electrical Remodeling

Having been initiated, AF may be brief or sustained. A variety of factors may act as perpetuators, ensuring the persistence of AF for longer periods. One is persistence of

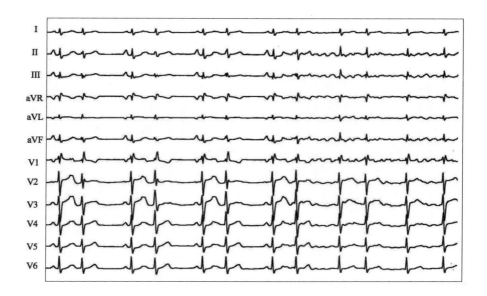

Figure 3.8

Typical ECG of focal atrial fibrillation, with atrial ectopic beats initiating a run of atrial fibrillation.

the triggers and initiators that induce AF,[121] but at some point, AF persists even in their absence. Persistence here may result from electrical and structural remodeling, characterized by atrial dilatation and shortening of the atrial ERP.[93, 122] This combination, along with other remodeling changes, possibly facilitates the appearance of multiple reentrant wavelets and results in atrial fibrillation being self-perpetuating. This is supported by observations in a goat model using an automatic fibrillator to repeatedly reinduce atrial fibrillation. Initially, the induced atrial fibrillation terminated spontaneously. However, after repeated inductions, the episodes became progressively more sustained until they become persistent, giving rise to the adage "atrial fibrillation begets atrial fibrillation."[122]

In patients with recurring paroxysmal or persistent atrial fibrillation, these factors promoting or perpetuating atrial fibrillation should be present for some time after reversion. In an experimental model, interposed periods of sinus rhythm prevented further remodeling so that subsequent atrial fibrillation episodes did not become persistent.[123] Atrial refractory periods were found to have normalized in 2 to 7 days.[117, 123] Clinically, repeated prompt cardioversion has been demonstrated to progressively reduce the total time that patients are in atrial fibrillation and progressively increase the time between cardioverted episodes.[124] This is attributable to prevention of long-lasting atrial fibrillation episodes and its attendant remodeling, suggesting that prompt restoration of sinus rhythm is associated with a better chance of maintaining sinus rhythm.[124, 125]

TREATMENT OF ATRIAL ARRHYTHMIAS

Treatment of atrial arrhythmias is based on two concepts: (1) rate control, where the ventricular rate is controlled with no commitment to restore or maintain sinus rhythm, usually applied to atrial fibrillation and sometimes atrial flutter, and (2) rhythm control, where restoration and/or maintenance of sinus rhythm is attempted.

The first-line treatment of atrial arrhythmias is still pharmacologic in most cases, with a variety of antiarrhythmic drugs available. However, a detailed discussion of pharmacologic treatment is beyond the scope of this chapter. This section will focus briefly on the only curative therapy currently available—catheter ablation.

Importance of Treating Atrial Arrhythmias

Patients with atrial arrhythmias are often symptomatic. These include palpitations, fatigue, lightheadedness, chest discomfort, dyspnea, presyncope, or more rarely, syncope. Often the symptoms vary with ventricular rate, duration of arrhythmia, or concomitant heart disease. The presence of structural heart disease may cause the arrhythmias to be poorly tolerated.

Of greater importance are their potentially dangerous consequences. Atrial arrhythmias that are persistent and associated with a fast ventricular response may lead to a tachycardia-mediated cardiomyopathy, which can result in severe left ventricular dysfunction, but is reversible if treated.[126-129] Atrial flutter and atrial fibrillation are associated with an increased incidence of thromboembolic events.[80, 83, 84, 130] The importance of anticoagulation to reduce the risk of stroke and other thromboembolic events cannot be overstated.[14, 93]

Catheter Ablation

Catheter ablation has been demon strated to be effective and safe for the treatment of cardiac arrhythmias. Unlike antiarrhythmic drugs, it offers the only means of achieving a permanent cure for arrhythmias, and is the best therapy for drug-refractory arrhythmias. Although associated with a small procedural risk, successful ablation enables antiarrhythmic drugs to be stopped, thus avoiding their potentially adverse effects.

Knowledge of the mechanisms of atrial arrhythmias, as discussed in the previous sections, has greatly facilitated this procedure. Conversely, the availability of new endocardial mapping systems has improved our understanding of these arrhythmias.

Focal Atrial Tachycardia

Regardless of whether the arrhythmia is caused by abnormal automaticity, triggered activity, or microreentry, focal atrial tachycardia is ablated by targeting the site of origin. The activation time at such sites are significantly earlier than the onset of the surface P-wave, and the electrograms are often fractionated and prolonged.[15, 21, 38] High-density or electroanatomical mapping can facilitate successful ablation.

Using pooled data from 514 patients, the success rate for catheter ablation of focal atrial tachycardia was 86%, with a recurrence rate of 8%.[131] Left atrial origins accounted for 18%, while 10% had multiple foci.

Cavotricuspid Isthmus-Dependent Flutter

The characterization of the flutter circuit and its dependence on the cavotricuspid isthmus make this region the ideal target for ablation. Unlike focal atrial tachycardia, the ablation lesion is not focal, but a line with the objective of transmural transection of all the myocardium between the tricuspid annulus and the inferior vena cava.[47-49, 132] However, termination of the arrhythmia alone is not considered an appropriate endpoint, as conduction will often persist across the isthmus, with resultant high recurrence rate.[133] Therefore, present endpoint requires the confirmation of bidirectional conduction block across the cavotricuspid isthmus,[134, 135] with an acceptable recurrence rate of < 10%.[132] However, the main long-term problem is the occurrence of atrial fibrillation, which can reach an incidence of up to 30%.[15, 132] It is conceivable that atrial flutter can cause significant atrial remodeling, resulting in predisposition to atrial fibrillation.

Noncavotricuspid Isthmus-Dependent Flutter

Regardless of right or left atrial origin, and whether spontaneous or lesion-related, the principles of ablation are similar to typical atrial flutter. Successful ablation requires the identification of a critical portion of the reentrant circuit where it can be interrupted by a focal or linear lesion.[55-57] High-density or electroanatomic mapping can greatly facilitate ablation, enabling detailed characterization of the circuit and regions of scarring or conduction block. To minimize recurrence, the linear lesions should be complete and extend between two electrically inert structures. The demonstration of bidirectional conduction block is again important.[136-138]

Atrial Fibrillation

Catheter ablation for atrial fibrillation has evolved significantly, guided by improved understanding of its pathophysiology. Early techniques were based on the surgical maze procedure, creating linear lesions in the atria to prevent multiple-wavelet reentry.[139] However, the technical difficulty and high complication rate of this procedure precluded its wide acceptance. The subsequent observation that pulmonary veins could be the source of atrial fibrillation and the demonstration that elimination of these foci could cure the arrhythmia dramatically increased enthusiasm for catheter ablation.[100] Initially, only the pulmonary veins were targeted, but with the demonstration of nonpulmonary foci,[103] and increased understanding of abnormal atrial substrate, the ablation procedure has been modified to incorporate left atrial linear lesions at various locations, particularly the roof,[137] and mitral isthmus connecting the mitral annulus and the left inferior pulmonary vein.[138] In patients with persistent atrial fibrillation, further ablation to modify the substrate may be needed.[140, 141] A different approach involves the ablation of complex fractionated electrograms.[142]

Concurrently, advances in technology have facilitated the procedure, including use of a circular catheter for pulmonary vein mapping,[143] use of intracardiac ultrasound,[144] and the availability of electroanatomic or nonfluoroscopic mapping systems.[145] The success rate has been variable. A worldwide survey of 8745 patients from 181 centers showed a success rate of 52% (ranging from 15–77%) of patients becoming asymptomatic without any antiarrhythmic drugs, with 24% requiring a repeat procedure.[146] Lastly, cure of atrial fibrillation by catheter ablation has been shown, although not in randomized trials, to be associated with a reduction in mortality and morbidity from heart failure and thromboembolism.[129, 147, 148]

CONCLUSION

Recognition of the prognostic significance of atrial arrhythmias and enhanced understanding of their mechanisms has brought this field to prominence. Based on knowledge of these mechanisms, new drugs can be developed to target these arrhythmias specifically. Recent advances in mapping and catheter ablation techniques and technology have led to improved definition and understanding of these arrhythmias, and may offer the prospective of a reliable and permanent cure.

◇◇◇◇◇◇◇◇◇◇◇◇

REFERENCES

1. Hoffman BF, Rosen MR. Cellular mechanisms for cardiac arrhythmias. *Circ Res* 1981; 49:1-15
2. Waldo AL, Wit AL. Mechanisms of cardiac arrhythmias. *Lancet* 1993; 341:1189-1193
3. Jones SB, Euler DE, Randall WC, et al. Atrial ectopic foci in the canine heart: Hierarchy of pacemaker automaticity. *Am J Physiol Heart Circ Physiol* 1980; 238:H788-H793
4. Podrid PJ, Kowey PR. *Cardiac arrhythmia: Mechanisms, diagnosis and management.* Baltimore, Williams & Wilkins 1995
5. Cranefield PF, Aronson RS. Initiation of sustained rhythmic activity by single propagated action potentials in canine cardiac Purkinje fibers exposed to sodium-free solution or to ouabain. *Circ Res* 1974; 34:477-481

6.   Cranefield PF. Action potentials, afterpotentials and arrhythmias. *Circ Res* 1977; 41:415-425

7.   Aronson RS, Hairman RJ, Gough WB. Delayed after-depolarization and pathologic states. In Rosen MR, Janse MJ, Wit AL (eds).: *Cardiac Electrophysiology: A Textbook*. Mt Kisco, NY: Futura Publishing Co 1990; 303-332

8.   Mines GR. On circulating excitations in heart muscles and their possible relation to tachycardia and fibrillation. *Trans R Soc Can* 1914; 4:43-52

9.   Frame LH, Page RL, Boyden PA, et al. Circus movement in the canine atrium around the tricuspid ring during experimental atrial flutter and during reentry in vivo. *Circulation* 1987; 76:1155-1175

10. Waldo AL. Mechanisms of atrial fibrillation, atrial flutter and ectopic atrial tachycardia – a brief review. *Circulation* 1987; 75-III:37-40

11. Allesie MA, Bonke FEM, Schopman FJG. Circus movement in rabbit atrial muscle as a mechanism of tachycardia. III. The "leading circle" concept: A new model of circus movement in cardiac tissue without the involvement of an anatomical obstacle. *Circ Res* 1977; 41:9-18

12. Spach MS, Miller WT Jnr, Geselowitz DB, et al. The discontinuous nature of propagation in normal canine cardiac muscle: Evidence for recurrent discontinuities of intracellular resistance that affect the membrane currents. *Circ Res* 1981: 48:39-54

13. Hoffman BF. Circus movement in the AV ring. In Rosen MR, Janse MJ, Wit AL (eds): *Cardiac Electrophysiology: A Textbook*. Mt Kisco, NY: Futura Publishing Co 1990; 573-587

14. Saoudi N, Cosio F, Waldo A, et al. A classification of atrial flutter and regular atrial tachycardia according to electrophysiological mechanisms and anatomical bases. A statement from a Joint Expert Group from the Working Group of Arrhythmias of the European Society of Cardiology and the North American Society of Pacing and Electrophysiology. *Eur Heart J* 2001: 22:1162-1182

15. Blomstrom-Lundqvist C, Scheinman MM, Aliot EM, et al. ACC/AHA/ESC guidelines for the management of patients with supraventricular arrhythmias--executive summary: a report of the American College of Cardiology/American Heart Association Task Force on Practice Guidelines and the European Society of Cardiology Committee for Practice Guidelines (Writing Committee to Develop Guidelines for the Management of Patients With Supraventricular Arrhythmias). *Circulation* 2003; 108:1871-1909

16. Boineau JP, Canavan TE, Schuessler RBm et al. Demonstration of a widely distributed atrial pacemaker complex in the human heart. *Circulation* 1988; 77:1221-1237

17. Morillo CA, Klein GJ, Thakur RK, et al. Mechanism of "inappropriate" sinus tachycardia: role of sympathovagal balance. *Circulation* 1994; 90:873-877

18. Bauernfeind RA, Amat YL, Dhingra RC, et al. Chronic non-paroxysmal sinus tachycardia in otherwise healthy persons. *Ann Intern Med* 1979; 91:702-710

19. Cossu SF, Steinberg JS. Supraventricular tachyarrhythmias involving the sinus node: Clinical and electrophysiologic characteristics. *Prog Cardiovasc Dis* 1998; 41:51-63

20. Krahn AD, Yee R, Klein GJ, et al. Inappropriate sinus tachycardia: evaluation and therapy. *J Cardiovasc Electrophysiol* 1995; 6:1124-1128

21. Chen SA, Chiang CE, Yang CJ, et al. Sustained atrial tachycardia in adult patients. Electrophysiological characteristics, pharmacological response, possible mechanisms, and effects of radiofrequency ablation. *Circulation* 1994; 90:1262-1278

22. Scheinman MM, Basy D, Hollenberg M. Electrophysiologic studies in patients with persistent atrial tachycardia. *Circulation* 1974; 50:266-273

23. Gillette PC, Garson A Jnr. Electrophysiologic and pharmacologic characteristics of automatic ectopic atrial tachycardia. *Circulation* 1977; 56:571-575

24. Rosen MR, Reder RF. Does triggered activity have a role in the genesis of cardiac arrhythmias? *Ann Intern Med* 1981; 94:794-801

25. Johnson NJ, Rosen MR. The distinction between triggered activity and other cardiac arrhythmias. In Brugada P, Wellens HJJ (eds): *Cardiac Arrhythmias: Where to go from here?* Mt Kisco, NY: Futura Publishing Co 1987; 129-145

26. Wu D, Amat-y-Leon F, Denes P, et al. Demonstration of sustained sinus and atrial reentry as a mechanism of paroxysmal supraventriclar tachycardia. *Circulation* 1975; 51:234-243

27. Coumel P, Flammang D, Attuel P, et al. Sustained intra-atrial reentrant tachycardia: Electrophysiologic study of 20 cases. *Clin Cardiol* 1979; 2:167-178

28. Haines DE, DiMarco JP,. Sustained intra-atrial reentrant tachycardia: Clinical, electrocardiographic and electrophysiologic characteristics and long-term follow-up. *J Am Coll Cardiol* 1990; 15:1345-1354

29. Sanders P, Hocini M, Jais P, et al. Characterization of focal atrial tachycardia using high-density mapping. *J Am Coll Cardiol* 2005; 46:2088-2099

30. Kalman JM, Olgin JE, Karch MR, et al. "Cristal tachycardias": origin of right atrial tachycardias from the crista terminalis identified by intracardiac echocardiography. *J Am Coll Cardiol* 1998; 31:451-459

31. Tada H, Nogami A, Naito S, et al. Simple electrocardiographic criteria for identifying the site of origin of focal right atrial tachycardia. *Pacing Clin Electrophysiol* 1998; 21:2431-2439

32. Kistler PM, Roberts-Thomson KC, Haqqani HM, et al. P-wave morphology in focal atrial tachycardia: development of an algorithm to predict the anatomic site of origin. *J Am Coll Cardiol* 2006; 48:1010-1017

33. Roberts-Thomson KC, Kistler PM, Kalman JM. Focal atrial tachycardia I: Clinical features, diagnosis, mechanisms and anatomic location. *Pacing Clin Electrophysiol* 2006; 29:643-652

34. Kistler PM, Sanders P, Fynn SP, et al. Electrophysiological and electrocardiographic characteristics of focal atrial tachycardia originating from the pulmonary veins: acute and long-term outcomes of radiofrequency ablation. *Circulation* 2003; 108:1968-1975

35. Kistler PM, Sanders P, Hussin A, et al. Focal atrial tachycardia arising from the mitral annulus: electrocardiographic and electrophysiologic characterization. *J Am Coll Cardiol* 2003; 41:2212-2219

36. Tang CW, Scheinman MM, Van Hare GF, et al. Use of P wave configuration during atrial tachycardia to predict site of origin. *J Am Coll Cardiol* 1995; 26:1315-1324

37. Shine KI, Kastor JA, Yurchak PM. Multifocal atrial tachycardia. Clinical and electrocardiographic features in 32 patients. *N Engl J Med* 1968; 279:344-349

38. Lesh MD, Van Hare GF, Epstein LM, et al. Radiofrequency catheter ablation of atrial arrhythmias: results and mechanisms. *Circulation* 1994; 89:1074-1089

39. Olgin JE, Kalman JM, Fitzpatrick AP, et al. Role of right atrial structures as barriers to conduction during human type I atrial flutter. Activation and entrainment mapping guided by intracardiac echocardiography. *Circulation* 1995; 92:1839-1848

40. Nakagawa H, Lazzara R, Khastgir T, et al. Role of the tricuspid annulus and the Eustachian valve/ridge on atrial flutter: relevance to catheter ablation of the septal isthmus and a new technique for rapid identification of ablation success. *Circulation* 1996; 94:407-424

41. Cosio FG, Arribas F, Palacios J, et al. Fragmented electrograms and continuous electrical activity in atrial flutter. *Am J Cardiol* 1986; 57:1309-1314

42. Cosio FG, Arribas F, Barbero JM, et al. Validation of double spike electrograms as markers of conduction delay or block in atrial flutter. *Am J Cardiol* 1988; 61:775-780

43. Olshansky B, Okumura K, Hess PG, et al. Demonstration of an area of slow conduction in human atrial flutter. *J Am Coll Cardiol* 1990; 15:833-841

44. Kalman JM, Olgin JE, Saxon LA, et al. Activation and entrainment mapping defines the tricuspid annulus as the anterior barrier in typical atrial flutter. *Circulation* 1996; 94:398-406

45. Arribas F, Lopez-Gil M, Nunez A, et al. The upper link of the common atrial flutter circuit. *Pacing Clin Electrophysiol* 1997; 20:2924-2929

46. Shah DC, Jais P, Haissaguerre M, et al. Three-dimensional mapping of the common atrial flutter circuit in the right atrium. *Circulation* 1997; 96:3904-3912

47. Cosio FG, Lopez-Gil M, Goicolea A, et al. Radiofrequency ablation of the inferior vena cava-tricuspid valve isthmus in common atrial flutter. *Am J Cardiol* 1993; 71:705-709

48. Saoudi N, Nair M, Abdelazziz A, et al. Electrocardiographic patterns and results of radiofrequency catheter ablation of clockwise type I atrial flutter. *J Cardiovasc Electrophysiol* 1996; 7:931-942

49. Tai CT, Chen SA, Chiang CE, et al. Electrophysiologic characteristics and radiofrequency catheter ablation in patients with clockwise atrial flutter. *J Cardiovasc Electrophysiol* 1996; 8:24-34

50. Cabrera JA, Sanchez-Quintana D, Ho SY, et al. The architecture of the atrial musculature between the orifice of the inferior caval vein and the tricuspid valve: the anatomy of the isthmus. *J Cardiovasc Electrophysiol* 1998; 14:1186-1195

51. Kalman JM, Olgin JE, Saxon LA, et al. Electrocardiographic and electrophysiologic characterization of atypical atrial flutter in man: use of activation and entrainment mapping and implications for catheter ablation. *J Cardiovasc Electrophysiol* 1997; 8:121-144

52. Cheng J, Scheinman MM. Acceleration of typical atrial flutter due to double-wave reentry induced by programmed electrical stimulation. *Circulation* 1998; 97:1589-1596

53. Cheng J, Cabeen WR, Scheinman MM. Right atrial flutter due to lower loop reentry: mechanism and anatomic substrates. *Circulation* 1999; 99:1700-1705

54. Yang Y, Cheng J, Bochoeyer A, et al. Atypical right atrial flutter patterns. *Circulation* 2001; 103:3092-3098

55. Shah DC, Jais P, Takahashi A, et al. Dual loop intra-atrial reentry in humans. *Circulation* 2000; 101:631-639

56. Nakagawa H, Shah N, Matsudaira K, et al. Characterization of reentrant circuit in macroreentrant right atrial tachycardia after surgical repair of congenital heart disease: isolated channels between scars allow "focal" ablation. *Circulation* 2001; 103:699-709

57. Triedman JK, Alexander ME, Berul CI, et al. Electroanatomic mapping of entrained and exit zones in

patients with repaired congenital heart disease and intra-atrial reentrant tachycardia. *Circulation* 2001; 103:2060-2065

58. Triedman JK, Saul JP, Weindling SN, et al. Radiofrequency ablation of intra-atrial reentrant tachycardia after surgical palliation of congenital heart disease. *Circulation* 1995; 91:707-714

59. Kall JG, Rubenstein DS, Kopp DE, et al. Atypical atrial flutter originating in the right atrial free wall. *Circulation* 2000; 101:270-279

60. Stevenson IH, Kistler PM, Spence SJ, et al. Scar-related right atrial macroreentrant tachycardia in patients without prior atrial surgery: electroanatomic characterization and ablation outcome. *Heart Rhythm* 2005; 2:594-601

61. Tai CT, Huang JL, Lin YK, et al. Noncontact three-dimensional mapping and ablation of upper loop reentry originating in the right atrium. *J Am Coll Cardiol* 2002; 40:746-753

62. Jais P, Shah DC, Haissaguerre M, et al. Mapping and ablation of left atrial flutters. *Circulation* 2000; 101:2928-2934

63. Ouyang F, Ernst S, Vogtmann T, et al. Characterization of reentrant circuits in left atrial macroreentrant tachycardia: critical isthmus block can prevent atrial tachycardia recurrence. *Circulation* 2002; 105:1934-1942

64. Marrouche NF, Natale A, Wazni OM, et al. Left septal atrial flutter: electrophysiology, anatomy and results of ablation. *Circulation* 2004; 109:2440-2447

65. Chugh A, Oral H, Lemola K, et al. Prevalence, mechanisms, and clinical significance of macroreentrant atrial tachycardia during and following left atrial ablation for atrial fibrillation. *Heart Rhythm* 2005; 2:464-471

66. Deisenhofer I, Estner H, Zrenner B, et al. Left atrial tachycardia after circumferential pulmonary vein ablation for atrial fibrillation: incidence, electrophysiological characteristics, and results of radiofrequency ablation. *Europace* 2006; 573-582

67. Haissaguerre M, Hocini M, Sanders P, et al. Catheter ablation of long-lasting persistent atrial fibrillation: clinical outcome and mechanisms of subsequent arrhythmias. *J Cardiovasc Electrophysiol* 2005; 16:1138-1147

68. Pappone C, Manguso F, Vicedomini G, et al. Prevention of iatrogenic atrial tachycardia after ablation of atrial fibrillation: a prospective randomized study comparing circumferential pulmonary vein ablation with a modified approach. *Circulation* 2004; 110:3036-3042

69. Gerstenfeld EP, Callans DJ, Dixit S, et al. Mechanisms of organized left atrial tachycardias occurring after pulmonary vein isolation. *Circulation* 2004; 110:1351-1357

70. Mesas CE, Pappone C, Lang CC, et al. Left atrial tachycardia after circumferential pulmonary vein ablation for atrial fibrillation: electroanatomic characterization and treatment. *J Am Coll Cardiol* 2004; 44:1071-1079

71. Chae S, Oral H, Good E, et al. Atrial tachycardia after circumferential pulmonary vein ablation of atrial fibrillation: mechanistic insights, results of catheter ablation, and risk factors for recurrence. *J Am Coll Cardiol* 2007; 50:1781-1787

72. Satomi K, Bansch D, Tilz R, et al. Left atrial and pulmonary vein macroreentrant tachycardia associated with double conduction gaps: a novel type of man-made tachycardia after circumferential pulmonary vein isolation. *Heart Rhythm* 2008; 5:43-51

73. Jais P, Sanders P, Hsu LF, et al. Flutter localized to the anterior left atrium after catheter ablation of atrial fibrillation. *J Cardiovasc Electrophysiol* 2006; 17:279-285

74. Wazni OM, Saliba W, Fahmy W, et al. Atrial arrhythmias after surgical maze: findings during catheter ablation. *J Am Coll Cardiol* 2006; 1405-1409

75. Magnano AR, Argenziano M, Dizon JM, et al. Mechanisms of atrial tachyarrhythmias following surgical atrial fibrillation ablation. *J Cardiovasc Electrophysiol* 2006; 17:366-373

76. Fuster V, Ryden LE, Cannom DS, et al. ACC/AHA/ESC guidelines for the management of patients with atrial fibrillation: a report of the American College of Cardiology/American Heart Association Task Force on Practice Guidelines and the European Society of Cardiology Committee for Practice Guidelines (Writing Committee to Revise the 2001 Guidelines for the Management of Patients With Atrial Fibrillation). *Circulation* 2006; 114:e257-e354

77. Feinberg WM, Blackshear JL, Laupacis A, et al. Prevalence, age distribution, and gender of patients with atrial fibrillation. Analysis and implications. *Arch Intern Med* 1995; 155:469-473

78. Go AS, Hylek EM, Phillips KA, et al. Prevalence of diagnosed atrial fibrillation in adults: national implications for rhythm management and stroke prevention: the anticoagulation and risk factors in atrial fibrillation (ATRIA) study. *JAMA* 2001; 285:2370-2375

79. Psaty BM, Manolio TA, Kuller LH, et al. Incidence of and risk factors for atrial fibrillation in older adults. *Circulation* 1997; 96:2455-2461

80. Wolf PA, Abbott RD, Kannel WB, et al. Atrial fibrillation: a major contributor to stroke in the elderly.

The Framingham Study. *Arch Intern Med* 1987; 147:1561-1564

81. Lloyd-Jones DM, Wang TJ, Leip EP, et al. Lifetime risk for development of atrial fibrillation: the Framingham Heart Study. *Circulation* 2004; 110:1042-1046

82. Kannel WB, Wolf PA, Benjamin EJ, et al. Prevalence, incidence, prognosis and predisposing conditions for atrial fibrillation: population-based estimates. *Am J Cardiol* 1998; 82:2N-9N

83. Wolf PA, Abbott RD, Kannel WB, et al. Atrial fibrillation as an independent risk factor for stroke: the Framingham Study. *Stroke* 1991; 22:983-988

84. Wolf PA, Dawber TR, Thomas HE, et al. Epidemiological assessment of chronic atrial fibrillation and risk of stroke: the Framingham Study. *Neurology* 1978; 28:973-977

85. Wang TJ, Larson MG, Levy D, et al. Temporal relations of atrial fibrillation and congestive heart failure and their joint influence on mortality: the Framingham Heart Study. *Circulation* 2003; 107:2920-2925

86. Benjamin EJ, Wolf PA, D'Agostino RB, et al. Impact of atrial fibrillation on the risk of death: the Framingham Heart Study. *Circulation* 1998; 98:946-952

87. Frustaci A, Chimenti C, Belloci F, et al. Histological substrate of atrial biopsies in patients with lone atrial fibrillation. *Circulation* 1997; 96:1180-1184

88. Bharti S, Lev M. Histology of the normal and diseased atrium. In: Fall RH, Podrid PJ, editors. *Atrial Fibrillation: Mechanism and Management.* New York: Raven Press. 1992:15-39

89. Pokharel S, van Geel PP, Sharma UC, et al. Increased myocardial collagen content in transgenic rats over-expressing cardiac angiotensin-converting enzyme is related to enhanced breakdown of N-acetyl-Ser-Asp-Lys-Pro and increased phosphorylation of Smad2/3. *Circulation* 2004; 110:3129-3135

90. Sanders P, Morton JB, Davidson NC, et al. Electrocal remodeling of the atria in congestive heart failure: electrophysiological and electroanatomic mapping in humans. *Circulation* 2003; 108:1461-1468

91. Morton JB, Sanders P, Vohra JK, et al. Effect of chronic right atrial stretch on atrial electrical modeling in patients with an atrial septal defect. *Circulation* 2003; 107:1775-1782

92. Kistler PM, Sanders P, Fynn SP, et al. Electrophysiologic and electroanatomical changes in the human atrium associated with age. *J Am Coll Cardiol* 2004; 44:109-116

93. Morillo CA, Klein GJ, Jones DL, et al. Chronic rapid atrial pacing. Structural, functional, and electrophysiological characteristics of a new model of sustained atrial fibrillation. *Circulation* 1995; 91:1588-1595

94. Ausma J, Wijffels M, Thone F, et al. Structural changes of atrial myocardium due to sustained atrial fibrillation in the goat. *Circulation* 1997; 96:3157-3163

95. Allesie M, Ausma J, Schotten U. Electrical, contractile and structural remodeling during atrial fibrillation. *Cardiovasc Res* 2002; 54:230-246

96. Everett TH, Li H, Mangrum JM, et al. Electrical, morphological and ultrastructural remodeling and reverse remodeling in a canine model of chronic atrial fibrillation. *Circulation* 2000; 102:1454-1460

97. Brundel BJ, Henning RH, Kampinga HH, et al. Molecular mechanisms of remodeling in human atrial fibrillation. *Cardiovasc Res* 2002; 54:315-324

98. Scherf D, Schaffer AI, Blumfeld S. Mechanism of flutter and fibrillation. *Arch Intern Med* 1953; 91:333-352

99. Jais P, Haissaguerre M, Shah DC, et al. A focal source of atrial fibrillation treated by discrete radiofrequency ablation. *Circulation* 1997; 95:572-576

100. Haissaguerre M, Jais P, Shah DC, et al. Spontaneous initiation of atrial fibrillation by ectopic beats originating in the pulmonary veins. *N Engl J Med* 1998; 339:659-666

101. Chen SA, Tai CT, Yu WC, et al. Right atrial focal atrial fibrillation: electrophysiologic characteristics and radiofrequency catheter ablation. *J Cardiovasc Electrophysiol* 1999; 10:328-335

102. Hsu LF, Jais P, Keane D, et al. Atrial fibrillation originating from persistent left superior vena cava. *Circulation* 2004; 109:828-832

103. Lin WS, Tai CT, Hsieh MH, et al. Catheter ablation of paroxysmal atrial fibrillation initiated by non-pulmonary vein ectopy. *Circulation* 2003; 107:3176-3183

104. Zipes DP, Knope RF. Electrical properties of the thoracic veins. *Am J Cardiol* 1972; 29:372-376

105. Nathan H, Eliakim M. The junction between the left atrium and the pulmonary veins. An anatomic study of human hearts. *Circulation* 1966; 34:412-422

106. Ho SY, Cabrera JA, Tran VH, et al. Architecture of the pulmonary veins: relevance to radiofrequency ablation. *Heart* 2001; 86:265-270

107. Jais P, Hocini M, Macle L, et al. Distinctive electrophysiological properties of pulmonary veins in patients with atrial fibrillation. *Circulation* 2002; 106:2479-2485

108. Oral H, Knight BP, Ozaydin M, et al. Segmental ostial ablation to isolate the pulmonary veins during atrial fibrillation: feasibility and mechanistic insights. *Circulation* 2002; 106:1256-1262

109. Kumagai K, Ogawa M, Noguchi H, et al. Electrophysiologic properties of pulmonary veins assessed using a multielectrode basket catheter. *J Am Coll Cardiol* 2004; 43:2281-2289

110. Takahashi Y, Iesaka Y, Takahashi A, et al. Reentrant tachycardia in pulmonary veins of patients with paroxysmal atrial fibrillation. *J Cardiovasc Electrophysiol* 2003; 14:927-932

111. Mansour M, Mandapati R, Berenfeld O, et al. Left-to-right gradient of atrial frequencies during acute atrial fibrillation in the isolated sheep heart. *Circulation* 2001; 103:2631-2636

112. Mandapati R, Skanes A, Chen J, et al. Stable microreentrant sources as a mechanism of atrial fibrillation in the isolated sheep heart. *Circulation* 2000; 101:194-199

113. Lazar S, Dixit S, Marchlinski FE, et al. Presence of left-to-right atrial frequency gradient in paroxysmal but not persistent atrial fibrillation in humans. *Circulation* 2004; 110:3181-3186

114. Sanders P, Berenfeld O, Hocini M, et al. Spectral analysis identifies sites of high-frequency activity maintaining atrial fibrillation in humans. *Circulation* 2005; 112:789-797

115. Sanders P, Nalliah CJ, Dubois R, et al. Frequency mapping of the pulmonary veins in paroxysmal versus permanent atrial fibrillation. *J Cardiovasc Electrophysiol* 2006; 17:965-972

116. Moe GK, Abildskov JA. Observations on the ventricular dysrhythmia associated with atrial fibrillation in the dog's heart. *Circ Res* 1964; 4:447-460

117. Allessie MA, Boyden PA, Camm AJ, et al. Pathophysiology and prevention of atrial fibrillation. *Circulation* 2001; 103:769-777

118. Cox JL, Canavan TE, Schuessler RB, et al. The surgical treatment of atrial fibrillation. II. Intraoperative electrophysiologic mapping and description of the electrophysiologic basis of atrial flutter and atrial fibrillation. *J Thorac Cardiovasc Surg* 1991; 101:406-426

119. Ramanna H, Hauer RN, Wittkampf FH, et al. Identification of the substrate of atrial vulnerability in patients with idiopathic atrial fibrillation. *Circulation* 2000; 101:995-1001

120. Nakao K, Seto S, Ueyama C, et al. Extended distribution of prolonged and fractionated right atrial electrograms predicts development of chronic atrial fibrillation in patients with idiopathic paroxysmal atrial fibrillation. *J Cardiovasc Electrophysiol* 2002; 13:996-1002

121. Hobbs WJ, Van Gelder IC, Fitzpatrick AP, et al. The role of atrial electrical remodeling in the progression of focal atrial ectopy to persistent atrial fibrillation. *J Cardiovasc Electrophysiol* 1999; 10:866-870

122. Wijffels M, Kirchhof C, Dorland R, et al. Atrial fibrillation begets atrial fibrillation: a study in awake, chronically instrumented goats. *Circulation* 1995; 92:1954-1968

123. Garratt CJ, Duytschaever M, Killian M, et al. Repetitive electrical remodeling by paroxysms of atrial fibrillation in the goat; no cumulative effect on inducibility or stability of atrial fibrillation. *J Cardiovasc Electrophysiol* 1999; 10:1101-1108

124. Timmermans C, Rodriguez LM, Smeets JL, et al. Immediate reinitiation of atrial fibrillation following internal atrial defibrillation. *J Cardiovasc Electrophysiol* 1998; 9:122-128

125. Yu WC, Lee SH, Tai CT, et al. Reversal of atrial electrical remodeling following cardioversion of long-standing atrial fibrillation in man. *Cardiovasc Res* 1999; 42:470-476

126. Shinbane JS, Wood MA, Jensen DN, et al. Tachycardia-induced cardiomyopathy: a review of animal models and clinical studies. *J Am Coll Cardiol* 1997; 29:709-715

127. Chiladakis JA, Vassilikos VP, Maounis TN, et al. Successful radiofrequency catheter ablation of automatic atrial tachycardia with regression of the cardiomyopathy picture. *Pacing Clin Electrophysiol* 1997; 20:953-959

128. Luchsinger JA, Steinberg JS. Resolution of cardiomyopathy after ablation of atrial flutter. *J Am Coll Cardiol* 1998; 32:205-210

129. Hsu LF, Jais P, Sanders P, et al. Catheter ablation for atrial fibrillation in congestive heart failure. *N Engl J Med* 2004; 351:2373-2383

130. Seidl K, Hauer B, Schwick NG, et al. Risk of thromboembolic events in patients with atrial flutter. *Am J Cardiol* 1998; 82:580-583

131. Hsieh MH, Chen SA. Catheter ablation of focal atrial tachycardia. In: Zipes DP, Haissaguerre M, eds. *Catheter ablation of arrhythmias.* Armonk, NY: Futura Publishing Co., Inc., 2002;185-204

132. Cosio FG, Pastor A, Nunez A, et al. Catheter ablation of typical atrial flutter. In: Zipes DP, Haissaguerre M, eds. *Catheter ablation of arrhythmias.* Armonk, NY: Futura Publishing Co., Inc., 2002;131-151

133. Saxon LA, Kalman JM, Olgin JE, et al. Results of radiofrequency ablation for atrial flutter. *Am J Cardiol* 1996; 77:1014-1016

134. Cosio FG. Atrial flutter update. *Card Electrophysiol Rev* 2002; 6:356-364

135. Cosio FG, Awamleh P, Pastor A, et al. Determining inferior vena cava-tricuspid isthmus block after typical atrial flutter ablation. *Heart Rhythm* 2005; 2:328-332

136. Jais P, Hocini M, Sanders P, et al. An approach to non-cavotricuspid isthmus dependent flutter. *J Cardiovasc Electrophysiol* 2005; 16:666-673

137. Hocini M, Jais P, Sanders P, et al. Techniques, evaluation and consequences of linear block at the left atrial

roof in paroxysmal atrial fibrillation: a prospective randomized study. *Circulation* 2005; 112:3688-3696

138. Jais P, Hocini M, Hsu LF, et al. Technique and results of linear ablation at the mitral isthmus. *Circulation* 2004; 110:2996-3002

139. Packer DL, Asirvatham S, Munger TM. Progress in nonpharmacologic therapy of atrial fibrillation. *J Cardiovasc Electrophysiol* 2003; 14:S296-S309

140. Hocini M, Sanders P, Jais P, et al. Techniques for curative treatment of atrial fibrillation. *J Cardiovasc Electrophysiol* 2004; 15:1467-1471

141. Haissaguerre M, Sanders P, Hocini M, et al. Catheter ablation of long-lasting persistent atrial fibrillation: critical structures for termination. *J Cardiovasc Electrophysiol* 2005; 16:1125-1137

142. Nademanee K, McKenzie J, Kosar E, et al. A new approach for catheter ablation of atrial fibrillation: mapping of the electrophysiological substrate. *J Am Coll Cardiol* 2004; 43:2044-2053

143. Haissaguerre M, Shah DC, Jais P, et al. Electrophysiological breakthroughs from the left atrium to the pulmonary veins. *Circulation* 2000; 102:2463-2465

144. Verma A, Marrouche NF, Natale A. Pulmonary vein antrum isolation: intracardiac echocardiography-guided technique. *J Cardiovasc Electrophysiol* 2004; 15:1335-1340

145. Pappone C, Rosanio S, Oreto G, et al. Circumferential radiofrequency ablation of pulmonary vein ostia: a new anatomic approach for curing atrial fibrillation. *Circulation* 2000; 102:2619-2628

146. Cappato R, Calkins H, Chen SA, et al. Worldwide survey on the methods, efficacy, and safety of catheter ablation for human atrial fibrillation. *Circulation* 2005; 111:1100-1105

147. Pappone C, Rosanio S, Augello G, et al. Mortality, morbidity, and quality of life after circumferential pulmonary vein ablation for atrial fibrillation: outcomes from a controlled nonrandomized long-term study. *J Am Coll Cardiol* 2003; 42:185-197

148. Nademanee K, Schwab MC, Kosar EM, et al. Clinical outcomes of catheter substrate ablation for high-risk patients with atrial fibrillation. *J Am Coll Cardiol* 2008; 51:843-849

CHAPTER 4

The Biology of Ventricular Dysrhythmias and Sudden Cardiac Death

Kurt C. Roberts-Thomson, MBBS, PhD, FRACP
William G. Stevenson, MD

INTRODUCTION

The term *ventricular dysrhythmia* encompasses a range of cardiac rhythms caused by a variety of mechanisms and with a spectrum of prognostic significance. These range from premature ventricular complexes (PVCs) in normal subjects to sudden cardiac death (SCD) due to ventricular tachyarrhythmias in subjects with and without structural heart disease.

The mechanism by which these occur is complex and often results from a confluence of a number of factors. These include the presence of an appropriate substrate, remodeling of the ventricular myocardial membrane properties, altered neurohormonal signaling, electrolyte abnormalities, myocardial ischemia, and a genetic predisposition to electrical instability.

Ventricular dysrhythmias may occur as a result of a variety of mechanisms: reentry, where a circuit revolves around a region of fixed or functional conduction block; triggered activity due to either early or delayed after-depolarizations; or abnormal automaticity. The underlying heart disease determines the arrhythmia substrate and thereby the likely mechanism. Ventricular tachycardia that is monomorphic typically has a fixed substrate, or focus, that produces repetitive depolarization of the ventricles in the same sequence. In contrast, polymorphic VT and ventricular fibrillation indicate a continually changing ventricular activation sequence, such that a fixed arrhythmia substrate is not required, although VF is often initiated by VT that has a substrate.

The mechanism of VF remains incompletely understood. Currently two theories exist: "the multiple wavelet VF" theory posits that the breakup of the initial circulating wavefront (rotor) into multiple wavelets causes and maintains VF;[1] alternatively, the other theory suggests that VF is the result of a high frequency rotor with breakup of its wavefronts as they traverse the myocardium or as the single rotor drifts through the myocardium.[2] Both mechanisms may occur.[3, 4] Electrophysiologic changes that accompany ventricular diseases can increase susceptibility to VF.

ARRHYTHMIC SUBSTRATES

Ischemic Heart Disease

Ventricular tachyarrhythmias related to coronary artery disease are the most common cause of SCD in the Western world. All patients with coronary disease are at risk for SCD, and most SCD occurs in patients without severe left ventricular dysfunction.

Acute Ischemia

Ischemia creates a complex milieau with hypoxia, hyperkalemia, acidosis, low levels of energy substrate, and local catcholamine release affecting the underlying myocardium. These conditions produce a number of electrophysiologic changes which predispose to the development of ventricular arrhythmias. Lysophosphoglyceride accumulation and elevated extracellular K+, likely resulting from efflux through ATP sensitive K+ channels, can cause significant depolarization of the resting membrane potential to between 50mV and 60mV.[5-7] There may be marked inhomogeneity of refractoriness between the central zone of ischemia and the border zone between ischemic and normal myocardium.[8, 9] Ischemia may also produce differences in action potential duration between the subendocardium and subepicardium.[10] Disruptions in gap junctions reduce cell-to-cell coupling and conduction velocity, creating heterogeneity in conduction and recovery that facilitate reentry.[11, 12] When reentry occurs, the circulating wavefronts can fragment resulting in ventricular fibrillation.[13, 14] As ischemia progresses, the region becomes inexcitable. Subacute arrhythmias, occurring 6–72 hours post-coronary occlusion, tend to be related to automaticity in injured Purkinje fibres.[15]

Infarct Scar Based Arrhythmias

Following infarction, myocardium is replaced by regions of fibrosis. In the border zone of the infarct, fibrosis produces inexcitable barriers interspersed with strands of viable myocardium. The viable cells and their orientation are deformed by the ingrowth of fibrous tissue producing poor cell-to-cell coupling and anisotropy. Consequently, fibrosis creates conduction slowing, macroscopic discontinuities in conduction, unidirectional block and reentry. In addition to the changes caused by fibrosis, conduction may also be affected by the downregulation and redistribution of gap junctions and reduced sodium current densities.[16-18] Heterogenous refractoriness also contributes to the potential for reentry that has been most frequently demonstrated as the mechanism of sustained ventricular tachycardia (VT) in patients with chronic ischemic heart disease.[19-21] However, focal activity is also seen, particularly as the initiating beat of VT.[22]

Recognition of the role of the infarct scar and border zone in ventricular arrhythmias has led to increasing interest in scar imaging. Wall motion abnormalities, magnetic resonance imaging (MRI) with assessement of regions of delayed gadolinium enhance-

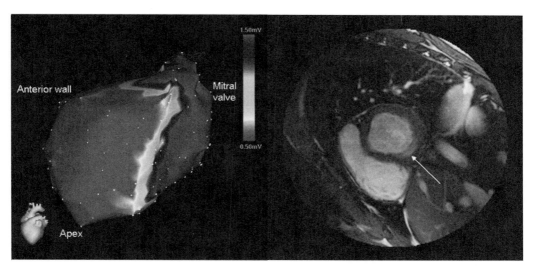

Figure 4.1

(Left Panel) A voltage map of the left ventricle in a patient with a prior anterior wall infarction. The map was created by sampling electrograms point by point with a catheter maneuvered around the ventricular endocardium. The electrogram voltage is color coded (see Color Plate 1) and plotted in the three-dimensional structure created by this electroanatomic mapping system (CARTO). The VT substrate is often contained within the scar or its border region, which can then be identified with further mapping and potentially targeted for catheter ablation. (Right Panel) Cardiac MRI in a different patient. This demonstrates delayed hyperenhancement (arrow) in the subendocardium of the anterior wall of the left ventricle, consistent with scar from a prior infarct.

ment and voltage mapping (Figure 4.1) have been used to delineate regions of scar from infarction or myopathic processes. MRI abnormalities show promise in risk prediction.

Nonischemic Cardiomyopathy

The 5-year mortality for dilated cardiomyopathy has been estimated at 20%, with SCD accounting for approximately one-third of deaths.[23, 24] Although VT and/or VF are considered the most common mechanism of SCD, bradyarrhythmias, pulmonary embolus, electromechanical dissociation, and other causes account for up 50% of SCD in patients with advanced heart failure.[25, 26] Although sustained monomorphic VT is much less frequent than in patient with prior infarction, areas of replacement fibrosis occur in some patients and create the substrate for reentry.[27] Mapping studies in patients presenting with VT have demonstrated that regions of fibrosis are frequently adjacent to the valve annuli and are often epicardial in location.[28, 29] Interstitial fibrosis also occurs, which promotes cellular uncoupling that facilitates reentry. Cardiomyopathies are accompanied by myocyte hypertrophy that has been associated with electrical remodeling with prolonged repolarization. They are enhanced by the dispersion of repolarization and altered calcium handling, factors that also predispose to triggered automaticity.[30] In addition to myocardial reentry and focal activity, these patients may have diseased conduction systems, predisposing to bundle branch reentrant VT, where reentry occurs involving the bundle branches.

Arrhythmogenic Right Ventricular Cardiomyopathy

Arrhythmogenic right ventricular cardiomyopathy is a potentially heritable condition characterized by the replacement of cardiomyocytes, primarily in the right ventricle, by fibrofatty tissue. The potential manifestations include right ventricular enlargement and dysfunction, electrocardiogram abnormalities and ventricular arrhythmias, including VT and VF. Because VT usually originates from the RV, it usually has left bundle branch morphology. SCD can be the first manifestation of the disease, often during exercise or stress, with an annual incidence of SCD to range from 0.08 to 9%.[31-34] The disease is frequently familial and typically involves autosomal dominant transmission. Approximately 50% of symptomatic individuals harbor a mutation in genes coding for one of the five major components of the cardiac desmosome: plakoglobin, desmoplakin, plakophilin-2, desmoglein-2, and desmocollin-2.[35] Mutations demonstrate incomplete penetrance and variable expressivity, implicating environmental factors and other genetic modifiers in the etiology.

The mechanism by which these mutations lead to fibrofatty replacement of the right ventricular myocardium has yet to be fully defined. A loss of myocyte adhesion provided by the desmosome,[36] increased adipogenesis because of desmosome mutations,[37] as well as increased apoptosis[38] have been suggested. These changes would contribute to the formation of fatty replacement and focal scarring in the right ventricle, providing the substrate for reentrant ventricular arrhythmias.

Hypertrophic Cardiomyopathy

The majority of individuals with hypertrophic cardiomyopathy (HCM) are asymptomatic, but the first manifestation can be SCD. In patients referred to tertiary centers, the annual mortality is as high as 6%,[39, 40] but community-based studies suggest a more benign disease with an annual mortality of approximately 1%.[41, 42] Ventricular tachyarrhythmias are an important cause of SCD. Ventricular arrhythmias are commonly seen with Holter studies reporting PVCs in approximately 60% of patients and nonsustained VT in 20–30% of patients.[43]

There are many factors which may contribute to the arrhythmic substrate of HCM. The disorganized myocardial cell arrangement,[44] the increased interstitial collagen and focal myocardial scarring (possibly related to ischemia due to abnormal microvasculature and diminished coronary flow relative to muscle mass) likely provide the substrate for reentrant ventricular arrhythmias.[45] Ischemia and arrhythmia may be provoked by dia-

Table 4.1   Risk Factors for Sudden Cardiac Death in Hypertrophic Cardiomyopathy

Major Risk Factors	Possible in Individual Patients
Cardiac arrest (VF)	AF
Spontaneous sustained VT	Myocardial ischemia
Family history of premature SCD	LV outflow tract obstruction
Unexplained syncope	High-risk mutation
LV thickness ≥ 30mm	Intense physical exertion
Abnormal exercise VT	
Nonsustained spontaneous	

AF = atrial fibrillation; BP = blood pressure; LV = left ventricular; VF = ventricular fibrillation; VT = ventricular tachycardia.

Modified with permission from Maron BJ, McKenna WJ, Danielson GK, et al. American College of Cardiology/European Society of Cardiology clinical expert consensus document on hypertrophic cardiomyopathy. A report of the American College of Cardiology Foundation Task Force on Clinical Expert Consensus Documents and the European Society of Cardiology Committee for Practice Guidelines. *J Am Coll Cardiol* 2003; 42: 1687-713.

stolic dysfunction, outflow tract obstruction, supraventricular tachycardias, or external factors such as physical exertion. Despite the heterogeneity of HCM, a number of clinical markers identify patients at increased risk of SCD (Table 4.1). While the genetic basis of this disease is well recognized, at this stage, the risk of sudden death can not be reliably inferred from the specific mutation, thus genotyping is not used for risk stratification.

Ventricular Tachycardia in the Structurally Normal Heart

Monomorphic VT may also occur in the absence of ventricular scar. Idiopathic and fascicular VT can occur in structurally normal hearts, often presenting with adrenergically mediated symptoms caused by PVCs or nonsustained VT, and rarely cause syncope. The majority of these patients have a good prognosis, although frequent or incessant tachycardias may cause cardiomyopathy.

Idiopathic VT

The most common type of idiopathic VT has a focal origin from the right ventricular outflow tract, often immediately below the pulmonary valve. VT has a left bundle branch block morphology and an inferior axis. While the majority arise from the RV outflow tract, up to 20% can originate from other sites, such as the LV outflow tract, coronary cusps,[46] pulmonary artery[47] and the junction of the anterior interventricular vein and great cardiac vein.[48]

The mechanism of these arrhythmias is thought to be caused by cyclic-AMP-mediated triggered activity. Clinical evidence for this comes from termination of the tachycardia by both calcium channel blockers and adenosine, and facilitation of its initiation by an acceleration of heart rate.[49, 50] One study demonstrated a somatic G-protein mutation,

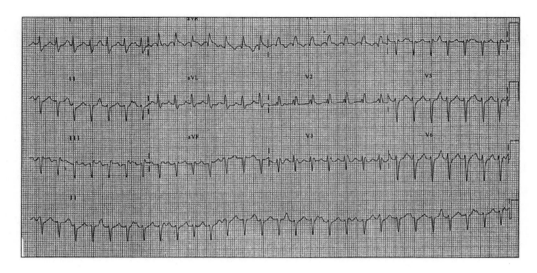

Figure 4.2

Idiopathic left fascicular VT. Note the AV dissociation, relatively narrow QRS, and right bundle branch morphology with left axis deviation.

which disrupts the normal regulation of intracellular cyclic-AMP content, in the outflow tract tachycardia.[51]

Left Fascicular VT

Idiopathic VT may also originate from the left ventricular septum, giving rise to a VT with a right bundle branch block and left superior axis morphology (Figure 4.2). This VT is often sensitive to verapamil and adenosine. The mechanism appears to be reentry involving the Purkinje network.[52, 53] The antegrade limb of the circuit appears to involve a slowly conducting region of the left ventricular septum with the posterior fascicle of the left bundle branch providing the retrograde limb.[54, 55] The left anterior fascicle may also be involved in a minority of patients and this usually gives rise to a VT with a right bundle branch block and right inferior axis morphology.

Genetic Syndromes

Mutations in genes coding for ion channel proteins, or proteins involved in ion channel function or trafficking to the membrane underlie the long QT, Brugada, and familial catecholaminergic polymorphic VT syndromes. These syndromes can present at any age, although many patients are relatively young, and have no evidence of structural heart

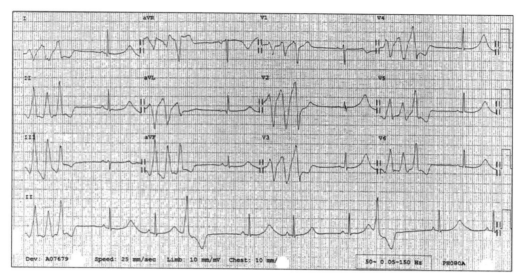

Figure 4.3

ECG of Long QT. Note the post pause potentiation of the QT interval and short runs of polymorphic VT.

disease. The ventricular arrhythmia is usually polymorphic VT or ventricular fibrillation causing syncope or cardiac arrest.

Long QT

The Long QT syndrome (LQTS) is a disease characterized by prolonged ventricular repolarization (Figure 4.3) and by the characteristic polymorphic VT, torsade de pointes (TdP). This may cause syncope and can degenerate into VF. At least eight mutations involving ion channel function have been identified (Table 4.2). Seven of these encode cardiac ion channel subunits and one encodes an anchoring protein. Inheritance occurs most commonly in an autosomal dominant pattern (Romano-Ward syndrome) and rarely in an autosomal recessive pattern, often associated with congenital deafness (Jervell Lange-Neilsen syndrome). Some phenotype-genotype correlations have emerged. Individuals affected by LQT1 mutations (I_{Ks} mutations) often have events during exercise, particularly swimming. Patients with LQT2 (I_{Kr} mutations) often have events during rest or emotion, particularly acoustic stimuli. LQT3 (I_{Na} mutations) patients are susceptible to events during rest and sleep.

The mechanism of TdP is complex and not completely understood. Transmural ion channel heterogeneities can cause regional action potential duration prolongation and hence large transmural repolarization gradients.[56] These gradients can result in unidirectional block and potentially reentry. In addition, early after-depolarizations (EADs) are

Table 4.2   Long QT Syndrome Subtypes

VARIANT	GENE	FUNCTION
LQT1	KCNQ1	IKs alpha subunit
LQT2	KCNH2	IKr alpha subunit
LQT3	SCN5A	INa alpha subunit
LQT4	ANK2	Targeting protein
LQT5	KCNE1	IKs beta subunit
LQT6	KCNE2	IKr beta subunit
LQT7	KCNJ2	IK1
LQT8	CACNA1C	ICa alpha subunit

enhanced when there is QT prolongation and can produce triggered beats that initiate TdP.[57] The short-long sequence seen at the onset of TdP, promotes the formation of EADs and potentiates these repolarization gradients.[58]

Brugada Syndrome
Brugada syndrome is a disease characterized by electrocardiogram abnormalities, right bundle branch block with J-point elevation in leads V1-V3 (Figure 4.4), and a predisposition to SCD.[59] The disease is transmitted in an autosomal dominant pattern. The syndrome is more common in Asian countries and clinical expression appears to be modified by gender, as 90% of affected individuals are male. The most common mutations identified have been in the cardiac sodium channel gene, SCN5A, but this accounts for a minority of cases. Ventricular arrhythmias are likely caused by the marked dispersion of repolarization across the ventricular wall which predisposes to the development of reentry.[60]

Familial Catecholaminergic Polymorphic VT
Familial catecholaminergic polymorphic VT is a rare disease characterized by polymorphic VT, without QT prolongation, in response to adrenergic stimulation, such as exercise, emotion, or isoproterenol. It usually presents in childhood and familial occurrence has been noted in about 30% of patients.[61] The disease may be transmitted as an autosomal dominant or autosomal recessive trait. Many of the autosomal dominant cases are caused by mutations in the cardiac ryanodine receptor (RyR2), which is responsible for the calcium-induced calcium release from the sarcoplasmic reticulum.[62] These mutations cause aberrant diastolic calcium release, activating delayed after-depolarizations (DADs) and producing ventricular arrhythmias. A very rare autosomal recessive type is caused by mutations in the gene encoding calsequestrin (CASQ2), a calcium binding protein in the sarcoplasmic reticulum. These mutations impair calcium binding and lead to diastolic calcium leak and DADs.[63] Ventricular ectopic beats appear predictably at heart rates around 120 bpm and the frequency and complexity increases with the heart rate, leading

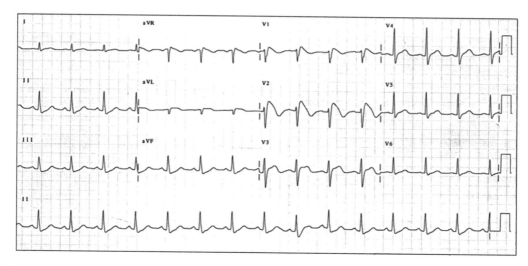

Figure 4.4

ECG of Brugada syndrome. Note the J point elevation in leads V1–V3.

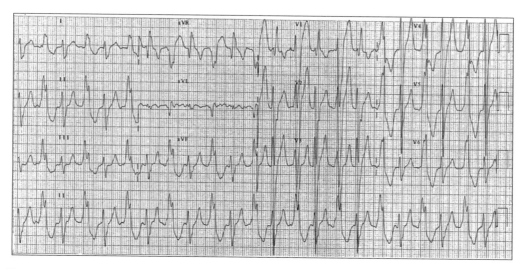

Figure 4.5

ECG of bidirectional VT in a patient with catecholaminergic polymorphic VT. Note the change in axis with alternating beats.

to bidirectional VT (Figure 4.5) and polymorphic VT. β-blocker therapy is beneficial, reducing sympathetic drive, however ICDs are often implanted as the mortality has been estimated at 30–50% by the age of 20–30 years.[64, 65]

Neurohormonal Factors in Arrhythmogenesis

Neurohormonal factors may influence both the triggers and substrate of ventricular arrhythmias. While the activation of the renin-angiotensin-aldosterone system (RAAS) and sympathetic nervous system are well defined in the development of heart failure, the role of these systems on the occurrence of SCD is less clear.

There are a number of mechanisms by which RAAS signaling may enhance the risk of ventricular dysrhythmias and SCD. The RAAS has been shown to participate in the development of cardiac fibroblast proliferation and increased collagen synthesis,[66] the induction of cardiomyocyte hypertrophy,[67] the generation of reactive oxygen species,[68] promotion of inflammation and fibrosis, and the modulation of active membrane properties.[69-76] Angiotensin II and aldosterone, two of the effectors of the RAAS, have direct effects on cardiac ion channels. Angiotensin II inhibits the transient outward K current (I_{TO})[77] and the delayed rectifier K currents,[78] as well as decreasing Na^+-K^+ ATPase,[79] and increasing the Cl^- current.[80] Aldosterone inhibits I_{TO} and increases L-type calcium $(I_{Ca,L})$ channel density.[81] Thus, the RAAS can alter both the arrhythmic substrate as well as the ionic properties of the cardiomyocyte membrane.

The role of the sympathetic nervous system in SCD post MI has been recognized for some time. Both β-blockers and left stellectomy, reduce mortality in patients post myocardial infarction.[82, 83] Cardiac sympathetic innervation is markedly heterogenous in the infarcted heart.[84] Infarction damages the sympathetic nerves and induces an exaggerated response to catecholamines, in the form of ventricular refractory period shortening and an enhanced inducibility of ventricular fibrillation.[85] This may relate to the nerve sprouting observed following injury to the sympathetic fibers. Cao et al.[86] examined transplanted hearts in patients with and without ventricular arrhythmias and found a higher density of nerve fibers in patients with ventricular arrhythmias. Infusion of nerve growth factor into the left stellate ganglion post infarct also has been shown to induce hyperinnervation and ventricular arrhythmias.[87] Regional sympathetic denervation has also been demonstrated in patients with ventricular arrhythmias without coronary artery disease.[88]

The effect of sympathetic stimulation on the heart is complex. In the normal ventricle, sympathetic stimulation shortens the action potential duration and reduces the dispersion of repolarization, reducing the arrhythmic risk.[89] However, in pathologic states, this stimulation is arrhythmogenic, possibly by enhancing the dispersion of repolarization, and may explain the benefits of β-blockers in reducing SCD in patients with coronary artery disease.

GENETIC PREDISPOSITION TO ARRHYTHMIAS

There is increasing evidence for a genetic influences on the risk of SCD independent of the sudden death syndromes discussed previously. Friedlander et al.[90] demonstrated that the rate of cardiac arrest in first degree relatives of arrest victims was 50% greater than in a control population and was independent of other factors of SCD. In the Paris Prospective study, SCD in a parent was associated with an 80% increase in risk for SCD in the child, despite controlling for conventional risk factors. When both parents had SCD the relative risk of SCD in the offspring was almost 9.[91]

There are likely to be a number of genetically determined factors that are associated with a response to certain stressors that influence arrhythmias. Splawski et al.[92] provided evidence for this, showing that a certain polymorphism in the SCN5A Na+ channel gene, commonly found in African Americans, was associated with an increased arrhythmic risk, but only in the presence of other proarrhythmic influences, such a QT prolonging drugs.

Allelic variation in a number of signaling systems have been proposed to enhance susceptibility to SCD. These include the myocardial membrane properties, myocardial substrate and triggers, and thrombotic cascades. Association studies have demonstrated an increased SCD risk in Finnish men with the A2 allele of the $PI^{A1/A2}$ polymorphism of glycoprotein IIIa.[93] Anvari et al.[94] showed an association with the plasminogen activator inhibitor type 1 4G/5G polymorphism. In patients with coronary artery disease and left ventricular dysfunction, combinations of polymorphisms, such as the DD allele of the angiotensin converting enzyme and the C allele of the angiotensin II receptor, have been found to be associated with an increased risk of malignant ventricular arrhythmias.[95]

The relationship between polymorphisms and phenotypes is complicated and our understanding of this area is continuously evolving. There are likely to be numerous genetic factors that contribute to the complex phenotypic manifestation of ventricular dysrhythmias. Some are likely to be known genes related to electrical stability, as well as those related to the progression of heart failure and the development of myocardial ischemia. In addition, genomic screening is likely to reveal novel variations in genes that contribute to ventricular dysrhythmias.

CONCLUSION

Significant progress has been made in the understanding of the mechanisms of ventricular dysrhythmias. While certain ventricular dysrhythmias are benign and important to recognize as such, many are life threatening. Risk prediction in individual patients is difficult due to the numerous and temporally heterogenous factors involved. In the future, a greater understanding of the biology, particularly of the genetic and molecular mechanisms, should improve identification and treatment of those at risk from SCD.

◇◇◇◇◇◇◇◇◇◇◇◇◇

REFERENCES

1. Weiss JN. Factors determining the transition from ventricular tachycardia to ventricular fibrillation. *Heart Rhythm* 2005 September;2(9):1008-10.
2. Jalife J, Berenfeld O. Molecular mechanisms and global dynamics of fibrillation: an integrative approach to the underlying basis of vortex-like reentry. *J Theor Biol* 2004 October 21;230(4):475-87.
3. Masse S, Downar E, Chauhan V, Sevaptsidis E, Nanthakumar K. Ventricular fibrillation in myopathic human hearts: mechanistic insights from in vivo global endocardial and epicardial mapping. *Am J Physiol Heart Circ Physiol* 2007 June;292(6):H2589-H2597.
4. Nash MP, Mourad A, Clayton RH, Sutton PM, Bradley CP, Hayward M, Paterson DJ, Taggart P. Evidence for multiple mechanisms in human ventricular fibrillation. *Circulation* 2006 August 8;114(6):536-42.
5. Clarkson CW, Ten Eick RE. On the mechanism of lysophosphatidylcholine-induced depolarization of cat ventricular myocardium. *Circ Res* 1983 May;52(5):543-56.
6. Kleber AG. Resting membrane potential, extracellular potassium activity, and intracellular sodium activity during acute global ischemia in isolated perfused guinea pig hearts. *Circ Res* 1983 April;52(4):442-50.
7. Trube G, Hescheler J. Inward-rectifying channels in isolated patches of the heart cell membrane: ATP-dependence and comparison with cell-attached patches. *Pflugers Arch* 1984 June;401(2):178-84.
8. Lazzara R, El-Sherif N, Hope RR, Scherlag BJ. Ventricular arrhythmias and electrophysiological consequences of myocardial ischemia and infarction. *Circ Res* 1978 June;42(6):740-9.
9. Janse MJ, Cinca J, Morena H, Fiolet JW, Kleber AG, de Vries GP, Becker AE, Durrer D. The "border zone" in myocardial ischemia. An electrophysiological, metabolic, and histochemical correlation in the pig heart. *Circ Res* 1979 April;44(4):576-88.
10. Gilmour RF, Jr., Zipes DP. Different electrophysiological responses of canine endocardium and epicardium to combined hyperkalemia, hypoxia, and acidosis. *Circ Res* 1980 June;46(6):814-25.
11. Wojtczak J. Contractures and increase in internal longitudianl resistance of cow ventricular muscle induced by hypoxia. *Circ Res* 1979 January;44(1):88-95.
12. Kaplinsky E, Ogawa S, Balke CW, Dreifus LS. Two periods of early ventricular arrhythmia in the canine

acute myocardial infarction model. *Circulation* 1979 August;60(2):397-403.
13. Pogwizd SM, Corr PB. Reentrant and nonreentrant mechanisms contribute to arrhythmogenesis during early myocardial ischemia: results using three-dimensional mapping. *Circ Res* 1987 September;61(3):352-71.
14. Janse MJ, van Capelle FJ, Morsink H, Kleber AG, Wilms-Schopman F, Cardinal R, d'Alnoncourt CN, Durrer D. Flow of "injury" current and patterns of excitation during early ventricular arrhythmias in acute regional myocardial ischemia in isolated porcine and canine hearts. Evidence for two different arrhythmogenic mechanisms. *Circ Res* 1980 August;47(2):151-65.
15. Friedman PL, Stewart JR, Wit AL. Spontaneous and induced cardiac arrhythmias in subendocardial Purkinje fibers surviving extensive myocardial infarction in dogs. *Circ Res* 1973 November;33(5):612-26.
16. Pu J, Boyden PA. Alterations of Na+ currents in myocytes from epicardial border zone of the infarcted heart. A possible ionic mechanism for reduced excitability and postrepolarization refractoriness. *Circ Res* 1997 July;81(1):110-9.
17. Peters NS, Green CR, Poole-Wilson PA, Severs NJ. Reduced content of connexin43 gap junctions in ventricular myocardium from hypertrophied and ischemic human hearts. *Circulation* 1993 September;88(3):864-75.
18. Smith JH, Green CR, Peters NS, Rothery S, Severs NJ. Altered patterns of gap junction distribution in ischemic heart disease. An immunohistochemical study of human myocardium using laser scanning confocal microscopy. *Am J Pathol* 1991 October;139(4):801-21.
19. De Bakker JM, van Capelle FJ, Janse MJ, Wilde AA, Coronel R, Becker AE, Dingemans KP, van Hemel NM, Hauer RN. Reentry as a cause of ventricular tachycardia in patients with chronic ischemic heart disease: electrophysiologic and anatomic correlation. *Circulation* 1988 March;77(3):589-606.
20. Pogwizd SM, Hoyt RH, Saffitz JE, Corr PB, Cox JL, Cain ME. Reentrant and focal mechanisms underlying ventricular tachycardia in the human heart. *Circulation* 1992 December;86(6):1872-87.
21. Chung MK, Pogwizd SM, Miller DP, Cain ME. Three-dimensional mapping of the initiation of nonsustained

ventricular tachycardia in the human heart. *Circulation* 1997 June 3;95(11):2517-27.

22. Pogwizd SM, Hoyt RH, Saffitz JE, Corr PB, Cox JL, Cain ME. Reentrant and focal mechanisms underlying ventricular tachycardia in the human heart. *Circulation* 1992 December;86(6):1872-87.

23. Dec GW, Fuster V. Idiopathic dilated cardiomyopathy. *N Engl J Med* 1994 December 8;331(23):1564-75.

24. Di LA, Secoli G, Perkan A, Gregori D, Lardieri G, Pinamonti B, Sinagra G, Zecchin M, Camerini F. Changing mortality in dilated cardiomyopathy. The Heart Muscle Disease Study Group. *Br Heart J* 1994 December;72(6 Suppl):S46-S51.

25. Kelly P, Coats A. Variation in mode of sudden cardiac death in patients with dilated cardiomyopathy. *Eur Heart J* 1997 May;18(5):879-80.

26. Tamburro P, Wilber D. Sudden death in idiopathic dilated cardiomyopathy. *Am Heart J* 1992 October;124(4):1035-45.

27. De Bakker JM, van Capelle FJ, Janse MJ, Tasseron S, Vermeulen JT, de JN, Lahpor JR. Slow conduction in the infarcted human heart. 'Zigzag' course of activation. *Circulation* 1993 September;88(3):915-26.

28. Soejima K, Stevenson WG, Sapp JL, Selwyn AP, Couper G, Epstein LM. Endocardial and epicardial radiofrequency ablation of ventricular tachycardia associated with dilated cardiomyopathy: the importance of low-voltage scars. *J Am Coll Cardiol* 2004 May 19;43(10):1834-42.

29. Hsia HH, Marchlinski FE. Characterization of the electroanatomic substrate for monomorphic ventricular tachycardia in patients with nonischemic cardiomyopathy. *Pacing Clin Electrophysiol* 2002 July;25(7):1114-27.

30. Tomaselli GF, Zipes DP. What causes sudden death in heart failure? *Circ Res* 2004 October 15;95(8):754-63.

31. Gemayel C, Pelliccia A, Thompson PD. Arrhythmogenic right ventricular cardiomyopathy. *J Am Coll Cardiol* 2001 December;38(7):1773-81.

32. Nava A, Bauce B, Basso C, Muriago M, Rampazzo A, Villanova C, Daliento L, Buja G, Corrado D, Danieli GA, Thiene G. Clinical profile and long-term follow-up of 37 families with arrhythmogenic right ventricular cardiomyopathy. *J Am Coll Cardiol* 2000 December;36(7):2226-33.

33. Fung WH, Sanderson JE. Clinical profile of arrhythmogenic right ventricular cardiomyopathy in Chinese patients. *Int J Cardiol* 2001 November;81(1):9-18.

34. Peters S, Peters H, Thierfelder L. Risk stratification of sudden cardiac death and malignant ventricular

arrhythmias in right ventricular dysplasia-cardiomyopathy. *Int J Cardiol* 1999 December 1;71(3):243-50.

35. Awad MM, Calkins H, Judge DP. Mechanisms of disease: molecular genetics of arrhythmogenic right ventricular dysplasia/cardiomyopathy. *Nat Clin Pract Cardiovasc Med* 2008 May;5(5):258-67.

36. Asimaki A, Syrris P, Wichter T, Matthias P, Saffitz JE, McKenna WJ. A novel dominant mutation in plakoglobin causes arrhythmogenic right ventricular cardiomyopathy. *Am J Hum Genet* 2007 November;81(5):964-73.

37. Garcia-Gras E, Lombardi R, Giocondo MJ, Willerson JT, Schneider MD, Khoury DS, Marian AJ. Suppression of canonical Wnt/beta-catenin signaling by nuclear plakoglobin recapitulates phenotype of arrhythmogenic right ventricular cardiomyopathy. *J Clin Invest* 2006 July;116(7):2012-21.

38. Nagata M, Hiroe M, Ishiyama S, Nishikawa T, Sakomura Y, Kasanuki H, Toyosaki T, Marumo F. Apoptotic cell death in arrhythmogenic right ventricular cardiomyopathy: a comparative study with idiopathic sustained ventricular tachycardia. *Jpn Heart J* 2000 November;41(6):733-41.

39. Spirito P, Seidman CE, McKenna WJ, Maron BJ. The management of hypertrophic cardiomyopathy. *N Engl J Med* 1997 March 13;336(11):775-85.

40. McKenna WJ, Behr ER. Hypertrophic cardiomyopathy: management, risk stratification, and prevention of sudden death. *Heart* 2002 February;87(2):169-76.

41. Maron BJ, Spirito P. Impact of patient selection biases on the perception of hypertrophic cardiomyopathy and its natural history. *Am J Cardiol* 1993 October 15;72(12):970-2.

42. Maron BJ, Peterson EE, Maron MS, Peterson JE. Prevalence of hypertrophic cardiomyopathy in an outpatient population referred for echocardiographic study. *Am J Cardiol* 1994 March 15;73(8):577-80.

43. Adabag AS, Casey SA, Kuskowski MA, Zenovich AG, Maron BJ. Spectrum and prognostic significance of arrhythmias on ambulatory Holter electrocardiogram in hypertrophic cardiomyopathy. *J Am Coll Cardiol* 2005 March 1;45(5):697-704.

44. Maron BJ, Roberts WC. Quantitative analysis of cardiac muscle cell disorganization in the ventricular septum of patients with hypertrophic cardiomyopathy. *Circulation* 1979 April;59(4):689-706.

45. Maron BJ, Wolfson JK, Epstein SE, Roberts WC. Intramural ("small vessel") coronary artery disease in hypertrophic cardiomyopathy. *J Am Coll Cardiol* 1986 September;8(3):545-57.

46. Ouyang F, Fotuhi P, Ho SY, Hebe J, Volkmer M, Goya M, Burns M, Antz M, Ernst S, Cappato R, Kuck KH. Repetitive monomorphic ventricular tachycardia originating from the aortic sinus cusp: electrocardiographic characterization for guiding catheter ablation. *J Am Coll Cardiol* 2002 February 6;39(3):500-8.

47. Tada H, Tadokoro K, Miyaji K, Ito S, Kurosaki K, Kaseno K, Naito S, Nogami A, Oshima S, Taniguchi K. Idiopathic ventricular arrhythmias arising from the pulmonary artery: prevalence, characteristics, and topography of the arrhythmia origin. *Heart Rhythm* 2008 March;5(3):419-26.

48. Daniels DV, Lu YY, Morton JB, Santucci PA, Akar JG, Green A, Wilber DJ. Idiopathic epicardial left ventricular tachycardia originating remote from the sinus of Valsalva: electrophysiological characteristics, catheter ablation, and identification from the 12-lead electrocardiogram. *Circulation* 2006 April 4;113(13):1659-66.

49. Iwai S, Cantillon DJ, Kim RJ, Markowitz SM, Mittal S, Stein KM, Shah BK, Yarlagadda RK, Cheung JW, Tan VR, Lerman BB. Right and left ventricular outflow tract tachycardias: evidence for a common electrophysiologic mechanism. *J Cardiovasc Electrophysiol* 2006 October;17(10):1052-8.

50. Kim RJ, Iwai S, Markowitz SM, Shah BK, Stein KM, Lerman BB. Clinical and electrophysiological spectrum of idiopathic ventricular outflow tract arrhythmias. *J Am Coll Cardiol* 2007 May 22;49(20):2035-43.

51. Lerman BB, Dong B, Stein KM, Markowitz SM, Linden J, Catanzaro DF. Right ventricular outflow tract tachycardia due to a somatic cell mutation in G protein subunitalphai2. *J Clin Invest* 1998 June 15;101(12):2862-8.

52. Nogami A, Naito S, Tada H, Taniguchi K, Okamoto Y, Nishimura S, Yamauchi Y, Aonuma K, Goya M, Iesaka Y, Hiroe M. Demonstration of diastolic and presystolic Purkinje potentials as critical potentials in a macroreentry circuit of verapamil-sensitive idiopathic left ventricular tachycardia. *J Am Coll Cardiol* 2000 September;36(3):811-23.

53. Ouyang F, Cappato R, Ernst S, Goya M, Volkmer M, Hebe J, Antz M, Vogtmann T, Schaumann A, Fotuhi P, Hoffmann-Riem M, Kuck KH. Electroanatomic substrate of idiopathic left ventricular tachycardia: unidirectional block and macroreentry within the purkinje network. *Circulation* 2002 January 29;105(4):462-9.

54. Nogami A, Naito S, Tada H, Taniguchi K, Okamoto Y, Nishimura S, Yamauchi Y, Aonuma K, Goya M, Iesaka Y, Hiroe M. Demonstration of diastolic and presystolic Purkinje potentials as critical potentials in a macroreentry circuit of verapamil-sensitive idio-

pathic left ventricular tachycardia. *J Am Coll Cardiol* 2000 September;36(3):811-23.

55. Ouyang F, Cappato R, Ernst S, Goya M, Volkmer M, Hebe J, Antz M, Vogtmann T, Schaumann A, Fotuhi P, Hoffmann-Riem M, Kuck KH. Electroanatomic substrate of idiopathic left ventricular tachycardia: unidirectional block and macroreentry within the purkinje network. *Circulation* 2002 January 29;105(4):462-9.

56. Antzelevitch C, Sicouri S, Litovsky SH, Lukas A, Krishnan SC, Di Diego JM, Gintant GA, Liu DW. Heterogeneity within the ventricular wall. Electrophysiology and pharmacology of epicardial, endocardial, and M cells. *Circ Res* 1991 December;69(6):1427-49.

57. Pelleg A, Hurt CM, Xu J. Reproducible induction of EADs and torsade de pointes. *Circulation* 1995 September 15;92(6):1666-7.

58. Liu J, Laurita KR. The mechanism of pause-induced torsade de pointes in long QT syndrome. *J Cardiovasc Electrophysiol* 2005 September;16(9):981-7.

59. Brugada P, Brugada J. Right bundle branch block, persistent ST segment elevation and sudden cardiac death: a distinct clinical and electrocardiographic syndrome. A multicenter report. *J Am Coll Cardiol* 1992 November 15;20(6):1391-6.

60. Yan GX, Antzelevitch C. Cellular basis for the Brugada syndrome and other mechanisms of arrhythmogenesis associated with ST-segment elevation. *Circulation* 1999 October 12;100(15):1660-6.

61. Leenhardt A, Lucet V, Denjoy I, Grau F, Ngoc DD, Coumel P. Catecholaminergic polymorphic ventricular tachycardia in children. A 7-year follow-up of 21 patients. *Circulation* 1995 March 1;91(5):1512-9.

62. Priori SG, Napolitano C, Tiso N, Memmi M, Vignati G, Bloise R, Sorrentino V, Danieli GA. Mutations in the cardiac ryanodine receptor gene (hRyR2) underlie catecholaminergic polymorphic ventricular tachycardia. *Circulation* 2001 January 16;103(2):196-200.

63. Viatchenko-Karpinski S, Terentyev D, Gyorke I, Terentyeva R, Volpe P, Priori SG, Napolitano C, Nori A, Williams SC, Gyorke S. Abnormal calcium signaling and sudden cardiac death associated with mutation of calsequestrin. *Circ Res* 2004 March 5;94(4):471-7.

64. Leenhardt A, Lucet V, Denjoy I, Grau F, Ngoc DD, Coumel P. Catecholaminergic polymorphic ventricular tachycardia in children. A 7-year follow-up of 21 patients. *Circulation* 1995 March 1;91(5):1512-9.

65. Swan H, Piippo K, Viitasalo M, Heikkila P, Paavonen T, Kainulainen K, Kere J, Keto P, Kontula K, Toivonen L. Arrhythmic disorder mapped to chromosome 1q42-q43 causes malignant polymorphic ventricular tachycardia in structurally normal hearts. *J Am Coll Cardiol* 1999 December;34(7):2035-42.

66. Crabos M, Roth M, Hahn AW, Erne P. Characterization of angiotensin II receptors in cultured adult rat cardiac fibroblasts. Coupling to signaling systems and gene expression. *J Clin Invest* 1994 June;93(6):2372-8.

67. Sadoshima J, Izumo S. Molecular characterization of angiotensin II--induced hypertrophy of cardiac myocytes and hyperplasia of cardiac fibroblasts. Critical role of the AT1 receptor subtype. *Circ Res* 1993 September;73(3):413-23.

68. Nakamura K, Fushimi K, Kouchi H, Mihara K, Miyazaki M, Ohe T, Namba M. Inhibitory effects of antioxidants on neonatal rat cardiac myocyte hypertrophy induced by tumor necrosis factor-alpha and angiotensin II. *Circulation* 1998 August 25;98(8):794-9.

69. Crabos M, Roth M, Hahn AW, Erne P. Characterization of angiotensin II receptors in cultured adult rat cardiac fibroblasts. Coupling to signaling systems and gene expression. *J Clin Invest* 1994 June;93(6):2372-8.

70. Allen IS, Cohen NM, Dhallan RS, Gaa ST, Lederer WJ, Rogers TB. Angiotensin II increases spontaneous contractile frequency and stimulates calcium current in cultured neonatal rat heart myocytes: insights into the underlying biochemical mechanisms. *Circ Res* 1988 March;62(3):524-34.

71. Bescond J, Bois P, Petit-Jacques J, Lenfant J. Characterization of an angiotensin-II-activated chloride current in rabbit sino-atrial cells. *J Membr Biol* 1994 June;140(2):153-61.

72. Kaibara M, Mitarai S, Yano K, Kameyama M. Involvement of Na(+)-H+ antiporter in regulation of L-type Ca2+ channel current by angiotensin II in rabbit ventricular myocytes. *Circ Res* 1994 December;75(6):1121-5.

73. Morita H, Kimura J, Endoh M. Angiotensin II activation of a chloride current in rabbit cardiac myocytes. *J Physiol* 1995 February 15;483 (Pt 1):119-30.

74. Ju H, Scammel-La FT, Dixon IM. Altered mRNA abundance of calcium transport genes in cardiac myocytes induced by angiotensin II. *J Mol Cell Cardiol* 1996 May;28(5):1119-28.

75. Obayashi K, Horie M, Xie LH, Tsuchiya K, Kubota A, Ishida H, Sasayama S. Angiotensin II inhibits protein kinase A-dependent chloride conductance in heart via pertussis toxin-sensitive G proteins. *Circulation* 1997 January 7;95(1):197-204.

76. Yu H, Gao J, Wang H, Wymore R, Steinberg S, McKinnon D, Rosen MR, Cohen IS. Effects of the renin-angiotensin system on the current I(to) in epicardial and endocardial ventricular myocytes from the canine heart. *Circ Res* 2000 May 26;86(10):1062-8.

77. Yu H, Gao J, Wang H, Wymore R, Steinberg S, McKinnon D, Rosen MR, Cohen IS. Effects of the renin-angiotensin system on the current I(to) in epicardial and endocardial ventricular myocytes from the canine heart. *Circ Res* 2000 May 26;86(10):1062-8.

78. Daleau P, Turgeon J. Angiotensin II modulates the delayed rectifier potassium current of guinea pig ventricular myocytes. *Pflugers Arch* 1994 July;427(5-6):553-5.

79. Hool LC, Whalley DW, Doohan MM, Rasmussen HH. Angiotensin-converting enzyme inhibition, intracellular Na+, and Na(+)-K+ pumping in cardiac myocytes. *Am J Physiol* 1995 February;268(2 Pt 1):C366-C375.

80. Morita H, Kimura J, Endoh M. Angiotensin II activation of a chloride current in rabbit cardiac myocytes. *J Physiol* 1995 February 15;483 (Pt 1):119-30.

81. Benitah JP, Perrier E, Gomez AM, Vassort G. Effects of aldosterone on transient outward K+ current density in rat ventricular myocytes. *J Physiol* 2001 November 15;537(Pt 1):151-60.

82. Timolol-induced reduction in mortality and reinfarction in patients surviving acute myocardial infarction. *N Engl J Med* 1981 April 2;304(14):801-7.

83. Schwartz PJ, Motolese M, Pollavini G, Lotto A, Ruberti U, Trazzi R, Bartorelli C, Zanchetti A. Prevention of sudden cardiac death after a first myocardial infarction by pharmacologic or surgical antiadrenergic interventions. *J Cardiovasc Electrophysiol* 1992;3(1):2-16.

84. Barber MJ, Mueller TM, Henry DP, Felten SY, Zipes DP. Transmural myocardial infarction in the dog produces sympathectomy in noninfarcted myocardium. *Circulation* 1983 April;67(4):787-96.

85. Inoue H, Zipes DP. Results of sympathetic denervation in the canine heart: supersensitivity that may be arrhythmogenic. *Circulation* 1987 April;75(4):877-87.

86. Cao JM, Fishbein MC, Han JB, Lai WW, Lai AC, Wu TJ, Czer L, Wolf PL, Denton TA, Shintaku IP, Chen PS, Chen LS. Relationship between regional cardiac hyperinnervation and ventricular arrhythmia. *Circulation* 2000 April 25;101(16):1960-9.

87. Cao JM, Chen LS, KenKnight BH, Ohara T, Lee MH, Tsai J, Lai WW, Karagueuzian HS, Wolf PL, Fishbein MC, Chen PS. Nerve sprouting and sudden cardiac death. *Circ Res* 2000 April 14;86(7):816-21.

88. Cao JM, Fishbein MC, Han JB, Lai WW, Lai AC, Wu TJ, Czer L, Wolf PL, Denton TA, Shintaku IP, Chen PS, Chen LS. Relationship between regional cardiac hyperinnervation and ventricular arrhythmia. *Circulation* 2000 April 25;101(16):1960-9.

89. Takei M, Sasaki Y, Yonezawa T, Lakhe M, Aruga M, Kiyosawa K. The autonomic control of the transmural dispersion of ventricular repolarization in anesthetized dogs. *J Cardiovasc Electrophysiol* 1999 July;10(7):981-9.

90. Friedlander Y, Siscovick DS, Weinmann S, Austin MA, Psaty BM, Lemaitre RN, Arbogast P, Raghunathan TE, Cobb LA. Family history as a risk factor for primary cardiac arrest. *Circulation* 1998 January 20;97(2):155-60.

91. Jouven X, Desnos M, Guerot C, Ducimetiere P. Predicting sudden death in the population: the Paris Prospective Study I. *Circulation* 1999 April 20;99(15):1978-83.

92. Splawski I, Timothy KW, Tateyama M, Clancy CE, Malhotra A, Beggs AH, Cappuccio FP, Sagnella GA, Kass RS, Keating MT. Variant of SCN5A sodium channel implicated in risk of cardiac arrhythmia. *Science* 2002 August 23;297(5585):1333-6.

93. Mikkelsson J, Perola M, Laippala P, Penttila A, Karhunen PJ. Glycoprotein IIIa Pl(A1/A2) polymorphism and sudden cardiac death. *J Am Coll Cardiol* 2000 October;36(4):1317-23.

94. Anvari A, Schuster E, Gottsauner-Wolf M, Wojta J, Huber K. PAI-I 4G/5G polymorphism and sudden cardiac death in patients with coronary artery disease. *Thromb Res* 2001 July 15;103(2):103-7.

95. Anvari A, Turel Z, Schmidt A, Yilmaz N, Mayer G, Huber K, Schuster E, Gottsauner-Wolf M. Angiotensin-converting enzyme and angiotensin II receptor 1 polymorphism in coronary disease and malignant ventricular arrhythmias. *Cardiovasc Res* 1999 September;43(2):879-83.

CHAPTER 5

The Biology of Congenital Heart Disease

Patrick J.S. Disney, MBBS, FRACP

INTRODUCTION

Adult congenital heart disease is one of the youngest subspecialties in adult cardiology but, like the patients, it is steadily growing and flourishing. A full coverage of the topic is beyond the scope of this book, but this chapter will highlight the important biologic issues faced by this very diverse group.

INCIDENCE AND CHANGING TRENDS

Congenital heart disease (CHD) is one of the most common forms of birth defects. The average estimated incidence is 8 per 1000 live births, but has ranged from 4 to 12 per 1000 in more recent studies of different populations.[1,2] If the bicuspid aortic valve is included, with an estimated frequency of 1.3%, then the incidence rises to 19 per 1000 births.[3] The actual incidence of congenital heart disease has likely not increased significantly since the mid-1950s, with advances in imaging and screening accounting for the slightly higher frequencies reported in the more current studies.

Ventricular septal defects (VSD) and bicuspid aortic valves are the most frequent forms of CHD, accounting for almost half of all defects. Tetralogy of Fallot, the most common cause of cyanotic congenital heart disease, accounts for approximately 5–10% of CHD. Not all forms of CHD are clinically significant—many VSDs will close spontaneously early in life and often will not require further follow-up. The significance of the clinically silent patent ductus arteriosus (PDA) detected on echocardiography is unknown.

The most dramatic change has been the survival of infants and children with increasingly complex forms of CHD, largely because of surgical advances. It is now likely that there are more adult survivors with CHD than children. Cardiac surgery has progressed rapidly from the first reported surgical closure of a PDA in 1939[4] through the first aortopulmonary shunt by Blalock and Taussig in 1945[5] to the complex intracardiac repair under circulatory arrest of Tetralogy of Fallot and the Fontan operation.[6]

Data from a large United Kingdom Grown Up Congenital Heart Unit[7] highlights the marked improvement in prognosis for what were almost universally fatal defects in childhood. For infants born with moderate congenital lesions, such as aortic coarctation, Ebstein's anomaly or Tetralogy of Fallot between 1940 and 1959, estimated one-year survival was 60%, compared with 90% for those born between 1980 and 89. The figures are even more impressive for those with complex defects such as pulmonary atresia, single ventricles or transposition of the great arteries—20% versus at least 85% one-year survival for the same time periods. The majority of these infants are now also living beyond childhood into adolescence and adulthood, thanks to ever-changing advances in surgical techniques and perioperative care. The impact of normal biological ageing processes in those with such abnormal cardiac physiology is largely unknown.

GENETICS AND RECURRENCE RISK

At present fewer than one in five patients with CHD have an identifiable genetic abnormality. Examples include Trisomy 21, which is commonly associated with atrioventricular septal defects (AVSD), and deletion 22q11, which has been found in many conotruncal abnormalities such as Tetralogy of Fallot, pulmonary atresia and truncus arteriosus.[8] The actual identification of the causal genes remains elusive, and the mere presence of the chromosomal abnormality does not guarantee CHD, as demonstrated by the finding that not all Trisomy 21 individuals have CHD.[9] However, this is an area of very active research. For example, animal models of Ch22q11 deletion have identified the Tbx1 gene as being critical in embryonic development of the pharyngeal pouches and cardiac development.[10] It is likely that future studies will reveal more of the critical genes and processes involved in normal and abnormal cardiac development. It is estimated that maternal exposure to environmental factors only accounts for approximately 2% of cases of CHD.

The risk of recurrence of CHD in offspring is particularly relevant as more individuals survive into their reproductive years. In a minority of cases, such as with the Ch22q11 deletion mentioned previously, there will be an identifiable autosomal inheritance pattern. In most cases however, the risk of passing on CHD seems to vary with the type of defect and the sex of the parent. The overall risk of recurrence is increased in most types of CHD, averaging 3–8%.[11] Generally the risk is increased in offspring of an affected mother with CHD as opposed to an affected father. A large contemporary study of more than 6000 fetal echocardiograms of families with a first-degree family history of CHD has reported a recurrence rate of 2.7%.[12] Offspring of an affected parent will usually have a quite different type of CHD than their parent. The exact concordance rate (probability of recurrence of the same type of CHD) in this study was 37%, although for AVSD this increased to 80%. The involvement of a clinical genetics service should be an intergral part of any prepregnancy counseling in most individuals with CHD, as well as fetal echocardiography, if available.

RESIDUA AND SEQUELAE

It is an unfortunate fact that very few forms of CHD can be regarded as curable. The exception is the ligated patent ductus arteriosus or isolated small VSD that is spontaneously closed. For almost all other defects, there are lifelong issues resulting from the abnormal cardiac anatomy, previous surgery/interventions or associated noncardiac diseases. These are commonly divided into either residua or sequelae. Residua are abnormalities that persist after an intervention, such as the electrical preexcitation seen with Ebstein's anomaly or systemic hypertension after repaired aortic coarctation. Sequelae refers to problems that are often an unwanted, but expected, result of surgery, such as the arrhythmias from atriotomy, or the degeneration of prosthetic material.

Arrhythmias

Arrhythmias are one of the most significant problems for adult survivors with CHD. These may be related to the intrinsic cardiac defect, such as Ebstein's anomaly and the commonly associated Wolff-Parkinson-White syndrome, or sequelae from surgery as with the atrial scars from the atriopulmonary variant of the Fontan operation. The majority of the burden falls on those who have moderate to complex CHD, although the simple atrial septal defect is at increased risk for atrial arrhythmias if repaired late. Table 5.1 outlines some of the arrhythmias associated with particular defects.

It soon becomes clear that almost all arrhythmias can be encountered in the CHD population and often multiple different arrhythmias can occur in the same individual. An obvious example is initial intracardiac repair of Tetralogy of Fallot, which often results in chronic, severe pulmonary regurgitation. Atrial fibrillation and intra-atrial reentrant arrhythmias are commonly seen because of the atriotomy scars, and ventricular tachycardia is increasingly common as right ventricular function deteriorates. A QRS duration of more than 180ms is reported as an independent risk factor for sudden death in the group with severe pulmonary regurgitation.[13] There does seem to be a mechanico-electrical relationship between the underlying cardiac function and the appearance of tachyarrhythmias in particular. When an arrhythmia is detected, appropriate correction of lesions causing significant volume or pressure overload is just as important as treatment directed at the arrhythmia itself.

Prompt recognition and treatment of arrhythmias in some defects is critical, as even atrial arrhythmias can lead to rapid deterioration in some groups. Atrial fibrillation is poorly tolerated in those with single ventricle physiology/Fontan operation, largely because of the important contribution of atrial contraction to pulmonary blood flow in the absence of a ventricular pump in the pulmonary circuit. Atrial flutter has been identified as a risk factor for sudden death in those with an atrial switch procedure for transposition of the great arteries.[14]

Table 5.1   Specific Arrhythmias and Cardiac Defects

ARRHYTHMIA	DEFECTS
Congenital sinus node dysfunction	Isomerism/Heterotaxy syndromes
Acquired sinus node dysfunction	TGA post atrial switch, Fontan
Congenital AV block	Atrioventricular septal defects, CCTGA
Accessory pathway	Ebstein's anomaly (including CCTGA)
Intra-atrial reentrant tachycardia	Fontan, TGA post atrial switch, Atriotomy scars
Atrial fibrillation	Fontan, Tetralogy of Fallot
Ventricular tachycardia	Tetralogy of Fallot, aortic stenosis

TGA – transposition of the great arteries, CCTGA – congenitally corrected transposition of the great arteries

*New onset event = myocardial infarction, sudden cardiac death, unstable angina, revascularization, stroke/transient ischemic attack, hospital stay for heart failure (heart failure), symptomatic aorto-iliac disease, end-stage renal disease.

Treatment options for arrhythmias are complicated by a number of different factors in this population. Implantation of pacemakers and of ablation catheters may be limited by venous access due to anomalies of venous anatomy. Baffles and conduits are prone to obstruction from pacing leads. It may not be possible to directly access the intracardiac structures percutaneously, such as with the extracardiac Fontan procedure, where the vena cavae are directly anastomosed to the pulmonary artery by conduits, completely bypassing the right atrium. Catheter ablation procedures are therefore more technically challenging, and generally have a lower long-term success rate compared to treatment of similar arrhythmias in those with normal cardiac anatomy. Epicardial pacing leads may be required where there is a risk of systemic thromboembolism.

While antiarrhythmic drug therapy still has a role, there are a number of limitations, not least because of the likelihood of very long-term treatment. As with catheter ablation techniques, response to drug therapy is generally less than in those without CHD. Amiodarone is commonly used due to its higher response rate, but is limited by the side effect profile—it has been reported that the risks of thyroid toxicity are higher in those with a Fontan operation.[15]

Sudden cardiac death is increased in the CHD cohort as compared to the general population, and is estimated at 0.9 per 1000 patient years.[16] The risk obviously varies with the type of underlying disorder, but those identified as being at particular risk include Tetralogy of Fallot, transposition of the great arteries, aortic coarctation and aortic stenosis. Implantable defibrillators (ICDs) are likely to have an increasing role in management, but as yet the indications for implantation are not as well developed as in the general population. There are no currently accepted guidelines for prophylactic ICD use in the CHD population.

Heart Failure

Heart failure is increasingly prevalent in the general adult population. There are internationally accepted guidelines on diagnosis and management, which are based on a wealth of randomized controlled clinical trials. Unfortunately, there is very limited data on heart failure in the CHD population, and there are many reasons why treatment algorithms generated from the non-CHD group cannot simply be applied to the heterogenous congenital population with heart failure.

There etiology of heart failure in the CHD population is multifactorial. Residual valvular stenosis or regurgitation, large septal defects or a systemic right ventricle or single ventricle physiology are the most common abnormalities encountered. The right ventricle appears to be able to adapt to an abnormal volume and pressure load for many years, but then there is a progressive decline in ventricular function with often clinical heart failure.

The most common example is the transposition defects, either simple transposition that has been repaired with an atrial switch (i.e., right ventricle left in the systemic position) and congenitally corrected transposition, again with a systemic right ventricle. Long-term studies have shown an increasing incidence of heart failure after the age of 30 years in this group.[17] Not only is the right ventricle not morphologically designed to act at systemic pressures like the left ventricle, but coexistent tricuspid regurgitation is common and places an extra volume load on the ventricle. Usually the tricuspid incompetence is a result of ventricular and annular dilatation, but occasionally is from intrinsic leaflet dysfunction. In the setting of more than moderate regurgitation, tricuspid valve repair or replacement should be considered early to hopefully prevent progressive ventricular dysfunction, even in the absence of symptoms.

A further potential cause of ventricular dysfunction in the systemic right ventricle is myocardial ischemia with a number of studies documenting ventricular perfusion defects in this group.[18, 19] Epicardial coronary artery disease does not appear to be more frequent in these individuals, and most likely this is the result of a combination of mismatched myocardial blood flow from a single right coronary artery to a hypertrophied systemic ventricle.

There is very limited data on the use of traditional heart failure medications such as angiotensin converting enzyme inhibitors (ACEIs), angiotensin receptor blockers (ARBs), or β-blockers for the systemic right ventricle. It has been postulated that there may not be the same degree of activation of the renin-angiotensin system, and this may explain the relatively disappointing results from the small randomized trials of ACEI/ARBs to date.[20] A small study has reported improvements in right ventricular volumes and ejection fraction with carvedilol in a group of transposition patients,[21] but further larger studies are required. The increased frequency of bradyarrhythmias in this group necessitates cautious β-blocker use.

Table 5.2   Long-Term Complications of Fontan Circulation

Atrial arrhythmias	Systemic venous collaterals
Systemic ventricular dysfunction	Plastic bronchitis
Pulmonary embolism	Protein-losing enteropathy
Pulmonary arteriovenous malformations	

An even more complicated situation is the single ventricle after a Fontan operation, where there is usually a single dominant systemic ventricle and effectively no pump for the pulmonary circulation. The long-term prognosis is also partially influenced by the morphology of the dominant ventricle, with a left ventricle faring better than a right ventricle in the systemic position. The Fontan procedure is associated with a number of potential chronic issues (Table 5.2), with MRI studies documenting reduced ventricular function compared to age-matched controls.[22] Studies have reported abnormalities of both pulmonary and systemic endothelial function in Fontan patients that may be caused by the loss of pulsatile flow in the pulmonary circuit.[23, 24] Reduced β-adrenergic reserve has also been reported because of a limited preload reserve in Fontan patients.[25] It is clear that there are important differences in cardiac physiology and neurohormonal controls between the Fontan and usual adult heart failure patient, and to date there have been no large reported clinical trials demonstrating long term benefits in this group. As with most other areas in adult congenital heart disease, more data from clinical trials is urgently required.

PREGNANCY

As more young women with CHD survive beyond their teenage years, there is an increasing expectation that cardiologists and obstetricians will help these women successfully deliver their own children. While pregnancy is certainly possible for most women with CHD, it is critical that the various risks are discussed before it is too late to make a choice.

Pregnancy is associated with an approximately 50% increase in blood volume, usually reaching a peak by 30 weeks gestation. In addition, the heart is required to adapt to changes in red cell mass, heart rate, systemic and pulmonary vascular resistance, and blood pressure. Rapid changes also occur at the time of labor and delivery, as well as in the early postpartum period. Any abnormality of cardiac function that restricts the heart's ability to adapt to these changes, will increase the risk of decompensation and complications. Some of the CHD defects associated with increased risk are listed in Table 5.3.

A study of almost 600 pregnancies in women with heart disease has reported that independent predictors of maternal cardiac complications during pregnancy were prior cardiac events or arrhythmias, poor functional class NYHA Class II, cyanosis, left heart obstruction, and systemic ventricular dysfunction.[26] Although not statistically significant

Table 5.3   Conditions Associated with High-Risk Pregnancy

Prosthetic heart valves
Severe obstructive cardiac lesions – AS,MS,CoA,RVOTO
Pulmonary hypertension – pulmonary artery pressure > 3/4 systemic pressure
Systemic ventricular dysfunction – EF < 40%
Poor functional class > NYHA II
Cyanosis
Marfans syndrome

AS – aortic stenosis, MS – mitral stenosis, CoA – coarctation of the aorta, RVOTO – right ventricular outflow tract obstruction

in this study, pulmonary hypertension is reported to have one of the highest rates of maternal mortality, approximately 30–50% in Eisenmenger's syndrome.[27]

The probability of fetal complications is also increased in CHD women, particularly in the presence of cyanosis, where there is only a 12% chance of a live birth if oxygen saturation is less than 85%.[28] Intrauterine growth retardation and preterm labor are also more common in this group.

Arrhythmias are a frequent complication in pregnant CHD women, and may have adverse effects on both mother and fetus. The relative risks and benefits of antiarrhythmic therapy must be carefully considered when deciding whether to continue or institute therapy during the pregnancy. DC cardioversion can be undertaken during all stages of pregnancy, with a seemingly low risk of harm to the fetus.[29]

Early identification of potential high-risk pregnancies and close communication between obstetrician and cardiologist ensures most women with CHD can safely deliver a healthy child.

CONCLUSION

Congenital heart disease is a rapidly expanding and changing field with many unique biologic issues. The long-term impact of normal biologic aging on a cardiovascular system that is abnormal from birth is unknown. More studies are required to determine if other therapies used in the non-CHD population are similarly useful, such as the use of the endothelin antagonist Bosentan in Eisenmenger's syndrome.[30] The increasing use of percutaneous procedures has revolutionized the treatment of many conditions such as septal defects and aortic coarctation, and percutaneous pulmonary valve replacement continues to evolve. Surgical techniques are constantly changing, which further alters the biologic substrate as with modifications to the Fontan operation. Cardiac imaging of CHD is discussed in another chapter, but clearly advances in echocardiography and MRI and, to a lesser extent computed tomography, have dramatically altered the follow-up and management of all forms of CHD. Three-dimensional imaging, tissue characterization, and flow mapping have provided new insights into cardiac function without the need for invasive catheterization. The hope is that the improved outcomes in childhood will be translated into long-term adult survival.

◇◇◇◇◇◇◇◇◇◇◇◇◇

REFERENCES

1. Ferenz Ch et al. The Baltimore-Washington Infant Study 1981-89. In: *Perspectives in Paediatric Cardiology*; NY Futura, 1997: 337-58

2. Robida A et al. Incidence of congenital heart disease in Quatari children. *Int J Cardiol* 1997; 60: 19-22.

3. Hoffman J, Kaplan S. The incidence of congenital heart disease. *J Am Coll Cardiol* 2002;39:1890-1900

4. Gross R, Hubbard J. Surgical ligation of a patent ductus arteriosus: report of first successful case. *JAMA* 1939; 112:729-31

5. Blalock A, Taussig H. The surgical treatment of malformations of the heart in which there is pulmonary stenosis or pulmonary atresia. *JAMA* 1945;128:189-202

6. Fontan F, Baudet E. Surgical repair of tricuspid atresia. *Thorax* 1971;26:240-48

7. Warnes C et al. Task Force 1: The changing profile of congenital heart disease in adult life. *J Am Coll Cardiol*. 2001; 37;1170-75

8. Renforth G, Wilson D Adults with congenital heart disease:a genetic perspective. In: *Diagnosis and Management of Adult Congenital Heart Disease*; Churchill Livingstone, 2003: 19-24

9. Sparkes R, Perloff J. Genetics, Epidemiology, Counselling, and Prevention. In: *Congenital Heart Disease in Adults*; W.B Saunders, Philadelphia, 1998: 165-188.

10. Merscher S et al. Tbx1 is responsible for cardiovascular defects in velo-cardiofacial/DiGeorge syndrome. *Cell* 2001;104:619-29

11. Burn J et al. Recurrence risks in offspring of adults with major heart defects: results from first cohort of British collaborative study. *Lancet* 1998;351:311-315

12. Gil H et al. Patterns of recurrence of congenital heart disease. *J Am Coll Cardiol* 2003;42:923-9

13. Gatzoulis M, Till J, Somerville J et al. Mechanico-electrical interaction in tetralogy of Fallot. QRS prolongation relates to right ventricular size and predicts malignant ventricular arrhythmias and sudden death. *Circulation* 1995;92:231-237

14. Gewillig M et al. Risk factors for arrhythmia and death after Mustard operation for simple transposition of the great arteries. *Circulation* 1991; 84(Supp III):187-192

15. Thorne S et al. Amiodarone-associated thyroid dysfunction. Risk factors in adults with congenital heart disease. *Circulation* 1999;100:149-154

16. Harris L, Balaji S. Arrhythmias in the adult with congenital heart disease. In: *Diagnosis and Management of Adult Congenital Heart Disease*; Churchill Livingstone, 2003:105-113

17. Graham T et al. Long term outcome in congenitally corrected transposition of the great arteries: a multi-institutional study. *J Am Coll Cardiol* 2000;36:255-61

18. Millane T et al. Role of ischaemia and infarction in late right ventricular dysfunction after atrial repair of transposition of the great arteries. *J Am Coll Cardiol* 2000;35:1661-68

19. Hornung T et al. Myocardial perfusion defects and associated systemic ventricular dysfunction in congenitally corrected transposition of the great arteries. *Heart* 1998;80:322-326

20. Dore A et al. Angiotensin receptor blockade and exercise capacity in adults with systemic right ventricles: a multicentre randomized placebo-controlled clinical trial. *Circulation* 2005;112(16):2411-6

21. Giardini A et al. A pilot study on the effect of carvedilol on right ventricular remodeling and exercise tolerance in patients with systemic right ventricle. *Int J Cardiol* 2007;114:241-246

22. Eicken A et al. Hearts late after Fontan operation have normal mass, normal volume, and reduced systolic function. *J Am Coll Cardiol* 2003;42:1061-5

23. Khambadkone S et al. Basal pulmonary vascular resistance and nitric oxide responsiveness late after Fontan-type operation. *Circulation* 2003;107:3204-3208

24. Jin S et al. Impaired vascular function in patients with Fontan circulation. *Int J Cardiol* 2007;120:221-226

25. Senzaki H et al. Ventricular afteload and ventricular work in Fontan circulation. *Circulation* 2002;105:2885-2892

26. Siu S et al. Prospective multicentre study of pregnancy outcomes in women with heart disease. *Circulation* 2001;104:515-521

27. Avila W et al. Maternal and fetal outcome in pregnant women with Eisenmenger's syndrome. *European Heart Journal* 1995;16:460-464

28. Presbitero P et al. Pregnancy in cyanotic congenital heart disease. *Circulation* 1994;89:2673-2676

29. lefroy D, Adamson D. Heart rhythm disorders. In: *Heart Disease in Pregnancy*. Blackwell Oxford 2007: 217-242

30. Galie N et al. Bosentan therapy in patients with Eisenmenger syndrome. *Circulation* 2006;114:48-54

Part II

Imaging Technologies in Cardiovascular Disease

CHAPTER 6
Echocardiography

Stuart Turner, MBBS, PhD, FRACP

INTRODUCTION

Echocardiography is the use of ultrasound to examine cardiac structure and function. Sound is a disturbance propagated through an elastic material. As such, it comprises regular compressions interspersed with rarefactions, with particle movement parallel to the direction of travel of the disturbance forming a longitudinal wave (Figure 6.1).

Sound Waves

Sound waves are characterized by their frequency and intensity (amplitude). Frequency is measured in Hertz (Hz) with one Hz equal to one oscillation (compression and rarefaction) per second. Frequencies greater than 20×10^3Hz (20kHz) cannot be perceived by the human ear and are termed *ultrasound*. Echocardiography uses sound frequencies greater than 1.5×10^6Hz (1.5MHz). Amplitude is a measure of displacement of elements within the tissue. The range of displacement values is large and is measured on a log scale (decibels).

Velocity of sound is dependent on the density and compressibility of the material through which it travels and represents a fixed value when the material is homogeneous. In cardiac tissue, it is 1540m/s. The wavelength of sound varies in direct proportion to

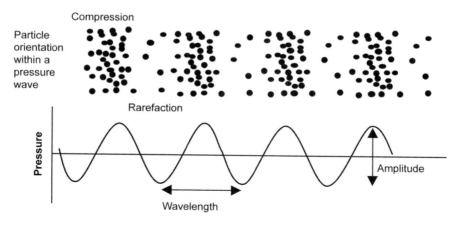

Figure 6.1

Particle orientation and a pressure time plot of a sound wave.

its velocity and inversely with its frequency. Wavelength determines resolution with shorter wavelengths producing better images. By increasing the frequency, the wavelength is reduced and the resolution is increased. The higher the frequency, the greater the interaction between the sound wave and the tissue, resulting in more attenuation and less penetration. The wavelength of ultrasound used for echocardiography is less than 0.5mm, which represents the best tradeoff between the competing requirements of resolution and penetration.

The Ultrasound Transducer

Diagnostic ultrasound is generated by piezoelectric crystals, which, because of their regular molecular structure, are able to transform electrical (voltage) oscillations into vibrations (sound). The crystal is also able to act as a sound receiver by reversing the process and producing electrical signals in response to reflected sound waves. A series of piezoelectric crystals and their associated electrodes comprise the working elements of an echocardiographic transducer. To collect sufficient echoes from cardiac structures, 99% of the transducer's time is spent in receive mode.

Image Production

Sound is reflected back to the transducer when a change in acoustic impedance occurs. This is usually at an interface between tissues of different densities. The greater the acoustic impedance, the more reflection occurs and the larger the amplitude of the returning echo. To form a two-dimensional (2D) image, three values must be measured in the returning echo: (a) time delay between transmission of an ultrasound pulse and the reception of the associated returning echoes (axial position); (b) direction of travel of the ultrasound pulse in relation to the transducer (lateral position); and (c) amplitude of the returning echo (grayscale intensity).

M-MODE ECHOCARDIOGRAPHY

Axial position is the distance of the tissue interface from the transducer along a straight beam of ultrasound called the scan line. The speed of sound in tissue is a fixed value, so once the time interval from ultrasound transmission to echo reception is accurately determined, precise distance can be calculated. When the movement of tissue interfaces along one scan line is plotted against time it is referred to as M mode.

TWO-DIMENSIONAL ECHOCARDIOGRAPHY

Lateral position is the horizontal coordinate of the tissue interface within the field of view. Scan lines are directed into the tissue at different angles from the transducer. This

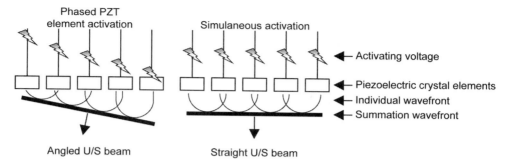

Figure 6.2

Electronic steering of an ultrasound beam.

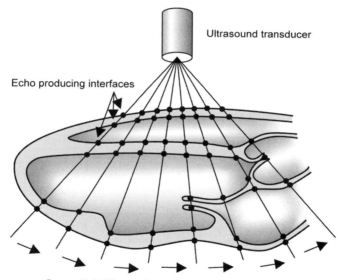

Figure 6.3

Typical, echo producing, acoustic interfaces of the heart.

allows a two-dimensional arch (scan plane) to be built up by stitching together multiple, sequential scan lines (Figure 6.3). Directing each scan line into the tissue at the correct angle is achieved electronically. The transducer comprises multiple individual piezoelectric crystal elements arranged in an array. The wavelets from each element summate to form a wave front of the scan line. The phased electrical activation of the elements allows the scan line to be steered along the appropriate angle (Figure 6.2). A single scan plane only records a brief snapshot of time within the cardiac cycle.

2D Cine Echocardiography

To produce a cine image (2D cine echocardiography or B Mode), the scan plane (and the individual scan lines that compose it) needs to be refreshed rapidly. In a typical system, each scan line takes 0.16msec (for a depth of 12.5cm) and the scan plane 24msec (assuming 150 scan lines). This allows a maximum refresh rate of 41 frames per second for the scan plane. With new beam forming and receiving technologies, as well as parallel processing, multiple scan lines can be read from a single ultrasound pulse, allowing substantially higher frame rates.

Doppler

Frequency is another property of ultrasound that can be used diagnostically. The transmitted frequency of ultrasound is dictated by a need for adequate resolution and penetration. As a transmitted ultrasound pulse strikes moving blood cell and tissue elements within the scan plane, the reflected echoes become Doppler shifted. In other words, the returning echo frequency is either higher or lower than the transmit frequency depending on whether the elements are moving toward or away from the transducer (Figure 6.4).

The magnitude of the shift is dependent on the velocity and angle of the elements relative to the transducer. Hence, Doppler information from returning echoes provides information about velocity and direction of blood flow and tissue movement. Velocities

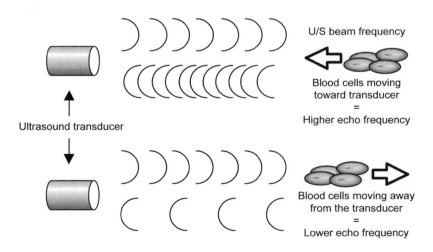

Figure 6.4

Doppler effect.

toward the transducer are recorded above the baseline and velocities away are recorded below on the spectral trace. Doppler information can be generated in a number of ways.

Continuous Wave

Continuous wave Doppler is acquired by sending a continuous beam of ultrasound into the tissue along a single scan line. The returning Doppler shifted echoes record a spectrum of velocities that are plotted against time (spectral trace). There is no limit to the magnitude of velocity that can be recorded with this method, however flow signals cannot be localized as the velocity spectrum is recorded along the entire scan line.

Pulse Wave

Pulse wave (PW) Doppler is acquired by only analyzing the Doppler shift from a specific point within the scan plane. This is achieved by receiving the echo signal after a time delay corresponding to the desired depth. This delay reduces the sampling rate and results in a phenomenon known as *aliasing*, which limits to the maximal detectable velocity (Nequist limit). In diagnostic echocardiography, this is usually no greater than 2m/s. PW is also recorded as a spectral trace.

Color Flow Mapping

Color flow mapping is an automated 2D version of pulse wave Doppler. This modality calculates blood velocity and direction at multiple points along a number of scan lines superimposed on a 2D echo image. The velocities and directions of blood flow are color encoded. Velocities away from the transducer are given an arbitrary color of blue and those towards it, red. Higher velocities are shown in progressively lighter shades of color. Above the Nequist velocity, color reversal occurs because of aliasing.

Tissue Doppler

Normally the high-amplitude, low-velocity tissue signals are filtered from Doppler traces to give a pure blood flow velocity. Reversing the filtering process yields a tissue velocity trace, which provides information regarding systolic and diastolic function. Velocity data can also be used to generate tissue strain (deformation) traces.

Tissue Harmonic Imaging

Tissue harmonic imaging (THI) utilises the phenomenon of propagation harmonics to improve 2D image quality. Harmonics are frequency overtones that occur because sound travels faster during the higher density compression phase than the low-density rarefaction phase (Figure 6.5). Harmonic frequencies increase as the ultrasound pulse penetrates deeper into the chest.[1] During harmonic imaging the transducer is tuned to "listen" only for harmonic echoes. This effectively filters out the surface clutter because harmonic frequencies are only formed deep to the surface layers. Two-dimensional harmonic imaging produces such an improvement in image quality it is now the standard cardiac imaging protocol.[2, 3]

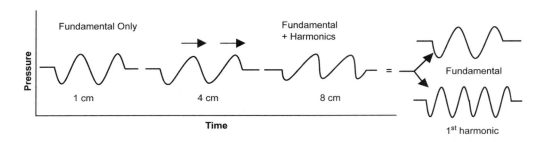

Figure 6.5

Harmonic overtones increase with depth of ultrasound penetration.

ECHO IMAGING MODALITIES

M Mode (Motion Mode)

M mode was the forerunner to 2D echocardiography and, as such, has a relatively limited role in the current era of high-quality, high-temporal resolution 2D echo.[4]

M mode displays a one-dimensional representation of cardiac structures transected by a single scan line. This scan line is continually updated, with each subsequent line of information added to the last to give a plot of cardiac motion over time. On an M-mode trace, the vertical axis records depth and the horizontal axis, time. As only a single scan line is in operation, the ultrasound pulse repetition frequency is very high (1000–2000 cycles per second compared to the 2D frame rate of 25–100), resulting in exceptional temporal resolution. Tissue interfaces are also better appreciated.

M mode yields the most information when the scan line cuts the heart perpendicular to its long axis. Hence, the M-mode examination is routinely performed from the parasternal position. The aorta lies anterior to the left atrium and M mode through these structures produces a square-shaped opening pattern of the aortic valve within the aortic root. The left atrium fills in systole and displaces the aorta anteriorly (Figures 6.6 and 6.7). Moving the M-mode cursor to cut the mitral valve leaflets at their tips, an *M*-shaped pattern is produced by the anterior leaflet. The posterior leaflet (when seen) creates a *W*-shaped pattern. This reflects the early passive diastolic filling, followed by diastasis, then active atrial filling (Figure 6.8). Finally, the basal LV cavity is transacted just beyond the tips of the mitral valve leaflets to provide a trace of the motion of the right ventricular free wall, the left ventricular antero-septum and the posterior wall (Figures 6.9 and 6.10).

The main uses of M mode currently are the timing of rapidly occurring events within the cardiac cycle, the assessment of valvular function and the measurement of cardiac dimensions. To obtain the most reliable information, the M-mode cursor should be accurately placed within a guiding 2D image. Significant overestimation of the left ventricular

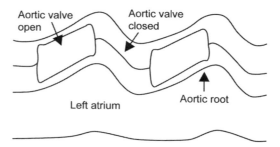

Figure 6.6

Diagram of aorta and left atrium M mode.

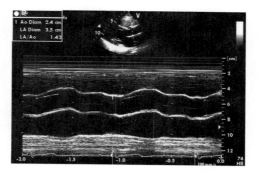

Figure 6.7

Typical normal aorta and left atrial M mode.

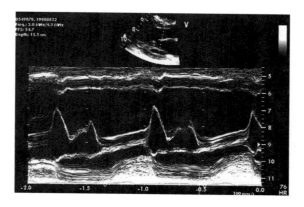

Figure 6.8

Normal left ventricular M mode at the mitral valve level.

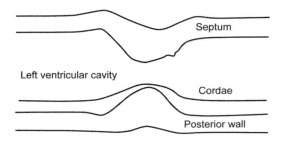

Figure 6.9

Diagram of the basal left ventricular cavity M mode.

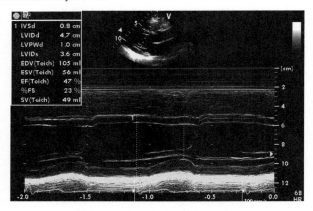

Figure 6.10

Normal M mode at the level of the basal LV cavity.

size commonly occurs when the M mode is taken obliquely through the LV cavity. LV dimensions taken directly from the 2D image have replaced M mode measurements in many institutions. M mode still provides useful information in a number of conditions and is a useful adjunct to 2D and Doppler findings.

2D (B Mode)

Two-dimensional echo allows a thorough assessment of cardiac structure and function, as well as guiding the placement of M mode, spectral, and Doppler cursors to regions of interest within the heart. The process of creating a 2D cine image has previously been discussed. Optimization of the image is achieved by making adjustments to the following controls:

- Depth—should be kept as shallow as possible to maximize frame rate.
- Focus—is the narrowest portion of the ultrasound beam, hence the area of highest resolution. This should be at the level of the greatest region of interest.

- Gain—adjusts the amplitude of the received echoes throughout the scan plane. If set too high, detail is lost, too low, and faint echoes may be missed.
- Time Gain Compensation—allows gain to be adjusted within the scan plan according to depth. This permits adjustment for depth attenuation to produce a uniform level of gain throughout the field of view.
- Dynamic Range (DR)—adjusts the amount of grey scale devoted to low-amplitude echoes. When the image quality is good, increasing the dynamic range will enhance tissue echotexture. Image clarity will be improved in poor quality echoes by decreasing the DR, which will suppress low-amplitude noise.
- Once the field of view has been optimized, it is used to "slice" the heart into a number of standardized cine images as detailed in the next section.

Doppler (PW, CW, CFM, TD)

Pulse wave Doppler (PWD) allows targeted assessment of blood flow at any point within the cardiac chambers or blood vessels. This data can then be used in hemodynamic equations to derive valve areas and calculate pressures and flows.[5] In the echo examination the PW sample, volume is routinely placed in the: (a) LV cavity in the four-chamber view, at the level of the tips of the mitral valve leaflets; (b) orifice of the right upper pulmonary vein; (c) left ventricular outflow tract; and (d) proximal descending aorta (Figure 6.11).

Continuous wave Doppler (CWD) is the most accurate way of assessing blood velocity when it is greater than the Nequist limit (approximately 2m/s). This primarily applies to high velocity outflow and regurgitation flows. In the echo examination, CW Doppler data

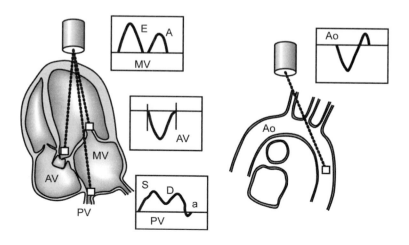

Figure 6.11

Pulse wave Doppler placement.

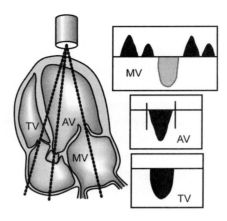

Figure 6.12

Continuous wave Doppler acquisition.

is routinely collected from: (a) the aortic outflow region in the four-chamber view; (b) over the mitral valve in the presence of mitral regurgitation; (c) over the tricuspid valve in the parasternal short-axis view and four-chamber view; and (d) over the pulmonary valve, if pulmonary stenosis is suspected (Figure 6.12).

Color flow Doppler is used primarily to detect the presence of valvular regurgitation and acquired and congenital shunts. It is mainly a qualitative examination tool. The color box area should be kept as small as practical to maintain adequate temporal resolution. In the echo examination, the CFD is routinely applied to each of the following structures, whenever they appear in the scan plane: (a) mitral, tricuspid, aortic, and pulmonary valves; (b) interatrial septum; (c) pulmonary veins; and (d) aortic arch. Color flow is best appreciated when the direction of flow is parallel to the scan lines.

Tissue Doppler (TD) imaging's role is limited to the assessment of longitudinal systolic and diastolic function of the left and right ventricle. The TD sample volume is positioned in much the same way as with PW. In a routine echo examination, the sample volume is placed within the tissue at the medial and lateral portions of the mitral annulus[6] (Figure 6.13).

Doppler Derived Hemodynamics

Stroke Volume

The area enclosed by a Doppler spectral trace is referred to as the *velocity time integral* (UTI) (velocity $\times$ time) and has the unit of distance (cm/sec $\times$ sec = cm). When the diameter of the orifice through which the blood is flowing is measured, cross-sectional area (CSA) can be calculated (CSA = $\varpi/2 \times D^2$). When a pulse wave Doppler trace is

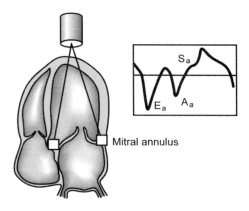

Mitral annulus

Figure 6.13

Tissue Doppler placement.

recorded from the same position as the CSA, a volume measurement can be derived using this formula:

$$Flow = VTI \times CSA$$

Hence, cardiac stroke volume can be measured at the level of the left and right outflow tracts as long as the 2D image is adequate to acquire accurate diameters.[7, 8] When heart rate is known, cardiac output can also be calculated.[5]

Pressure Gradient

The difference in pressure between two cardiac chambers can be used to assess valvular stenosis as well as calculate a pressure value for one chamber if the true pressure in the other chamber is known.[7] The pattern of change in a gradient over time can also provide valuable information. Fortunately, converting Doppler velocity data into pressure gradients is relatively simple and relies on the concept of conservation of energy—*in a closed system energy remains constant.* This means that the blood flow passing over a discrete stenosis must be the same as the flow of blood proximal to the stenosis. This can only occur if the velocity of blood flow increases over the stenosis. The extent of velocity increase is proportional to the severity of the stenosis. The simplified Bernoulli equation converts peak velocity across the stenosis into an accurate pressure gradient:

$$Pressure\ gradient = 4(v^2)$$

Where the pressure gradient is in mmHg and v is in m/s and measured by continuous or pulse wave Doppler at $< 20^0$ angle to the direction of flow. The results are valid for both peak and mean velocities.

Continuity Equation

Continuity equation is a variation of the stroke volume equation and relies on the principle of the conservation of mass—*in a closed system volumetric flow is constant at all points in the circuit*. This equation is predominately used to estimate aortic valve area in the presence of aortic stenosis.[9] In this setting, the equation can be expressed as flow proximal to the stenosis (left ventricular outflow tract) must equal flow across the stenosis:

$$CSA_{LVOT} \times VTI_{LVOT} = CSA_{AS} \times VTI_{AS}$$
or
$$CSA_{AS} = (CSA_{LVOT} \times VTI_{LVOT}) / VTI_{AS}$$

The data needed to solve this equation is the same as that to calculate LV stroke volume with the addition of the VTI from the continuous wave spectral trace through the aortic valve. All values should be in cm or cm^2 and the result will be a valve area also in cm^2. This equation corrects for changes in transvalvular gradient that may occur with LV impairment or aortic regurgitation.[10]

Pressure Half-Time

The pressure half-time is a useful measure of the change in pressure gradient over a valve during systole or diastole. It is defined as the time taken for the peak gradient to fall by half and has two important clinical uses. In mitral stenosis, a persistently high diastolic pressure gradient (prolonged P½t) implies severe stenosis.[11-13] In aortic regurgitation, a rapidly decaying pressure gradient (short P½t) implies equalization of LV and aortic pressures, indicating acute, severe aortic regurgitation.[14] Because Doppler measures velocity, and velocity is related to the square root of the pressure gradient, the equation for calculating the pressure half-time is:

$$P½t = \text{time elapsed from } V_{Peak} \text{ to } V_{Peak} / \sqrt{2}$$

Mitral valve area can be calculated using an empirically derived formula incorporating the P½t:

$$MVA = 220 / P½t.$$

This relationship is only valid in the absence of significant aortic regurgitation or LV diastolic impairment. In the setting of aortic regurgitation, a P½t value of < 300msec implies a clinically significant fall in the diastolic aortic–LV gradient.[15]

3D Echocardiography

Real time three-dimensional (3D) transthoracic echo has become a reality since 2004, with the introduction of matrix array transducers capable of electronically steering the ultrasound beam through a volume (as opposed to a slice) of cardiac tissue[16, 17] (Figure 6.14). Prior to this, 3D images could only be generated by integrating multiple 2D slices using offline processing.

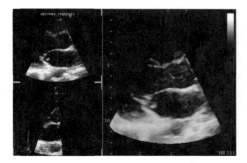

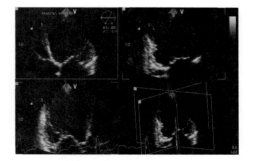

Figure 6.14

Parasternal long axis 3D slice showing aortic and mitral valves.

Figure 6.15

3D matrix transducers can also take multiple simultaneous images from a single precordial position (the apex in this example).

Currently, image acquisition is too slow to capture a volume containing the entire heart at an adequate frame rate. To obtain a full volume acquisition, four to six smaller, ECG-gated volumes are taken and spliced together.[18, 19]

The advantages of 3D include accurate estimation of left and right ventricular volumes with low inter- and intraobserver variability and high test–retest reliability,[18] unique views of the valves particularly with regard to mitral prolapse[20] and, finally, viewing irregular anatomical abnormalities (septal defects, atrial myxomas, thrombi).[19] Newer advances, such as quantitative left ventricular dyssynchony assessment, predict response to biventricular pacemaker implantation with a high level of accuracy.[21]

The matrix transducer is also capable of acquiring multiple images from a single precordial position (see Figure 6.15). This substantially reduces imaging time during stress echo.[22] Rapid, accurate calculation of ventricular volumes is also possible.[18]

Contrast

Saline microbubbles are the simplest contrast agent and are prepared by forcefully agitating saline between two syringes. A population of large unstable microbubbles are so formed and, when injected intravenously, strongly reflect ultrasound (Figure 6.16). Their size and very short half-life prevents them from crossing the pulmonary microcirculation. This property is utilized to scan for right to left shunts either at the level of the heart (atrial septal defects, patent foramen ovale) or lung (atrio-venous fistula).

Synthetically engineered microbubbles with a long half-life and of sufficiently small diameter to cross the lung capillaries became available in the 1990s.[23] These agents have found clinical utility for:

1. left ventricular cavity opacification[24] (LVO, Figure 6.17)
2. myocardial contrast echocardiography[25] (MCE)

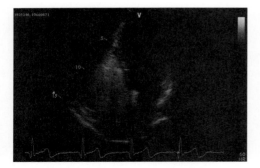

Figure 6.16

Agitated saline contrast confined to right sided chambers.

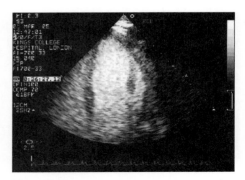

Figure 6.17

Transpulmonary contrast.

The agents consist of an albumin or synthetic outer shell containing a high-density gas to maintain bubble integrity. They behave in a similar manner to red blood cells in the circulation and act as blood flow tracers.[23] Their resonant frequency, by fortunate coincidence, is the same as diagnostic ultrasound, permitting a strong echo signal from low blood contrast concentrations. However, contrast bubbles are fragile and will rupture and rapidly dissipate at normal ultrasound amplitude intensities.

LVO is a simple technique involving a bolus injection of contrast agent that rapidly fills the LV cavity. The large amount of contrast permits normal amplitude scanning as destroyed microbubbles are rapidly replenished. LVO uses include accurate LV volume and regional wall motion assessment when the endocardial border cannot be seen, establishing the diagnosis of noncompaction, identifying intracavity masses, and diagnosing apical hypertrophic cardiomyopathy.[24]

MCE is more difficult because the contrast signal within low-volume microvessels must be differentiated from the tissue signal. To achieve a pure contrast signal, multi-pulse scanning is used to select for nonlinear resonance or high-order harmonics, which are both contrast specific.[26] Low-amplitude ultrasound is also required to limit contrast destruction within the scan plane.

Because a contrast signal is only present where there is flowing blood, MCE is useful for: (a) differentiation of scarred from hibernating myocardium;[26] (b) detecting vascular tumors;[24] and (c) stress echocardiography to improve sensitivity for ischemia.[27]

Not only can the absence of flow be measured but also regions of reduced perfusion. By using a high-amplitude ultrasound pulse, or flash, contrast within the scan plane is destroyed. Following the flash, underperfused areas take longer to replenish with blood and this can be quantified on a time intensity curve relative to normal myocardial segments.[28]

IMAGING TECHNIQUES

Transthoracic Echo

Transthoracic echo (TTE) makes selective use of all echocardiographic modalities (primarily 2D, Doppler, and color flow mapping) to comprehensively assess cardiac structure and function, both quantitatively and qualitatively. Standardized views and Doppler protocols have been established to maximize the diagnostic yield.[29] The TTE study is performed with a streamlined exam technique designed to minimize the constraints imposed by the chest wall and ensure accuracy and reproducibility.

Coupling gel is applied to the transducer to exclude air and maximize the transmission of ultrasound from the probe to the patient. A combination of tilting, angulation, and rotation of the transducer head against the skin permits the scan plane to be aligned correctly with respect to the axes and pertinent structures of the heart.

Acoustic windows through the precordium are limited to positions where the heart and vessels are in direct contact with the chest cavity without overlying lung or bone. In practice, this limits transthoracic scanning to four regions: parasternal, apical, subcostal, and suprasternal (Figure 6.18). The parasternal and apical regions are scanned with the patient in the left lateral decubitus position to maximize heart-chest wall contact, whereas the subcostal and suprasternal regions are scanned in the supine position to optimize transducer positioning.

From these positions the heart can be examined along its long and short axes to give the following standardized 2D views:

a. Parasternal; long axis (Figures 6.19 and 6.20), RV inflow (Figures 6.21 and 6.22), and short axis (Figures 6.23–6.27)

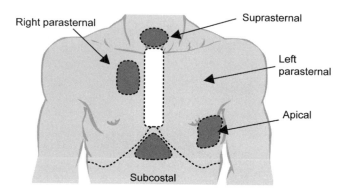

Figure 6.18

Transthoracic echocardiographic windows.

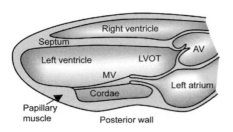

Figure 6.19

Diagram of the 2D parasternal long-axis view.

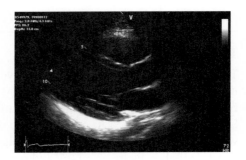

Figure 6.20

Normal 2D parasternal 2D long-axis view.

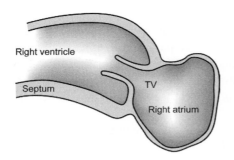

Figure 6.21

Diagram of the 2D parasternal long-axis view of the right ventricle.

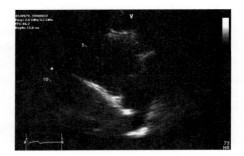

Figure 6.22

Normal 2D parasternal long-axis view of the right ventricle.

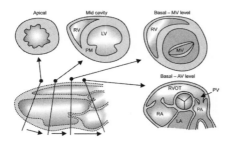

Figure 6.23

Diagram of the 4 2D parasternal short-axis views in relation to the long-axis view.

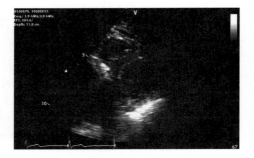

Figure 6.24

Normal 2D parasternal apex short-axis view.

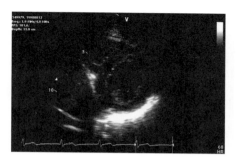

Figure 6.25

Normal 2D parasternal midcavity short-axis view.

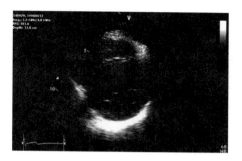

Figure 6.26

Normal 2D parasternal mitral valve short-axis view.

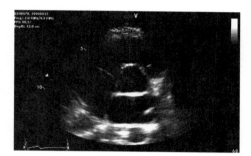

Figure 6.27

Normal 2D parastenal aortic valve short-axis view.

b. Apical; 4 chamber ('5' chamber), 2 chamber, 3 chamber / long axis (Figures 6.28–6.31)

c. Subcostal; 4 chamber, short axis, IVC, aorta

d. Suprasternal; aortic arch, right main pulmonary artery, left atrium (Figures 6.32 and 6.33)

Two-dimensional images form the backdrop for the targeted application of M mode, PW and CW Doppler, zoom, and color Doppler.

The actual position of the heart within the chest is variable between individuals; hence, the correct position of the transducer on the chest wall is the one that results in the appropriate 2D view. In general, the parasternal views can be found to the left of the sternum anywhere between the second and fifth intercostal spaces. The apical views are usually optimal at the maximal apical impulse. Poor parasternal and apical images can be improved by deep expiration to minimize lung tissue artifacts.

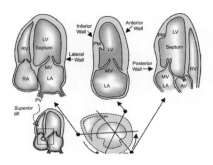

Figure 6.28

Diagram of the 5 2D apical views in relation to the short-axis view.

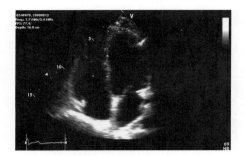

Figure 6.29

Normal 2D apical 4-chamber view.

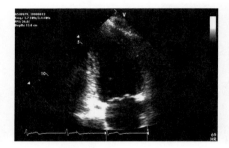

Figure 6.30

Normal 2D apical 2-chamber view.

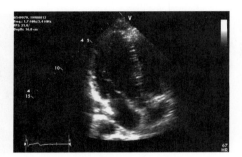

Figure 6.31

Normal apical long-axis (3-chamber) view.

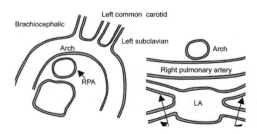

Figure 6.32

Diagram of the 2 2D suprasternal views of the aorta and associated structures.

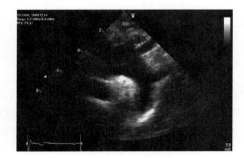

Figure 6.33

Normal 2D suprasternal long-axis view of aorta.

Transesophageal Echo (TEE)

TEE allows an echo transducer to be positioned within millimeters to a few centimeters of the base of the heart—the region encompassing the major vascular communications, the valves, and the atria. This position also eliminates chest wall artifacts. Higher frequencies can be used (7MHz and higher) because tissue penetration is less important. All echo modalities are available including 3D.[20] Hence, TEE is a simple method of acquiring images with three times greater resolution and with minimal artifacts.

A motorized transducer able to rotate the scan plane 180 degrees is mounted at the tip of an endoscope similar to a gastroscope. The patient is fasted and sedated, and his pharynx is anesthetized with local anesthetic. Images of the heart and vessels are obtained from the midesophagus to the fundus of the stomach by physically anteflexing and retroflexing the endoscope tip and mechanically rotating the transducer. The main risks associated with TEE are aspiration, sedation-related hypoxia, and esophageal injury.

Because the esophagus runs parallel to the long axis of the body and the heart is tilted approximately 45 degrees to this axis, the most useful scan plan angles are 45 ($\pm$ 20) degrees and 135 ($\pm$ 20) degrees, to take in short and long axis cuts of the heart respectively.

The standard TEE views are similar to the equivalent TTE views and can be inverted on the screen to assume the same orientation.

TEE is complementary to TTE and is used to image structures at the base of the heart in more detail. The aortic and mitral valves, the left atrial appendage, the interatrial septum, the pulmonary veins, and the thoracic aorta in particular are seen with much greater clarity.[30]

SPECIFIC INDICATIONS

Transthoracic Echocardiography

TTE has the advantage over most imaging modalities because it involves no ionizing radiation or bulky equipment and, as a consequence, can be frequently repeated and can be taken directly to the patient. Even with suboptimal patient positioning, diagnostic images can be obtained in most situations. TTE has the greatest clinical utility for investigating the following symptoms or findings: (a) chest pain; (b) dysponea; (c) murmurs; (d) palpitations; (e) syncope; (f) hypotension; (g) embolic event; (h) suspected endocarditis; and (i) suspected procedural complications

In asymptomatic patients TTE is indicated for: (a) abnormal CXR/ECG; (b) family history of inheritable cardiac disease; (c) known aortic enlargement; (d) chronic valvular regurgitation; (e) precardiotoxic chemotherapy; (f) postvalve replacement; and (g) hypertension—systemic or pulmonary.

In certain emergency situations echocariographic diagnoses can be life saving: (a) pericardial tamponade;[31] (b) acute aortic dissection;[32] (c) acute myocardial infarct with a nondiagnostic ECG;[33] (d) myocardial infarct complications;[34, 35] (e) endocarditis complications;[36] (f) heart failure of unknown cause;[37] and (g) acute pulmonary emboli.[38]

The main drawback of TTE is its dependence on operator skill and the semisubjective nature of image reporting, often resulting in interobserver and intraobserver disagreement.

Transesophageal Echocardiography

TEE is indicated whenever the basal structures of the heart need to be seen in more detail. Although very safe, it is inherently more risky and time consuming than TTE and is reserved for higher yield or more serious indications than TTE. Proven indications include: (a) suspected endocarditis/endocarditis complications; (b) suspected cardiac source of emboli; (c) mitral valve prolapse; (d) suspected left atrial appendage thrombus; (e) aortic dissection; (f) suspected prosthetic valve complications; (g) atrial septal defects; and (h) poor TTE acoustic windows.

Interoperative TEE is now considered standard management for valve repair and replacement surgery as well as for ventricular and atrial septal repairs. It is being used increasingly for coronary bypass surgery and other forms of major surgery where the patient is at risk of coronary ischemia.[39] It is also commonly used for percutaneous closure in those with an atrial septal defect or patent foramen ovale.

TEE and TTE should be considered complementary as they produce separate diagnostic information. TTE is largely quantitative, TEE largely qualitative. In the case of prosthetic valve acoustic shadowing both examination modalities are required to view the ventricular and atrial sides of the valve.

ASSESSMENT OF SYSTOLIC LV FUNCTION

The quantification of left ventricular systolic function is the most commonly requested indication for echocardiography. Not only does systolic function determine prognosis, but it is used to guide pharmacologic and device therapy and measure response to treatment. Systolic function is a shorthand way of referring to myocardial contractility and can be considered on a regional or global level.

Global Systolic Function

Global contractility is not a fixed entity and is largely dependent on preload and afterload, heart rate, adrenergic tone, and myocardial perfusion. From a qualitative point of view, contractility is appreciated as the extent of myocardial thickening. This is manifest as the degree of reduction in LV volume from the end of diastole to the end of systole and can be expressed as:

$$(EDV-ESV) / EDV$$

This equation is commonly referred to as the *ejection fraction* (EF) and is a useful measure of contractility because it controls change in systolic volume (stroke volume) for variations in preload (end diastolic volume) and has been extensively validated.[40]

EF can be determined in one of four ways by echocardiography:

Visual estimate: Usually formed by looking at the three apical images and the parasternal short axis. Effective and reliable when performed by those with experience.

M mode: Is a one-dimensional measurement and requires substantial geometric assumptions of the LV shape, which are usually not met when the EF is reduced.

2D: Involves manually tracing endocardial borders at end systole and diastole in the four-chamber and two-chamber views. This 2D information is converted to volumetric data using algorithms with geometric assumptions.[41] The model most commonly used is the Simpson's rule (or disk summation method), which divides the LV into a series of disks to control for regional wall motion abnormalities (Figures 6.34 and 6.35).

3D: Involves semiautomated endocardial tracking to create an accurate cast of the LV cavity at end systole and diastole. It is the most accurate technique as no geometric models or assumptions are required.[18]

When there is a poorly defined endocardium and/or off axis cuts through the long axis of the LV, EF calculations are often inaccurate.

Other indices of systolic function are also commonly obtained during routine echocariography. *E point septal separation (EPSS)* is a well-established M-mode technique that simply involves the measurement of the minimum separation of the anterior mitral leaflet from the intraventricular septum in early diastole. An EPSS > 7mm indicates both an enlarged LV and reduced early mitral inflow. These findings usually occur in the presence of significant systolic impairment. An abnormal EPSS may also indicate aortic regurgitation. *Systolic mitral annular velocity (S_a),* as measured by tissue Doppler of either the septal or lateral annulus, is an index of longitudinal LV function and is normally >10cm/s [42] (see Figure 6.13). This index of systolic function is thought to be sensitive to systolic impairment because the longitudinally oriented myocardium includes the endocardium, which is the first myocardial layer to become impaired.

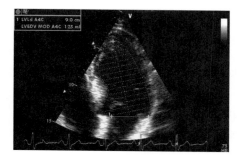

Figure 6.34

Simpson's disk summation method—calculating diastolic volume.

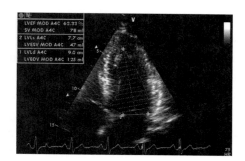

Figure 6.35

Simpson's disk summation method—calculating systolic volume and ejection fraction.

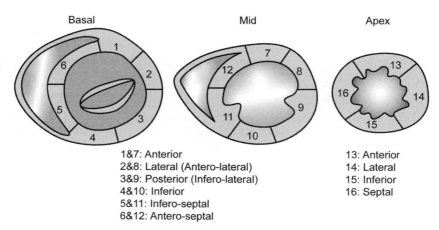

Basal   Mid   Apex

1&7: Anterior   13: Anterior
2&8: Lateral (Antero-lateral)   14: Lateral
3&9: Posterior (Infero-lateral)   15: Inferior
4&10: Inferior   16: Septal
5&11: Infero-septal
6&12: Antero-septal

Figure 6.36

16 segment LV model to describe regional systolic function.

Regional Systolic Function

Regional function becomes impaired primarily due to ischemic heart disease. Septal function may also be altered in the presence of right ventricular disease, conduction abnormalities, pericardial disease, and hypertrophic cardiomyopathy. A 16-segment model of the LV has been established to standardize the description of regional function.[43] There are six basal, six mid, and four apical segments (Figure 6.36). Regional motion is assessed qualitatively according to the following scale:

Hypokinetic: thickening reduced by 50% or more
Akinetic: no thickening
Dyskinetic: outward motion during systole

The presence of impaired regional systolic function only implies irreversible tissue death when evidence of scarring is present (thinning, increased echodensity).[44] In the absence of scarring, reduced regional function may also indicate stunning or hibernation. The infero-basal segment may often appear hypokinetic in the absence of disease.[45]

ASSESSMENT OF LV DIASTOLIC FUNCTION/ FILLING PRESSURES

Diastolic left ventricular impairment is present in virtually all forms of structural heart disease and is commonly present in the elderly, even when structural disease appears absent.[46] There is a gradient of diastolic impairment with the higher grades associated with elevated diastolic left atrial pressures at rest and the lower grades with higher left atrial (LA) pressures only with exertion or not at all.[47]

Increased diastolic LA pressure is transmitted to the pulmonary veins, causing secondary pulmonary hypertension and the respiratory symptoms of cardiac failure. The assessment of diastolic function is an important element of the echocardiographic examination because: (a) systolic and diastolic heart failure are usually clinically indistinguishable but require substantially different management strategies; (b) echo is the best modality for the assessment of diastolic function; and (c) symptoms and prognosis is more strongly correlated to diastolic than systolic impairment.[48]

Diastolic function can be measured both indirectly (2D, M mode) and directly (pulse wave, tissue, and color Doppler). No single parameter of diastolic function should be used in isolation. Rather, an integrated approach should be used, whereby all parameters are measured and integrated to produce a comprehensive picture.

M Mode

A B bump–delayed mitral valve closure is the only M-mode measure of diastolic function still in routine use. It is a qualitative indication of elevated LV end diastolic pressure.[49]

2D Echo

The presence of specific disease states detected by 2D can indirectly suggest the presence of diastolic impairment. Concentric left ventricular hypertrophy, cardiac amyloid, and hypertrophic cardiomyopathy are examples of pathology usually associated with elevated LV filling pressures, particularly when LA enlargement is present.

PW Doppler Mitral Inflow

Recordings of mitral inflow are taken from the apical four-chamber view with the PW sample volume at the level of the mitral leaflet tips. This is the point of greatest inflow velocity and laminar flow. In the normal state there is a biphasic inflow velocity pattern, with the E-wave to A-wave ratio greater than 1.0 but less than 2.5. The time for the E-wave to decelerate to diastasis is between 150 and 240ms. The isovolumic relaxation time (time from aortic valve closure to mitral valve opening) is 60 to 90ms.[50]

Diastolic function deteriorates, and left atrial pressure rises, because of a progressive reduction in left ventricular compliance. This may be the result of the disease state and is independent of systolic function or may be the result of the compensatory Frank-Starling mechanism that occurs during systolic heart failure. A sequence of changes in is observed as LV compliance deteriorates: (a) reduction in compliance in early diastole only, with preserved mean LA pressure; (b) reduced LV compliance throughout diastole with compensatory increase in LA pressure; and (c) loss of LV compliance with a substantial increase in LA pressure. The first of these stages is marked by a delayed diastolic relaxation pattern involving the loss of E-wave height, a reduction of the E/A ratio to <0.7, an

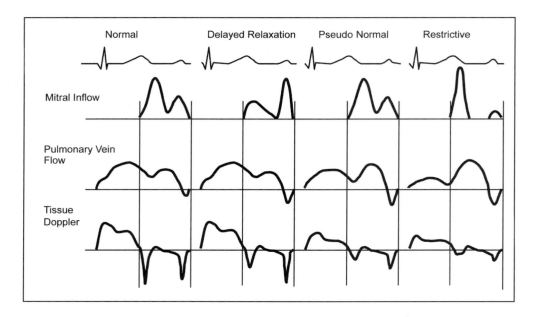

Figure 6.37

Diastolic parameters with increasing left ventricular filling pressure /diastolic impairment.

increase in E-wave deceleration time and a prolongation of the IVRT. The last of these stages, the restrictive filling pattern is characterized by an increase in E-wave height with a fall in A-wave height, an E/A ratio >2.5, a decrease in the E-wave deceleration time (<150ms) and shortening of the IVRT. The pseudo-normalized pattern is intermediate between these extremes (Figure 6.37). It is the result of the delayed diastolic relaxation pattern being modified by increased filling pressure. This can be distinguished from a truly normal filling pattern by repeating the measurement during the valsalva maneuver, which transiently reduces LA pressure to reveal delayed relaxation.[33]

PW Doppler Pulmonary Veins

Recordings of pulmonary vein flow are taken in the apical four-chamber view with the sample volume placed at the point of greatest color flow (usually the right upper PV). The longitudinal length of the heart essentially remains constant throughout the cardiac cycle so, as the ventricles contact and shorten longitudinally, the atria are forced to expand. The opposite occurs when the ventricles relax. As a consequence, the period of greatest blood velocity from the pulmonary veins (S-wave) is during ventricular systole when the atria are forcefully elongated, or "sucking" blood from the veins. Diastolic flow wave (D-wave) occurs as the ventricles relax and the atrio-ventricular valves open. This creates a direct line of flow from the veins to the enlarging ventricular cavities. Finally, the atria contract and a small amount of reverse flow into the veins occurs (A-wave). Normally the S-wave is greater than or equal to the D-wave and the A-wave has a velocity of less than 25cm/s.[51]

As the pressure in the left atrium increases, less pulmonary vein flow occurs during systole (blunted S-wave) and a compensatory increase in diastolic flow is present (accentuated D-wave). There is also an increase in the velocity and duration of reverse flow during atrial contraction (see Figure 6.37). These changes parallel the changes of mitral inflow and can be used to distinguish the pseudo-normal from normal mitral inflow pattern.

Tissue Doppler Mitral Annulus

Recordings of mitral annular velocity are taken in the apical four-chamber view with the sample volume placed at the level of the lateral and/or the medial annulus. The normal diastolic velocity of the mitral annulus is the opposite in direction but similar in pattern to mitral inflow, with the Ea velocity being greater than the Aa velocity. As the left ventricle becomes less compliant, the Ea velocity progressively decreases (see Figure 6.37). Unlike mitral inflow, however, tissue Doppler is volume independent and does not exhibit a pseudo-normalized pattern. The empirically derived formula E/Ea bears a linear relationship with left atrial pressure such that values > 15 are associated with progressively greater LA pressure and values < 9 indicate normal pressure.[52] Unlike other measures of diastolic function, this relationship is independent of disease state, heart rate, and the presence of atrial fibrillation.[6, 42]

Color Doppler M Mode

This is performed by placing an M-mode cursor through the apex and midpoint of the mitral valve in the four-chamber view and recording a colortrace during diastole. The leading edge slope of the E-wave color profile is the propagation velocity of blood entering the LV. The less compliant the LV, the slower this velocity: <45cm/s indicates impaired diastolic relaxation. This value is also independent of the presence of atrial fibrillation.[53]

TRANSTHORACIC ECHOCARDIOGRAPHY IN SPECIFIC CARDIAC CONDITIONS

Transthoracic echocardiography (TTE) is a valuable adjunct in the diagnosis and management of practically all forms of cardiac disease. It is most commonly requested to assess the extent of LV impairment in the setting of ischemic heart disease and to assess valve function. In most echo departments these 2 indications account for 70–80% of all echocardiogram requests. The various modalities that constitute the TTE examination have differing levels of importance depending on the indication—LV impairment is heavily dependent on high-quality 2D images, whereas valve disease relies on accurate Doppler assessment.

Ischemic Heart Disease

Ischemia may be acute, resulting in one of the spectrum of coronary syndromes, or chronic, leaving a legacy of impaired segmental wall function and/or infarct-related complications.

Impaired regional wall motion and myocardial thickening, in the setting of chest pain, are the hallmarks of reduced myocardial perfusion. The number of affected myocardial segments and their degree of hypokinesis have a direct bearing on prognosis, hence, on triage. When these echo features are not present, an ischemic cause for the symptoms can be reliably excluded.[54] Furthermore, echocardiography can frequently detect diseases responsible for nonischemic chest pain (pericarditis, aortic dissection, mitral valve prolapse, HOCM, pulmonary embolism).[55]

Myocardial infarction causes varying degrees of tissue death and scarring, which extends from the endocardium to the epicardium. Full thickness infarction is associated with a highly echogenic, permanently thinned (<6mm) region of myocardium corresponding to a coronary territory (Figures 6.38–6.40).[37] Full thickness infarction is prone to aneurysm formation, which may be a true aneurysm (wide neck, Figures 6.41 and 6.42) or pseudo-aneurysm when a LV free wall rupture is contained by the pericardium (narrow neck).[35] Aneurysms, or any moderate sized area of akinetic myocardium, form a substrate for thrombus formation. This most commonly occurs when the cardiac apex is involved.[34]

Partial thickness infarction is associated with varying degrees of hypokinesis. Large regions of impaired LV function are associated with findings of heart failure (LV enlargement, elevated left atrial filling pressures, pulmonary hypertension, mitral regurgitation, dilated inferior cava).[37]

Most infarct complications are heralded by acute onset heart failure and are rapidly diagnosed by a targeted bedside echo examination. Common complications include

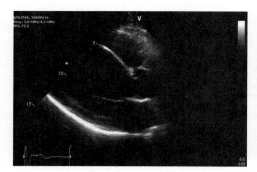

Figure 6.38

Anterior infarct with scar, parasternal view.

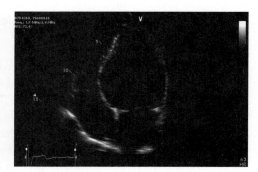

Figure 6.39

Anterior infarct with scar, apical 4-chamber view.

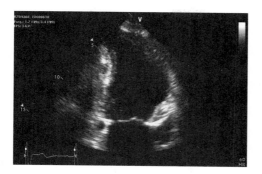

Figure 6.40

Anterior infarct with scar.

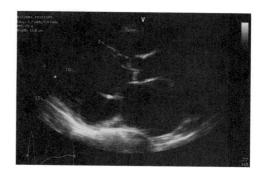

Figure 6.41

Inferior aneurysm, parasternal view.

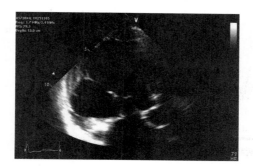

Figure 6.42

Inferior aneurysm, apical long-axis view.

postero-lateral papillary muscle rupture associated with flail mitral valve leaflets, inter-ventricular septal rupture and pericardial effusion/tamponade.

Valvular Heart Disease

The echo assessment of valve disease involves establishing a diagnosis, finding an etiol-ogy for the diagnosis, determining severity, assessing hemodynamic load imposed by the lesion, and identifying other pathologies commonly associated with the diagnosis.[56]

AORTIC VALVE

Stenosis: Calcific degeneration of the aortic valve is the most common cause of stenosis. It is predominantly found in those older than 65 years, but usually at younger ages when a bicuspid aortic valve is present (Figures 6.46 and 6.47). The first step in establishing

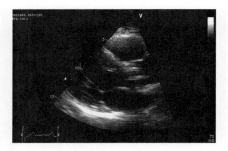

Figure 6.43

Degeneratvie aortic stenosis with heavily
sclerosed leaflets and left ventricular
hypertrophy.

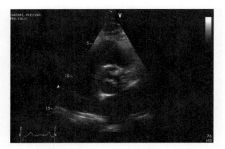

Figure 6.44

Degenerative aortic stenosis, parasternal short-
axis view.

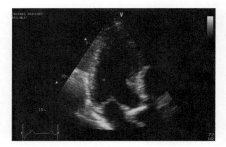

Figure 6.45

Degenerative aortic stenosis, apical 3-chamber
view.

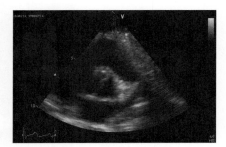

Figure 6.46

Sclerotic bicuspid aortic valve (closed),
parasternal short-axis view.

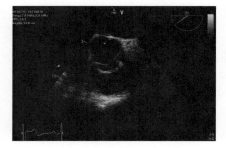

Figure 6.47

Bicuspid aortic valve without stenosis
(open), Transesophageal image. The left and
noncoronary cusps are fused (raphe).

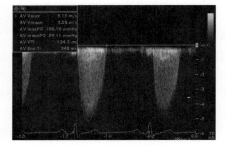

Figure 6.48

Continuous wave Doppler of severe aortic
stenosis (peak gradient 106mmHg).

the diagnosis is to obtain high-quality 2D images of the valve from the parasternal long (Figure 6.43) and short-axis views (Figure 6.44). These images provide immediate information regarding the presence of a bicuspid valve, associated aortic root abnormalities (aortic dilatation, coarctation), degree of degenerative changes and leaflet excursion. Severe aortic stenosis can be excluded in the presence of minimally restricted leaflet motion; however, stenosis can often be overestimated when the valve is severely calcified.

A CW Doppler cursor is placed over the valve from the apical 4 and long-axis views (Figure 6.48) as well as the suprasternal and right parasternal view (patient in right lateral decubitus position). The spectral trace with the greatest velocity is chosen for analysis. Peak and mean pressure gradients are calculated. The continuity equation is used to determine valve area.[9, 57]

Pathologies associated with aortic stenosis include aortic regurgitation, left ventricular hypertrophy, diastolic impairment, atrial enlargement, and pulmonary hypertension.

Valve area calculations in the setting of LV impairment may be artificially low because there is insufficient force of ejection to adequately open the aortic valve. In this situation, it is best to recalculate valve area after increasing the stroke volume with a dobutamine infusion.[58] If the valve area increases, then fixed aortic stenosis is not present.

Regurgitation: Aortic regurgitation may be caused by either intrinsic valve pathology or secondary to disease of the aortic root (particularly involving the sino-tubular junction). Intrinsic valve abnormalities include calcific degeneration, bicuspid aortic valve, endocarditis, and rheumatic heart disease. Common root abnormalities include hypertensive dilatation, aortic dissection, Marfan syndrome, and ankylosing spondylitis.

M mode provides indirect evidence of AR. High frequency anterior mitral leaflet fluttering occurs if it is in the path of the regurgitation jet. Premature closure of the mitral valve is present if diastolic LV pressure increases rapidly.

Two-dimensional examination frequently fails to show a valvular abnormality; however, aortic root disease and LV volume overload (increased end diastolic LV volume with preserved end systolic volume) are often apparent. TEE may be required to diagnose endocarditis and aortic root abscess.

Color flow Doppler is the modality with the highest level of diagnostic accuracy for aortic regurgitation.[59] AR is seen as a turbulent jet extending into the LVOT throughout diastole (Figures 6.49–6.53). The spectral trace of CW Doppler can be used to determine the pressure half-time across the valve (Figure 6.54).[14]

The best indicators of severe AR are: (a) an AR jet width of >60% of the LVOT diameter in the parasternal long-axis view (see Figure 6.50); (b) pan-diastolic flow reversal in the proximal descending aorta on the suprasternal view (Figure 6.55); and (c) dense spectral envelope during CW Doppler (see Figure 6.54).[15]

Acute AR, usually as a result of endocarditis, is associated with a normal-sized, hyperdynamic LV with high filling pressures and, usually, severe pulmonary hypertension. The pressure half-time will usually be <300msec.[14] Chronic, clinically significant

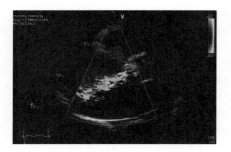

Figure 6.49

Severe aortic regurgitation directed over the anterior mitral valve leaflet. The left ventricle is moderately enlarged. (See Color Plate 2.)

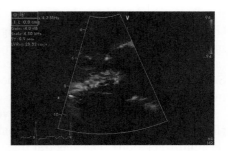

Figure 6.50

Zoomed view of the vena contracta (arrows) in severe aortic regurgitation. (See Color Plate 3.)

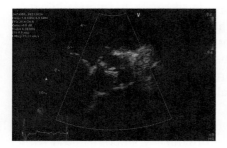

Figure 6.51

Central jet of aortic regurgitation seen from the short-axis view. (See Color Plate 4.)

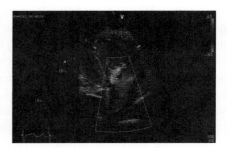

Figure 6.52

Apical 4-chamber view of aortic regurgitation mixing with mitral inflow. (See Color Plate 5.)

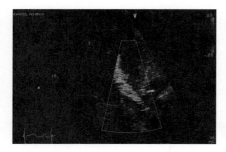

Figure 6.53

Apical long-axis view of severe aortic regurgitation during diastasis. (See Color Plate 6.)

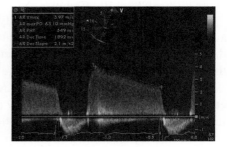

Figure 6.54

Continuous wave Doppler of severe chronic aortic regurgitation.

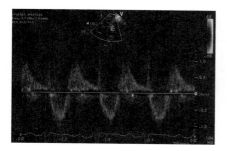

Figure 6.55

Pulse wave Doppler of pan-diastolic aortic flow reversal in severe aortic regurgitation.

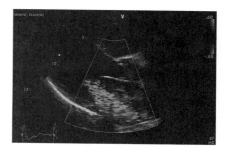

Figure 6.56

Long-axis view of severe mitral regurgitation. The jet occupies most of the atrium, has a wide vena contracta and proximal flow acceleration. (See Color Plate 7.)

AR is associated with an enlarged LV with normal end systolic volumes and preserved filling pressures. When chronic AR begins to decompensate, the end systolic volume and filling pressures increase.

MITRAL VALVE

Regurgitation: To maintain patency the mitral valve relies on normal leaflet anatomy and, just as importantly, the mitral apparatus (cordae, papillary muscles, annulus, and underlying ventricular myocardium). Impairment of any one or combination of these components will result in malcoaptation and regurgitation.

Common intrinsic valve diseases include age-related degeneration, myxomatous degeneration/redundancy (Figure 6.60), endocarditis (Figure 6.61), rheumatic heart disease, congenital clefts, and medication/carcinoid-related valvulopathy. Common mitral apparatus diseases include LV enlargement, ischemic papillary impairment,[60] cordal rupture (degenerative or endocarditis), and hypertrophic obstructive cardiomyopathy.

M mode can directly image some pathologies causing MR. With HOCM and mitral prolapse, M mode is a sensitive modality for the detection of systolic anterior motion of the mitral valve and atrial leaflet buckling respectively.

Two-dimensional echo is capable of identifying all pathologies that contribute to regurgitation. TEE is commonly required to achieve sufficient resolution to confirm a diagnosis (e.g., endocarditis, clefts) or to determine the extent of disease (prolapse, cordal rupture). Three-dimensional TEE is now capable of producing high-resolution images of mitral prolapse.[61] These 3D images assist in planning the surgical approach and assessing the adequacy of mitral valve repair with a greater level of clarity than has previously been possible.[62]

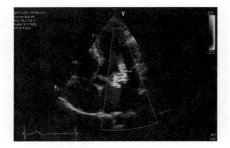

Figure 6.57

Apical 4-chamber view of severe mitral
regurgitation due to posterior leaflet pathology.
(See Color Plate 8.)

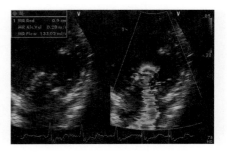

Figure 6.58

Zoomed 4-chamber view of severe mitral
regurgitation showing a wide vena contracta and
a pronounced PISA. (See Color Plate 9.)

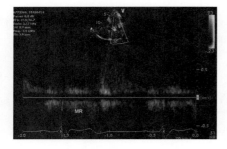

Figure 6.59

Systolic flow reversal in the pulmonary veins
as recorded by pulse wave Doppler is a sign of
moderate to severe mitral regurgitation. (See
Color Plate 10.)

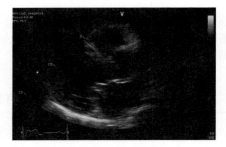

Figure 6.60

Parasternal long-axis view of posterior
mitral leaflet prolapse due to myxomatous
degeneration.

Color Doppler is the principle modality for diagnosis and quantification of mitral
regurgitation (Figures 6.56–6.58).[11] The direction of the regurgitation jet often provides
confirmation of the type of mitral pathology. Left ventricular enlargement displaces the
leaflets apically, resulting in a central jet. Degenerative changes involving both leaflets
will also produce central regurgitation. With the other regurgitant mitral diseases, the jet
is usually directed away from the diseased valve (see Figure 6.57), apart from myocardial
ischemia involving one papillary muscle. In this situation, abnormal leaflet restriction
occurs keeping it half open and the jet is directed behind the involved leaflet (usually
posterior).[60] Any jet entrained along the atrial wall will have less area than a central jet
of similar volume. Blood exiting the ventricle via the mitral valve defect will begin to
accelerate and is visualized on color flow Doppler as a proximal isovelocity surface area

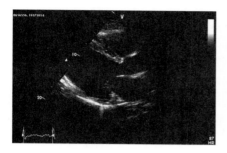

Figure 6.61

Vegetation on the atrial side of the posterior mitral leaflet.

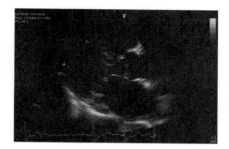

Figure 6.62

Long-axis view of moderate mitral stenosis with typical deformity of the anterior leaflet, left atrial and right ventricular enlargement.

(PISA) within the LV cavity (see Figure 6.58).[63] There is a direct correlation between PISA area and regurgitation volume.[64]

The best indicators of severe MR are: (a) the area of the MR jet is > 50% of the LA area (central jets only);[65] (b) the narrowest point of the MR jet (vena contracta) is > 6mm; (c) a dense CW spectral trace; (d) systolic flow reversal in the pulmonary veins (Figure 6.59);[66] (e) a large PISA radius (> 0.9cm, see Figure 6.58).

Acute MR is usually to the result of cordae rupture, papillary muscle rupture/ ischemia, and endocarditis. There is usually a normal-size, hyperdynamic LV, often with a deceptively small MR jet and high LA filling pressures, as well as severe pulmonary hypertension.

Chronic, hemodynamicaly significant MR is always associated with an enlarged left atrium and usually an enlarged LV with preserved end systolic volumes. As the ventricle decompensates the pulmonary pressures and end systolic dimensions increase. Chronic severe MR is better tolerated than AR because, in MR, the regurgitant fraction is pumped out against pulmonary venous pressures not systemic pressures.

Stenosis: Mitral stenosis is an uncommon finding because it is primarily the result of rheumatic fever, which has largely been eradicated in Western societies. Occasionally, it may be the result of excessive annular calcification or occur as a congenital abnormality.

With rheumatic stenosis, the scarring process begins at the leaflet tips and progresses to involve the remainder of the leaflets. At the commisures the leaflets are progressively bound together like two zippers being drawn closed. A variable amount of calcification and cordal scarring also occurs (Figures 6.62 and 6.63).

M mode clearly demonstrates the degree of leaflet thickening, the reduction of leaflet excursion and loss of mid-diastolic dip. Two-dimensional echo of the valve in the long-axis view demonstrates doming of the leaflet tips (see Figure 6.62). In the short-axis

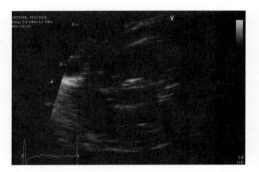

Figure 6.63

Zoomed short-axis view of moderate mitral stenosis
showing commissural fusion, leaflet thickening, and
calcification.

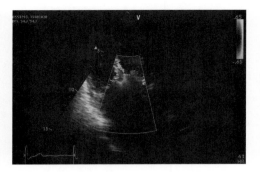

Figure 6.64

Apical 3-chamber view showing flow acceleration/
aliasing as blood crosses the stenosed mitral valve.
(See Color Plate 11.)

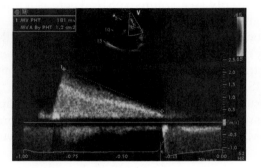

Figure 6.65

Continuous wave Doppler trace in mitral stenosis
showing the pressure half-time technique of valve area
calculation. The patient is in atrial fibrillation.

view, the narrowed orifice of the valve caused by commissural fusion is appreciated (see
Figure 6.63).[12] The degree of leaflet thickening, calcification, and cordal retraction and
scarring can also be determined.[67]

In addition, 2D echo can also detect the presence of abnormalities caused by excessive left atrial pressure, these being: left atrial enlargement, right ventricular hypertrophy/
enlargement, and IVC dilatation.

Continuous wave Doppler through the mitral valve in the four-chamber view is used to
calculate the pressure half-time of mitral inflow and mean transvalvular gradient (Figure
6.65).[13] CW over the tricuspid valve is used to calculate pulmonary artery systolic pressure. Color flow Doppler may show turbulent flow across the valve and a PISA effect
within the left atrium (Figure 6.64). Mitral regurgitation is frequently present.

The severity of mitral stenosis is determined by the calculated valve area (severe < 1cm²) mean transvalvular gradient (severe > 15mmHg) and pulmonary systolic pressure. The pressure half-time valve area calculation is invalid in the presence of moderate or more aortic regurgitation.[12] Direct 2D planimetry of the mitral orifice at the leaflet tips is an acceptable alternative technique for the determination of valve area.

TRICUSPID VALVE

Regurgitation: The tricuspid valve comprises three leaflets (anterior, septal, and posterior) and is positioned more apically than the mitral valve. Tricuspid stenosis is rare, as opposed to regurgitation, which can usually be detected to some degree in most studies. The Doppler analysis of tricuspid regurgitation, be it pathologic or not, is also the best technique to calculate pulmonary systolic pressure.

Mechanistically, pathologic regurgitation is either the result of intrinsic valve disease (endocarditis, myxomatous degeneration/prolapse, pacing leads/catheters, carcinoid, Ebstein anomaly) or abnormal function of the tricuspid valve apparatus, including the annulus (right ventricular enlargement, pulmonary hypertension, ischemic papillary muscle impairment, arrhythmogenic right ventricular dysplasia). Of all the causes of TR, right ventricular enlargement causing annular dilatation and functional regurgitation is the most common.

Two-dimensional imaging is capable, in most instances, of detecting the pathologic process responsible for regurgitation. Ebstein anomaly, resulting in extreme apical displacement of the tricuspid valve often with the septal leaflet bound to the septum, is one of the more obvious abnormalities detectable by 2D imaging (Figures 6.68 and 6.69). Right ventricular enlargement is difficult to confidently diagnose because there is substantial variability in RV shape between individuals. ARVD and endocarditis can also be a challenge.

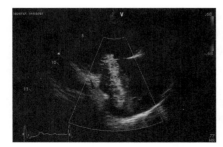

Figure 6.66

Parasternal right ventricular inflow view of severe tricuspid regurgitation. (See Color Plate 12.)

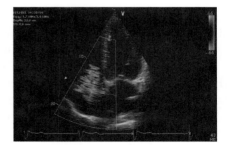

Figure 6.67

Four-chamber view of severe tricuspid regurtiation. (See Color Plate 13.)

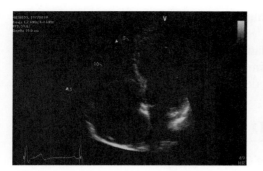

Figure 6.68

Ebstein's anomaly, note apical displacement of the septal leaflet and atrialization of the right ventricle.

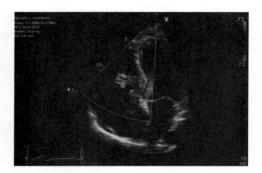

Figure 6.69

Severe tricuspid regurgitation in Ebstein's anomaly with jet directed behind the relatively immobile septal leaflet. (See Color Plate 14.)

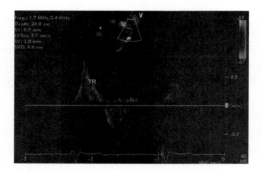

Figure 6.70

Reversal of hepatic vein flow in severe tricuspid regurgitation. (See Color Plate 15.)

As with the other forms of valvular regurgitation, color flow Doppler is the cornerstone of tricuspid regurgitation assessment. Central color jets indicate RV enlargement, whereas eccentric jets are more commonly associated with intrinsic valve pathology.

The best indicators of severe TR are: (a) a large TR jet area within the right atrium (Figures 6.66 and 6.67); (b) a wide vena contracta (Figure 6.67); (c) a dense CW spectral trace; (d) systolic flow reversal in the hepatic veins (Figure 6.70); and (e) a large PISA radius.

Because TR is often secondary to rather than the cause of RV enlargement, the true cause of an enlarged right ventricle should always be sought. The most common etiologies are: (a) passive pulmonary hypertension from high left-sided filling pressures; (b) intrinsic pulmonary hypertension, usually related to airways disease or pulmonary emboli; and (c) left to right shunting, particularly undiagnosed atrial septal defects.

Continuous wave Doppler assessment of the tricuspid valve should always be per-formed (even in the absence of regurgitation on color flow) for assessment of pulmonary pressures.[68, 69] The peak velocity of TR gives the gradient between the RV and RA during systole. Right atrial pressure can be calculated based on IVC diameter. When RA pres-sure has been calculated, it is added to the TR-derived pressure gradient to yield the right ventricular systolic pressure, which is the same as pulmonary artery systolic pressure (in the absence of pulmonary stenosis).

PASP = RVSP = 4(TR vel)^2 + RAP
RAP = 5mmHg when IVC diameter < 2.5cm + > 50% collapse with inspiration
RAP = 10mmHg when IVC diameter < 2.5cm + ≤ 50% collapse with inspiration
RAP = 15mmHg when IVC diameter > 2.5cm + < 50% collapse with inspiration
RAP ≥ 20mmHg when IVC and hepatic veins are dilated with no collapse

The calculation of PASP may be significantly underestimated in the presence of severe tricuspid regurgitation because of the rapid rise in right atrial pressure, which will reduce the gradient across the valve.

PULMONARY VALVE

Clinically significant pulmonary valve disease is uncommon. The pulmonary valve can exhibit congenital stenosis as well as supra and subvalvular stenosis caused by congenital webs. Regurgitation most commonly occurs in the context of endocarditis. Lesser degrees of eccentric pulmonary regurgitation can be mistaken for ventricular septal defects. Accu-rately diagnosing pulmonary valve pathology can be difficult because the valve is often poorly seen both with transthoracic and with esophageal echocardiography.[70]

Cardiomyopathies

The etiologies of myocardial disease (cardiomyopathies) are divided into three broad categories: primary, inflammatory, and secondary.[71] Echocardiography is regarded as a class 1 diagnostic test for those with suspected cardiomyopathy because it is capable of establishing the diagnosis, disease severity, associated complications, prognosis, and response to therapy.

Primary cardiomyopathies have a strong genetic component, usually incompletely elucidated, and include: (a) dilated; (b) hypertrophic; (c) restrictive, arrhythmic; and (d) unclassified (primarily noncompaction).

Inflammatory cardiomyopathies include all diseases, both infectious and noninfec-tious, resulting in inflammation of the myocardium and associated structures excluding the endocardium. This category primarily features the viral cardiomyopathies.

Secondary cardiomyopathies are acquired myopathic diseases of known origin and include: (a) ischemic; (b) hypertensive; (c) valvular; (d) alcoholic; (e) metabolic; (f) peripartum; and (g) muscular dystrophy associated.

From an echocardiographic perspective, most cardiomyopathies are associated with features of cardiac failure: raised left atrial pressures, left atrial enlargement, pulmonary hypertension, and venous congestion. Phenotypically the preceding disease states result in left ventricular dilatation, hypertrophy, or restriction.

DILATED CARDIOMYOPATHY

Dilated cardiomyopathy (DCM) is the phenotype associated with most cardiomyopathies. Its two salient features are left ventricular enlargement (Figures 6.71 and 6.72) and impaired systolic function.[72] The degree of enlargement varies greatly. It is important for the end-diastolic dimensions to be indexed for body surface area to prevent false positive diagnoses. As the left ventricle enlarges and remodels, it becomes more spherical, the mitral annulus dilates, and the papillary muscles are displaced apically. As a consequence, functional mitral regurgitation is usually present.

Systolic impairment also varies greatly and may be preserved at rest, even in the presence of LV enlargement. In this situation stress echocardiography is often useful. Systolic dysfunction may be overestimated in the presence of left bundle branch block. Regional wall motion abnormalities are frequently present in the absence of ischemic heart disease and, unless scar tissue corresponding to a coronary territory is present, an ischemic cause of DCM cannot reliably be established by echocardiography. Conversely, a globally hypokinetic LV without regional wall motion impairment can still have an ischemic cause.

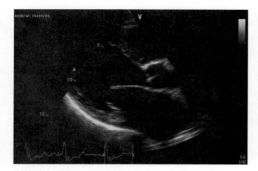

Figure 6.71

Ideopathic dilated cardiomyopathy. Note enlarged left atrium and spherical shape of the left ventricle.

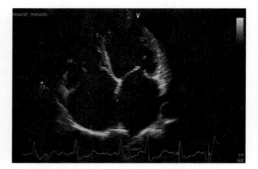

Figure 6.72

Apical view showing right ventricular and atrial enlargement.

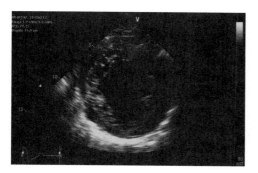

Figure 6.73

Dilated cardiomyopathy caused by noncompaction, particularly evident through the septum and inferior wall.

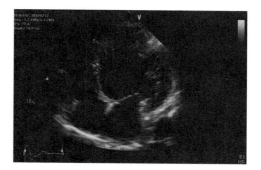

Figure 6.74

Four-chamber view of noncompaction showing spherical left ventricular shape.

Other echocardographic features that provide clues to the underlying cause of DCM are frequently present. Noncompaction[73] is the most obvious and is characterized by: (a) prominent segmental endocardial trabeculations (noncompacted myocardium) involving the apex, lateral, and inferior walls; (b) a noncompacted layer at least twice the thickness of the compacted layer (Figure 6.73); and (c) spherical remodelling of the left ventricle (Figure 6.74).

End-stage hypertensive cardiomyopathy is usually associated with persistent concentric left ventricular hypertrophy. Acute viral cardiomyopathy often has severe systolic impairment but only mild LV dilatation. Differentiating valvular DCM caused by mitral regurgitation from DCM of another cause with functional mitral regurgitation can often be difficult. Mitral valvular DCM is usually associated with well-defined mitral valve pathology and less-pronounced systolic impairment.

Poor prognostic features of DCM include an ejection fraction < 30%, a restrictive mitral valve diastolic flow pattern unresponsive to antifailure treatment, and a moderate to severely increased end diastolic and systolic volumes.[50]

HYPERTROPHIC CARDIOMYOPATHY

Hypertrophic cardiomyopathy (HCM) is primarily the phenotype of a group of spontaneous or inherited, autosomal dominant mutations of cardiac myosin, actin, and troponin. An identical picture may also be apparent in those with either inborn errors of metabolism (Fabry's disease) or hypertensive heart disease of the elderly.

There are three elements to the echocardiographic diagnosis of hypertrophic cardiomyopathy. The first is the presence of inappropriate myocardial hypertrophy (Figures 6.75 and 6.76). This is usually regional with the anteroseptum most commonly affected and the

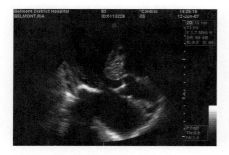

Figure 6.75

Hypertrophic obstructive cardiomyopathy with a septal thickness of 3cm.

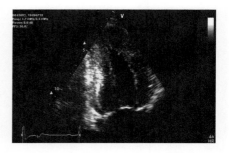

Figure 6.76

Apical hypertrophic cardiomyopathy without obstruction.

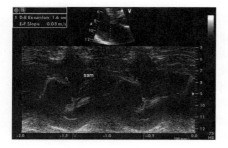

Figure 6.77

M mode showing systolic anterior motion of the mitral valve in HOCM.

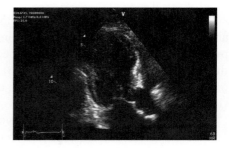

Figure 6.78

Apical long-axis view of HOCM with SAM of the cordae (arrow).

posterior wall spared, however apical (Figure 6.76) and concentric forms are occasionally seen.[74] Traditionally, a septal wall thickness of > 1.3cm and a septal to posterior wall thickness ratio of 1.3:1 have been used as diagnostic criteria. Care must be exercised in the presence of a posterior infarct and right ventricular hypertrophy, which can cause a similar ratio.

The second element is the presence of dynamic left ventricular outflow tract obstruction (outflow obstruction may also occur in the mid LV cavity). LVOTO is established by first excluding the presence of aortic stenosis by 2D analysis, then placing a continuous wave Doppler cursor through the LVOT. When dynamic obstruction is present a dagger-shaped spectral trace is seen with high outflow velocities occurring late in systole, as the fall in LV volume permits the hypertrophied septum to obstruct the LVOT (Figure 6.80).

The third element is the presence of systolic anterior movement (SAM) of the mitral valve, commonly associated with mitral regurgitation. SAM occurs as a result of abnormal anterior displacement of the papillary muscles combined with a Venturi suction effect

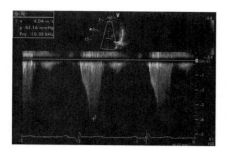

Figure 6.79

Dagger shaped continous wave Doppler indicating dynamic LV outflow obstruction. (See Color Plate 16.)

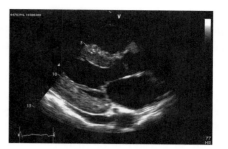

Figure 6.80

Amyloid restrictive cardiomyopathy with characteristic "speckled" echotexture and generalized myocardial thickening.

produced by the LVOTO. This results in the anterior mitral valve leaflet being dragged into the LVOT and impinging on the septum during systole (Figures 6.77 and 6.78). Loss of mitral valve coaptation frequently produces a posteriorly directed, late systolic mitral regurgitation jet.

The second two elements may not be present at rest and may only appear with an increase in septal contractility or a reduction in diastolic filling. Postectopic beats and the valsalva maneuver can provoke LVOTO. Stress echo is another useful modality to determine the relative contributions of LVOTO and diastolic impairment in those with hypertrophic cardiomyopathy and reduced exercise capacity.

The prognosis of HCM is directly related to degree of septal thickening and, to a lesser degree, to the presence of resting LVOTO.[75] Rapid atrial fibrillation reduces filling time, exacerbating outflow obstruction and commonly results in acute decompensated heart failure.

Athletes may have adaptive LV hypertrophy, but, in contrast to hypertrophic cardiomyopathy, will never exhibit LVOTO and will have entirely normal diastolic function and usually substantially greater LV diastolic volumes. Acquired HCM in the hypertensive elderly is not uncommonly associated with LVOTO.

RESTRICTIVE CARDIOMYOPATHY

Restrictive cardiomyopathy is manifest as diastolic heart failure with or without systolic impairment and LV thickening. It is the phenotype of inflammatory, infiltrative, and storage diseases but is also commonly seen in hypertensive heart disease and restrictive heart disease of the elderly. The common factor is abnormally stiffened myocardium with reduced diastolic compliance.[76] In Western societies, amyloidosis, sarcoidosis, hemachromatosis, and radiation exposure should all be considered as differential diagnoses.

The echocardiographic hallmarks are: (a) impaired diastolic function, often in the presence of normal or mildly reduced systolic function; (b) biatrial enlargement, often substantial; and (c) abnormal myocardial echotexture with or without thickening, commonly involving the right ventricle.

Cardiac amyloid is apparent as a speckled, often grossly thickened, myocardium (Figure 6.80). Thickening of the mitral valve leaflets is also present. Sarcoidosis often manifests regional wall motion abnormalities and scarring, which do not conform to coronary territories.

Restriction can be differentiated from constriction[77] by: (a) reduced tissue Doppler velocity; (b) no respiratory variation in mitral/tricuspid inflow velocities; (c) pulmonary hypertension; and (d) atrial enlargement.

Infective Endocarditis

Infective endocarditis (IE) is broadly defined as *infection of the cardiovascular endothelium* but also extends to include prosthetic material within the heart. IE predominantly involves the cardiac valves and usually requires some form of endothelial damage, often in the form of preexisting valvular pathology to gain a foothold. Those with bicuspid aortic valves, mitral valve prolapse, degenerative valve disease, ventricular septal defects, and aortic coarctation are particularly at risk when exposed to bacteraemia in the absence of antibiotic prophylaxis. The immunosuppressed, the elderly, and intravenous drug users are also at higher risk even in the absence of overt valve pathology.

Echocardiography is the test of choice for suspected endocarditis as it is the only modality with sufficient sensitivity to detect the hallmark of the disease, which is the vegetation.[30] However, echocardiographic features alone are insufficient and ideally blood cultures positive for an IE associated organism are also required. When clinical suspicion of IE is present, transthoracic echo is performed first. Although not as sensitive as transesophageal echo, TTE is still capable of detecting larger vegetations and, more importantly, can quantitate the hemodynamic significance of IE complications (valvular regurgitation, intracardiac fistulae, pericardial effusions). TEE is used when the diagnosis remains in doubt, if prosthetic valves are present or abscess formation is suspected. Its sensitivity is 20–50% greater than TTE and is regarded as the gold standard test for IE.[78]

The echocardiographic examination aims to uncover the presence and consequences of vegetations. Vegetations are conglomerations of platelets, fibrin, red cells, and the infective organism and are usually present in vast numbers. Vegetations can grow very rapidly and repeat testing is indicated if clinical suspicion remains high after a negative examination.

Vegetations are relatively echo-lucent, attach to the free, upstream edge of the valve (Figures 6.81 and 6.82), and have independent motion. Prolapse and high frequency fluttering of the vegetation is common when valve tissue destruction and regurgitation are present. In the case of prosthetic valves, vegetations involve the sewing ring and cause dehiscence. Vegetations may extend to involve the leaflets of bio-prosthetic valves.[79]

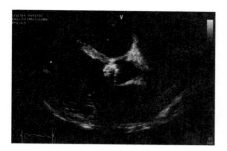

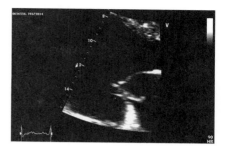

Figure 6.81

Large vegetation on right coronary cusp of the aortic valve. There was associated severe aortic regurgitation—note enlarged LV cavity.

Figure 6.82

Zoomed parasternal long-axis view of a moderate sized vegetation involving the posterior mitral valve leaflet.

Abscesses commonly occur around the aortic root and can extend into the aortic/mitral fibrosa secondarily involving the anterior mitral leaflet or creating an aortic to left atrial fistula. Vegetations can be seeded via a regurgitation jet to a downstream valve.[36]

The size of the vegetation has been correlated with its embolic risk and overall complication rate with lesions > 11 mm being the most prone to embolization. The type of organism and site of the vegetation are also important predictors of complications. *Staphylococcus aureus* is regarded as the most destructive organism. A small vegetation causing cordal rupture of the mitral apparatus can result in life-threatening mitral regurgitation.

Because vegetations start as small lesions, it is important that each valve is examined by panning the scan plane across the entire valve with and without color flow Doppler, in as many views as possible. The use of the zoom function is also an important way of increasing resolution.

Other cardiac abnormalities can be mistaken for vegetations and include myxomatous prolapse of the mitral valve, degenerative changes of the aortic valve, mitral annulus calcification, atrial myxomas, thrombi, and scanning artefacts. Old sterile vegetations may also be present and are usually small and echogenic with reduced mobility.[80]

Pericardial Disease

Disease of the pericardium may be either primary (usually inflammatory) or secondary as a result of myocardial rupture or aortic dissection. Any form of pericardial disease can cause varying degrees of pericardial effusion, pericardial constriction, or both (effusive-constrictive).[81] Excess pericardial fluid may result in tamponade.

The most common forms of primary pericardial disorders include: (a) viral and idiopathic; (b) postcardiac surgery; (c) uraemia; (d) connective tissue disease; (e) malignancy; (f) radiotherapy; (g) para-pneumonic; (h) hypothyroidism; (i) postinfarct (Dressler) syndrome; and (j) tuberculosis.

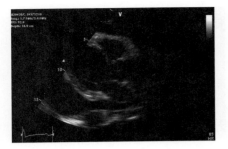

Figure 6.83

Large pericardial effusion, long-axis orientation. Note fluid between the aorta and posterior wall that differentiates it from a pleural effusion.

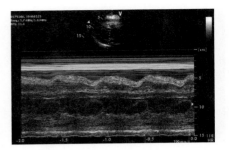

Figure 6.84

M mode showing diastolic collapse of the right ventricular free wall indicating high extracardiac pressure.

When pericardial disease is present or suspected, echocardiography provides the means to diagnose, monitor, and detect tamponade and/or constriction as well as to assist with aspiration.[82]

The hemodynamic features of clinically significant pericardial disease occur because a noncompliant pericardium, whether it is from constriction or tamponade, will restrict filling in all four cardiac chambers. Furthermore, increased filling of the right ventricle, during inspiration, will be at the expense of reduced LV filling. Hence, all forms of hemodynamically significant pericardial disease will feature increased inspiratory right-sided flow velocities, (over the tricuspid [Figure 6.88] and pulmonary valve and in the pulmonary trunk) associated with reduced left-sided flow velocities (mitral [Figure 6.86] and aortic valves and pulmonary veins).[83]

The visceral and parietal pericardial layers normally only separate in systole and this is best appreciated in the parasternal view below the posterior wall by either M mode or 2D. Echo free space above the right ventricle, in the absence of an increase in posterior fluid, represents pericardial fat. It is often difficult to measure the thickness of the pericardium because it is such a strong reflector. Using M mode with low gain settings is the best technique.

Pericardial effusions are commonly associated with pericardial disease and the amount of pericardial space is directly related to the volume of fluid. The accurate assessment of fluid volume is less important than its hemodynamic effect and should only be described as small, medium, or large. A slowly accumulating but large effusion will often show no evidence of tamponade in contrast to a small, rapid-onset effusion. As an effusion enlarges, it is seen along the medial and lateral aspects of the heart and, finally, in front of the right ventricular free wall (Figures 6.83, 6.85, and 6.86). Loculated effusions are not uncommon following surgery.

Tamponade hemodynamics occur when the pressure of fluid within the pericardium exceeds the passive filling pressures of the cardiac chambers. With increasing pressure

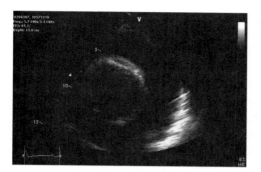

Figure 6.85

Large pericardial effusion completely surrounding the heart in this parasternal short-axis view.

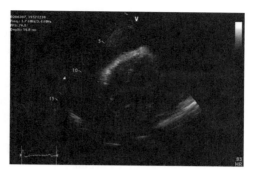

Figure 6.86

Large effusion with 4cm separating the visceral from the parietal pericardium.

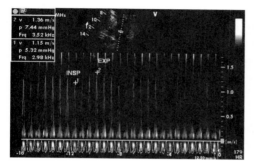

Figure 6.87

Mitral inflow Doppler at slow sweep speed showing reduced inspiratory LV filling in pericardial disease.

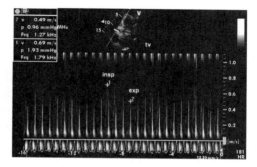

Figure 6.88

Tricuspid inflow velocities showing reduced RV inflow during expiration in a patient with pericardial disease.

the most compliant chambers with the lowest passive filling pressures (right atrium and ventricle) begin to collapse in early diastole. This is best appreciated by M mode of the RV free wall (Figure 6.84) and outflow tract. RA collapse is clearly seen on 2D. Right-sided filling pressures rise and the IVC dilates. A reciprocal respiratory variation of inflow velocities between the left and right cardiac chambers occurs as already detailed. The variation in velocity, from inspiration to expiration, over the tricuspid valve usually exceeds 25%. Pericardial drainage should only be performed if there is > 1cm of fluid over the RV free wall. The presence of the pericardiocentesis needle within the pericardial space can be confirmed by injecting agitated saline.

Constrictive pericarditis is an infrequent sequelae of any form of inflammatory pericarditis. It is usually progressive but on occasion can be transient, particularly if the inflammation resolves. Constriction is usually difficult to diagnose and ultimately rests on a combination of clinical, echocardiographic, radiologic, and catheterization criteria.[77] Two-dimensional and M-mode echo can often demonstrate a thickened pericardium (> 2mm). M mode often shows an abrupt posterior wall descent in early diastole as well as a diastolic septal bounce. Doppler reveals a restrictive mitral inflow pattern in association with a normal mitral annulus tissue velocity profile. In common with other pericardial diseases, an exaggerated variation of both tricuspid and mitral inflow is present, with tricuspid inflow greatest in inspiration and mitral in expiration. Usually > 25% variation in inflow during respiration is evident. The IVC and hepatic vessels are usually dilated. Effusive-constrictive pericarditis is present when Doppler abnormalities and elevated right-sided filling pressures remain following pericardiocentesis.

Diseases of the Aorta

The thoracic aorta is easily visualized by both transthoracic and transesophageal echocardiography. TEE in particular is capable of producing high-resolution images of all but the aortic arch and is the test of choice when life-threatening aortic pathology is suspected.[84]

Common aortic pathologies include: (a) dissection; (b) aneurysm; (c) dilatation; (d) atheroma; and (e) intramural hematoma. These are most commonly found in those with poorly treated hypertension, aortic stenosis, giant cell arteritis, Marfan's syndrome, and, occasionally, ischemic stroke. Diseases that result in loss of the sino-tubular junction are usually associated with aortic regurgitation.

Transthoracic echo can image the ascending aorta and arch via the parasternal and suprasternal windows. The descending aorta can usually be seen in the subcostal view. Transesophageal echo cannot image the arch from the brachiocephalic to the left subclavian artery because of shadowing from the trachea.

Aortic dilatation usually involves the proximal aorta where the systolic pressure waves and valvular turbulence are greatest. The annulus is spared but the sinuses, STJ, and ascending aorta are usually all affected. In the case of Marfan's, the process often begins in early adulthood and is commonly associated with aortic regurgitation. Aortic root replacement should be considered in all forms of aortic dilatation when the ascending aorta reaches 55mm diameter to avoid dissection and/or rupture.

Aortic aneurysms are discrete outpouchings of the aorta usually associated with atheroma. They commonly contain thrombus and have the potential to dissect or rupture. They should also be surgically corrected at 55mm or greater.

Valsalva sinus aneurysms are congenital areas of weakness, which may elongate to more than 50mm. The most common type arises from the right coronary sinus with a windsock appearance into the right atrium. Complications include rupture and right heart failure, as well as aortic regurgitation.

Aortic dissection is divided into Stanford type A lesions, which involve the aortic arch, and type B lesions, which are confined to the descending aorta. When suspected,

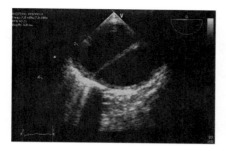

Figure 6.89

TEE image of chronic aortic dissection with a band of endothelium dividing the thoracic aorta into a true and false lumen.

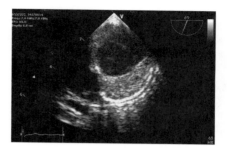

Figure 6.90

At the proximal end of the dissection the false lumen is larger than the true lumen and contains thrombus and spontaneous echo contrast.

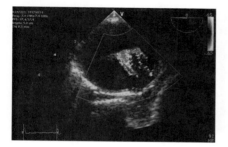

Figure 6.91

Surgically constructed fenestrations ensure equalization of pressure between the lumens. (See Color Plate 17.)

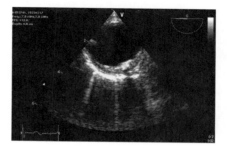

Figure 6.92

Crescentic, stable aortic atheroma with evidence of calcification.

a thorough inspection of the aorta requires TEE.[32] This will also permit examination for the potential dissection complications: aortic regurgitation and pericardial effusion.[85] The dissection flap (Figure 6.89) appears as a linear echo, usually lying parallel to the wall of the aorta. Blood flow within the false lumen is usually sluggish and often exhibits spontaneous echo contrast (Figure 6.90). Color flow Doppler will confirm high-velocity flow in the true lumen, as well as flow between the lumen (Figure 6.91).

Aortic atheroma is often an incidental finding in those with multiple cardiovascular risk factors. In those with an ischemic stroke, it is a potential source of emboli.[86, 87] Atheroma may be complex with mobile components or crescentic with a smooth, laminated appearance (Figure 6.92). Atheroma may be the site of dissection, dilatation, and aneurysm formation.

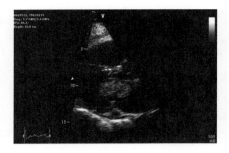

Figure 6.93

Large left atrial myxoma prolapsing through the mitral valve in this parasternal long-axis view.

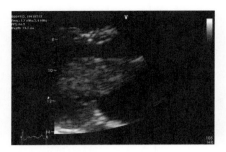

Figure 6.94

Zoomed view of the myxoma showing heterogeneous echotexture.

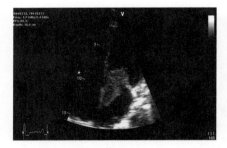

Figure 6.95

Atrial myxoma in the 4-chamber view showing attachment to the midinteratrial septum.

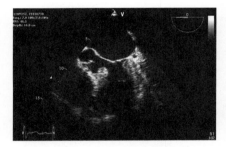

Figure 6.96

Unusually large fibroelastoma attached to the septum in a patient with left ventricular hypertrophy (TEE image).

Masses and Emboli

The most common cardiac tumors are myxomas, papillary fibroelastomas, and lipomas, all of which are benign. They must be differentiated from scan artifacts, normal cardiac structures, and thrombi.

Myxomas usually arise from the *fossa ovalis* within the left atrium. However, they may occur anywhere within the heart. They have a heterogeneous appearance and can often occupy the majority of the atrium, causing obstruction to mitral inflow (Figures 6.93–6.95). They are not uncommonly the cause of systemic emboli.[88]

Fibroelastomas generally arise from the downstream side of valves and rarely exceed 2cm in diameter. They have an irregular shape and may be confused with vegetations (Figure 6.96). Size and degree of mobility are linked to embolic potential.[89]

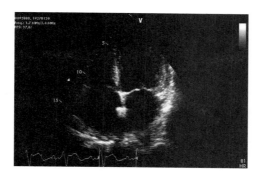

Figure 6.97

Lipomatous interatrial septum.

Lipomas occur in the form of lipomatous hypertrophy of the interatrial septum.[90] This produces a grossly thickened, echogenic septum with sparing of the *fossa ovalis* (Figure 6.97). This form of tumor is usually an incidental finding as is not associated with pathology.[91]

All tumors and suspected tumors should be examined in multiple planes, with and without color flow Doppler. The site of myxoma attachment should be ascertained whenever possible. Transesophageal echo should routinely be utilized to thoroughly assess tumor anatomy and as a high-resolution guide to surgery. If doubt remains regarding the nature of the mass, the use of transpulmonary contrast will assist in determining the presence of vascularity, which rules out thrombus.

Intracardiac thrombi most commonly occur in the left atrial appendage, generally in the setting of atrial fibrillation (less commonly atrial flutter). The atrial appendage is poorly imaged by TTE. TEE is the only reliable method of assessing the appendage for the presence of thrombus. The high-resolution TEE images will usually show pectinate muscles within the appendage and these should not be confused with thrombi. They have no independent motion and are present throughout the appendage. Thrombi are usually rounded structures associated with spontaneous echo contrast. Pulse wave Doppler of the emptying velocity of the appendage is commonly low (< 2.5cm/sec) when thrombus is present or is likely to occur.

Left ventricular thrombus is found predominantly in areas of akinesis, dyskinesis, or aneurysm of the apex, but may also be found in aneurysms elsewhere in the heart. LV thrombus can be laminated and of low embolic potential or freely mobile with high embolic likelihood. Thrombus is almost never present in the absence of regional wall motion abnormality.

IVC thrombus can lodge in any of the right heart chambers when in transit to the pulmonary arteries. Within the right atrium, thrombus may be seen migrating across a patent foramen ovale. Large thrombi can sometimes be seen within the left or right pulmonary arteries. In those with a systemic embolus, a patent foramen ovale,[92] established by agitated saline contrast, is circumstantial evidence for the existence of paradoxical embolism and indicates the need for more aggressive anticoagulation or PFO closure.

◇◇◇◇◇◇◇◇◇◇◇◇

REFERENCES

1. Thomas, J. D. and D. N. Rubin (1998). "Tissue harmonic imaging: why does it work?" *J Am Soc Echocardiogr* 11(8): 803-8.
2. Senior, R., P. Soman, et al. (1999). "Improved endocardial visualization with second harmonic imaging compared with fundamental two-dimensional echocardiographic imaging." *Am Heart J* 138(1 Pt 1): 163-8.
3. Tranquart, F., N. Grenier, et al. (1999). "Clinical use of ultrasound tissue harmonic imaging." *Ultrasound Med Biol* 25(6): 889-94.
4. Anderson, B. (2007). Echocardiography: the Normal Examination and Echocardiographic Measurements. Australia, MGA Graphics.
5. Quinones, M. A., C. M. Otto, et al. (2002). "Recommendations for quantification of Doppler echocardiography: a report from the Doppler Quantification Task Force of the Nomenclature and Standards Committee of the American Society of Echocardiography." *J Am Soc Echocardiogr* 15(2): 167-84.
6. Sohn, D. W., I. H. Chai, et al. (1997). "Assessment of mitral annulus velocity by Doppler tissue imaging in the evaluation of left ventricular diastolic function." *J Am Coll Cardiol* 30(2): 474-80.
7. Currie, P. J., D. J. Hagler, et al. (1986). "Instantaneous pressure gradient: a simultaneous Doppler and dual catheter correlative study." *J Am Coll Cardiol* 7(4): 800-6.
8. Moulinier, L., T. Venet, et al. (1991). "Measurement of aortic blood flow by Doppler echocardiography: day to day variability in normal subjects and applicability in clinical research." *J Am Coll Cardiol* 17(6): 1326.33.
9. Taylor, R. (1990). "Evolution of the continuity equation in the Doppler echocardiographic assessment of the severity of valvular aortic stenosis." *J Am Soc Echocardiogr* 3(4): 326.30.
10. Callahan, M. J., A. J. Tajik, et al. (1985). "Validation of instantaneous pressure gradients measured by continuous-wave Doppler in experimentally induced aortic stenosis." *Am J Cardiol* 56(15): 989-93.
11. Blumlein, S., A. Bouchard, et al. (1986). "Quantitation of mitral regurgitation by Doppler echocardiography." *Circulation* 74(2): 306.14.
12. Loperfido, F., F. Laurenzi, et al. (1987). "A comparison of the assessment of mitral valve area by continuous wave Doppler and by cross sectional echocardiography." *Br Heart J* 57(4): 348-55.
13. Faletra, F., A. Pezzano, Jr., et al. (1996). "Measurement of mitral valve area in mitral stenosis: four echocardiographic methods compared with direct measurement of anatomic orifices." *J Am Coll Cardiol* 28(5): 1190-7.
14. Samstad, S. O., L. Hegrenaes, et al. (1989). "Half-time of the diastolic aortoventricular pressure difference by continuous wave Doppler ultrasound: a measure of the severity of aortic regurgitation?" *Br Heart J* 61(4): 336.43.
15. Evangelista, A., H. G. del Castillo, et al. (2000). "Strategy for optimal aortic regurgitation quantification by Doppler echocardiography: agreement among different methods." *Am Heart J* 139(5): 773-81.
16. Sheikh, K., S. W. Smith, et al. (1991). "Real-time, three-dimensional echocardiography: feasibility and initial use." *Echocardiography* 8(1): 119-25.
17. Shung, K. K. (2002). "The principle of multidimensional arrays." *Eur J Echocardiogr* 3(2): 149-53.
18. Hibberd, M. G., M. L. Chuang, et al. (2000). "Accuracy of three-dimensional echocardiography with unrestricted selection of imaging planes for measurement of left ventricular volumes and ejection fraction." *Am Heart J* 140(3): 469-75.
19. Monaghan, M. J. (2006). "Role of real time 3D echocardiography in evaluating the left ventricle." *Heart* 92(1): 131-6.
20. Roelandt, J. R., F. J. ten Cate, et al. (1994). "Ultrasonic dynamic three-dimensional visualization of the heart with a multiplane transesophageal imaging transducer." *J Am Soc Echocardiogr* 7(3 Pt 1): 217-29.
21. Kapetanakis, S., M. T. Kearney, et al. (2005). "Real-time three-dimensional echocardiography: a novel

technique to quantify global left ventricular mechanical dyssynchrony." *Circulation* 112(7): 992-1000.

22. Sugeng, L., J. Kirkpatrick, et al. (2003). "Biplane stress echocardiography using a prototype matrix-array transducer." *J Am Soc Echocardiogr* 16(9): 937-41.

23. Blomley, M. J., J. C. Cooke, et al. (2001). "Micro-bubble contrast agents: a new era in ultrasound." *Bmj* 322(7296): 1222-5.

24. Main, M. L. and P. A. Grayburn (1999). "Clinical applications of transpulmonary contrast echocardiography." *Am Heart J* 137(1): 144-53.

25. Monaghan, M. J. (2003). "Contrast echocardiography: from left ventricular opacification to myocardial perfusion. Are the promises to be realised?" *Heart* 89(12): 1389-90.

26. Sieswerda, G. T., L. J. Klein, et al. (2004). "Quantitative evaluation of myocardial perfusion in patients with revascularized myocardial infarction: comparison between intravenous myocardial contrast echocardiography and 99mTc-sestamibi single photon emission computed tomography." *Eur J Echocardiogr* 5(1): 41-50.

27. Otani, K., T. Toshida, et al. (2004). "Adenosine triphosphate stress myocardial contrast echocardiography detects coronary artery stenosis with greater sensitivity than wall-motion abnormality measurements." *J Am Soc Echocardiogr* 17(12): 1275-80.

28. Wei, K., M. Ragosta, et al. (2001). "Noninvasive quantification of coronary blood flow reserve in humans using myocardial contrast echocardiography." *Circulation* 103(21): 2560-5.

29. Cheitlin, M. D., W. F. Armstrong, et al. (2003). "ACC/AHA/ASE 2003 Guideline Update for the Clinical Application of Echocardiography: summary article. A report of the American College of Cardiology/American Heart Association Task Force on Practice Guidelines (ACC/AHA/ASE Committee to Update the 1997 Guidelines for the Clinical Application of Echocardiography)." *J Am Soc Echocardiogr* 16(10): 1091-110.

30. Yvorchuk, K. J. and K. L. Chan (1994). "Application of transthoracic and transesophageal echocardiography in the diagnosis and management of infective endocarditis." *J Am Soc Echocardiogr* 7(3 Pt 1): 294-308.

31. Feigenbaum, H., J. A. Waldhausen, et al. (1965). "Ultrasound Diagnosis of Pericardial Effusion." *Jama* 191: 711-4.

32. Erbel, R., F. Alfonso, et al. (2001). "Diagnosis and management of aortic dissection." *Eur Heart J* 22(18): 1642-81.

33. Moller, J. E., K. Egstrup, et al. (2003). "Prognostic importance of systolic and diastolic function after acute myocardial infarction." *Am Heart J* 145(1): 147-53.

34. Jugdutt, B. I. and C. A. Sivaram (1989). "Prospective two-dimensional echocardiographic evaluation of left ventricular thrombus and embolism after acute myocardial infarction." *J Am Coll Cardiol* 13(3): 554-64.

35. Jiang, L., J. A. Vazquez de Prada, et al. (1995). "Quantitative three-dimensional reconstruction of aneurysmal left ventricles. In vitro and in vivo validation." *Circulation* 91(1): 222-30.

36. Bayer, A. S., A. F. Bolger, et al. (1998). "Diagnosis and management of infective endocarditis and its complications." *Circulation* 98(25): 2936.48.

37. Palmieri, V., B. Dahlof, et al. (1999). "Reliability of echocardiographic assessment of left ventricular structure and function: the PRESERVE study. Prospective Randomized Study Evaluating Regression of Ventricular Enlargement." *J Am Coll Cardiol* 34(5): 1625-32.

38. Chan, K. L., P. J. Currie, et al. (1987). "Comparison of three Doppler ultrasound methods in the prediction of pulmonary artery pressure." *J Am Coll Cardiol* 9(3): 549-54.

39. Kuhl, H. P. and P. Hanrath (2004). "The impact of transesophageal echocardiography on daily clinical practice." *Eur J Echocardiogr* 5(6): 455-68.

40. Quinones, M. A., A. D. Waggoner, et al. (1981). "A new, simplified and accurate method for determining ejection fraction with two-dimensional echocardiography." *Circulation* 64(4): 744-53.

41. Schiller, N. B., P. M. Shah, et al. (1989). "Recommendations for quantitation of the left ventricle by two-dimensional echocardiography. American Society of Echocardiography Committee on Standards, Subcommittee on Quantitation of Two-Dimensional Echocardiograms." *J Am Soc Echocardiogr* 2(5): 358-67.

42. Zamorano, J., D. R. Wallbridge, et al. (1997). "Noninvasive assessment of cardiac physiology by tissue Doppler echocardiography. A comparison with invasive haemodynamics." *Eur Heart J* 18(2): 330-9.

43. Cerqueira, M. D., N. J. Weissman, et al. (2002). "Standardized myocardial segmentation and nomenclature for tomographic imaging of the heart. A statement for healthcare professionals from the Cardiac Imaging Committee of the Council on Clinical Cardiology of the American Heart Association." *Int J Cardiovasc Imaging* 18(1): 539-42.

44. Eaton, L. W., J. L. Weiss, et al. (1979). "Regional cardiac dilatation after acute myocardial infarction:

recognition by two-dimensional echocardiography." *N Engl J Med* 300(2): 57-62.

45. Feigenbaum, H., W. F. Armstrong, et al., Eds. (2004). *Echocardiography*. Philadelphia, Lippincott, Williams & Wilkins.

46. Nishimura, R. A. and A. J. Tajik (1997). "Evaluation of diastolic filling of left ventricle in health and disease: Doppler echocardiography is the clinician's Rosetta Stone." *J Am Coll Cardiol* 30(1): 8-18.

47. Appleton, C. P., J. M. Galloway, et al. (1993). "Estimation of left ventricular filling pressures using two-dimensional and Doppler echocardiography in adult patients with cardiac disease. Additional value of analyzing left atrial size, left atrial ejection fraction and the difference in duration of pulmonary venous and mitral flow velocity at atrial contraction." *J Am Coll Cardiol* 22(7): 1972-82.

48. Camm, A. J., T. F. Luscher, et al., Eds. (2006). *The ESC Textbook of Cardiovascular Medicine*. Oxford, Blackwell Publishing.

49. St. John Sutton, M., Ed. (1996). *Textbook of Echocardiography and Doppler in Adults and Children*. Oxford, Blackwell Science.

50. Hansen, A., M. Haass, et al. (2001). "Prognostic value of Doppler echocardiographic mitral inflow patterns: implications for risk stratification in patients with chronic congestive heart failure." *J Am Coll Cardiol* 37(4): 1049-55.

51. Nishimura, R. A., M. D. Abel, et al. (1990). "Relation of pulmonary vein to mitral flow velocities by transesophageal Doppler echocardiography. Effect of different loading conditions." *Circulation* 81(5): 1488-97.

52. Ommen, S. R., R. A. Nishimura, et al. (2000). "Clinical utility of Doppler echocardiography and tissue Doppler imaging in the estimation of left ventricular filling pressures: A comparative simultaneous Doppler-catheterization study." *Circulation* 102(15): 1788-94.

53. Garcia, M. J., N. G. Smedira, et al. (2000). "Color M-mode Doppler flow propagation velocity is a preload insensitive index of left ventricular relaxation: animal and human validation." *J Am Coll Cardiol* 35(1): 201-8.

54. Peels, C. H., C. A. Visser, et al. (1990). "Usefulness of two-dimensional echocardiography for immediate detection of myocardial ischemia in the emergency room." *Am J Cardiol* 65(11): 687-91.

55. Horowitz, R. S., J. Morganroth, et al. (1982). "Immediate diagnosis of acute myocardial infarction by two-dimensional echocardiography." *Circulation* 65(2): 323-9.

56. Zoghbi, W. A., M. Enriquez-Sarano, et al. (2003). "Recommendations for evaluation of the severity of native valvular regurgitation with two-dimensional and Doppler echocardiography." *J Am Soc Echocardiogr* 16(7): 777-802.

57. Bermejo, J., R. Odreman, et al. (2003). "Clinical efficacy of Doppler-echocardiographic indices of aortic valve stenosis: a comparative test-based analysis of outcome." *J Am Coll Cardiol* 41(1): 142-51.

58. deFilippi, C. R., D. L. Willett, et al. (1995). "Usefulness of dobutamine echocardiography in distinguishing severe from nonsevere valvular aortic stenosis in patients with depressed left ventricular function and low transvalvular gradients." *Am J Cardiol* 75(2): 191-4.

59. Perry, G. J., F. Helmcke, et al. (1987). "Evaluation of aortic insufficiency by Doppler color flow mapping." *J Am Coll Cardiol* 9(4): 952-9.

60. Grigioni, F., M. Enriquez-Sarano, et al. (2001). "Ischemic mitral regurgitation: long-term outcome and prognostic implications with quantitative Doppler assessment." *Circulation* 103(13): 1759-64.

61. Pua, E. C., S. F. Idriss, et al. (2004). "Real-time 3D transesophageal echocardiography." *Ultrason Imaging* 26(4): 217-32.

62. Scohy, T. V., F. J. Cate, et al. (2008). "Usefulness of Intraoperative Real-Time 3D Transesophageal Echocardiography in Cardiac Surgery." *J Card Surg* 23(6): 784-6.

63. Bargiggia, G. S., L. Tronconi, et al. (1991). "A new method for quantitation of mitral regurgitation based on color flow Doppler imaging of flow convergence proximal to regurgitant orifice." *Circulation* 84(4): 1481-9.

64. Iwakura, K., H. Ito, et al. (2006). "Comparison of orifice area by transthoracic three-dimensional Doppler echocardiography versus proximal isovelocity surface area (PISA) method for assessment of mitral regurgitation." *Am J Cardiol* 97(11): 1630-7.

65. Chao, K., V. A. Moises, et al. (1992). "Influence of the Coanda effect on color Doppler jet area and color encoding. In vitro studies using color Doppler flow mapping." *Circulation* 85(1): 333-41.

66. Enriquez-Sarano, M., K. S. Dujardin, et al. (1999). "Determinants of pulmonary venous flow reversal in mitral regurgitation and its usefulness in determining the severity of regurgitation." *Am J Cardiol* 83(4): 535-41.

67. Erbel, R., P. Schweizer, et al. (1985). "Sensitivity of cross-sectional echocardiography in detection of impaired global and regional left ventricular function: prospective study." *Int J Cardiol* 7(4): 375-89.

68. Yock, P. G. and R. L. Popp (1984). "Noninvasive estimation of right ventricular systolic pressure by Doppler ultrasound in patients with tricuspid regurgitation." *Circulation* 70(4): 657-62.

69. Stephen, B., P. Dalal, et al. (1999). "Noninvasive estimation of pulmonary artery diastolic pressure in patients with tricuspid regurgitation by Doppler echocardiography." *Chest* 116(1): 73-7.

70. Zipes, D. P., P. Libby, et al., Eds. (2005). *Braunwald's Heart Disease.* Philadelphia, Elsevier Saunders.

71. Richardson, P., W. McKenna, et al. (1996). "Report of the 1995 World Health Organization/International Society and Federation of Cardiology Task Force on the Definition and Classification of cardiomyopathies." *Circulation* 93(5): 841-2.

72. Rihal, C. S., R. A. Nishimura, et al. (1994). "Systolic and diastolic dysfunction in patients with clinical diagnosis of dilated cardiomyopathy. Relation to symptoms and prognosis." *Circulation* 90(6): 2772-9.

73. Agmon, Y., H. M. Connolly, et al. (1999). "Noncompaction of the ventricular myocardium." *J Am Soc Echocardiogr* 12(10): 859-63.

74. Shapiro, L. M. and W. J. McKenna (1983). "Distribution of left ventricular hypertrophy in hypertrophic cardiomyopathy: a two-dimensional echocardiographic study." *J Am Coll Cardiol* 2(3): 437-44.

75. Lakkis, N. M., S. F. Nagueh, et al. (1998). "Echocardiography-guided ethanol septal reduction for hypertrophic obstructive cardiomyopathy." *Circulation* 98(17): 1750-5.

76. Klein, A. L. and A. J. Tajik (1991). "Doppler assessment of diastolic function in cardiac amyloidosis." *Echocardiography* 8(2): 233-51.

77. Hatle, L. K., C. P. Appleton, et al. (1989). "Differentiation of constrictive pericarditis and restrictive cardiomyopathy by Doppler echocardiography." *Circulation* 79(2): 357-70.

78. Khandheria, B. K. (1993). "Suspected bacterial endocarditis: to TEE or not to TEE." *J Am Coll Cardiol* 21(1): 222-4.

79. Durack, D. T., A. S. Lukes, et al. (1994). "New criteria for diagnosis of infective endocarditis: utilization of specific echocardiographic findings. Duke Endocarditis Service." *Am J Med* 96(3): 200-9.

80. Vuille, C., M. Nidorf, et al. (1994). "Natural history of vegetations during successful medical treatment of endocarditis." *Am Heart J* 128(6 Pt 1): 1200-9.

81. Maisch, B., P. M. Seferovic, et al. (2004). "Guidelines on the diagnosis and management of pericardial diseases executive summary; The Task force on the diagnosis and management of pericardial diseases of the European society of cardiology." *Eur Heart J* 25(7): 587-610.

82. Chandraratna, P. A. (1991). "Echocardiography and Doppler ultrasound in the evaluation of pericardial disease." *Circulation* 84(3 Suppl): I303-10.

83. Myers, R. B. and D. H. Spodick (1999). "Constrictive pericarditis: clinical and pathophysiologic characteristics." *Am Heart J* 138(2 Pt 1): 219-32.

84. Armstrong, W. F., D. S. Bach, et al. (1996). "Spectrum of acute dissection of the ascending aorta: a transesophageal echocardiographic study." *J Am Soc Echocardiogr* 9(5): 646.56.

85. Song, J. K., H. S. Kim, et al. (2001). "Different clinical features of aortic intramural hematoma versus dissection involving the ascending aorta." *J Am Coll Cardiol* 37(6): 1604-10.

86. Karalis, D. G., K. Chandrasekaran, et al. (1991). "Recognition and embolic potential of intraaortic atherosclerotic debris." *J Am Coll Cardiol* 17(1): 73-8.

87. Tunick, P. A. and I. Kronzon (2000). "Atheromas of the thoracic aorta: clinical and therapeutic update." *J Am Coll Cardiol* 35(3): 545-54.

88. Nomeir, A. M., L. E. Watts, et al. (1989). "Intracardiac myxomas: twenty-year echocardiographic experience with review of the literature." *J Am Soc Echocardiogr* 2(2): 139-50.

89. Sun, J. P., C. R. Asher, et al. (2001). "Clinical and echocardiographic characteristics of papillary fibroelastomas: a retrospective and prospective study in 162 patients." *Circulation* 103(22): 2687-93.

90. Fyke, F. E., 3rd, A. J. Tajik, et al. (1983). "Diagnosis of lipomatous hypertrophy of the atrial septum by two-dimensional echocardiography." *J Am Coll Cardiol* 1(5): 1352-7.

91. DePace, N. L., R. L. Soulen, et al. (1981). "Two dimensional echocardiographic detection of intraatrial masses." *Am J Cardiol* 48(5): 954-60.

92. Kerut, E. K., W. T. Norfleet, et al. (2001). "Patent foramen ovale: a review of associated conditions and the impact of physiological size." *J Am Coll Cardiol* 38(3): 613-23.

CHAPTER 7

Computerized Tomography

Christoph R. Becker, MD

DEVELOPMENT OF CARDIAC CT TECHNOLOGY

First attempts to image the heart by CT have been made from the moment when the bore of a CT gantry became wide enough to image the thorax. However, for imaging the heart and, in particular the coronary arteries, it is a prerequisite to have high spatial and temporal resolution available at the same time. The design of conventional CT scanners, with an x-ray source rotating around the body of the patient for long time, did not fulfil of any of these fundamental imaging requirements.

The first CT scanner particularly designed for these special requirements was the dynamic spatial reconstructor. The system consisted of 14 x-ray tubes allowing for the acquisition of 60 CT image frames per second. The dynamic spatial reconstructor claimed an area of 6m by 4.5m and had a total weight of 15 tons.[1] Apart from experimental and animal studies, the dynamic spatial reconstructor never made it to routine clinical cardiac examination, mainly because of the difficulties that arose from intensive postprocessing and the extensive radiation that went along with an investigation with this scanner.

The electron beam CT was the first commercially available dedicated cardiac CT system. In this system, electrons were accelerated by an electron gun and travelled through a vacuum funnel until they hit a tungsten target under the patient table. X-rays were produced in this system by avoiding any mechanical parts and images could be created in a very short time frame. Image acquisition was triggered by the ECG signal to the mid diastole phase of the cardiac cycle. For long time, slice thickness and temporal resolution of 3mm and 100ms respectively, were not achievable by any other CT system. The electron beam CT scanner has set the standard for the coronary calcium screening protocol up to now.[2]

Conventional CT systems over the years also improved their temporal resolution by faster gantry rotation speed. In general, to create an image in CT, x-ray projection data from at least 180 degrees of the gantry rotation cycle are necessary for image reconstruction. Therefore, with faster CT gantry rotation, temporal resolution improves accordingly. The fastest gantry rotation time currently available is 300ms, resulting in a temporal resolution of 150ms. The temporal resolution seems to be sufficient to image the heart and the coronary arteries in a slowly beating heart (60 beats per minute or fewer), without any motion artifacts in the diastolic phase of the cardiac cycle. Because of the significant centrifugal forces of the CT components on the gantry during rotation and because of mechanical limits, even shorter gantry rotations are difficult to implement.[3]

Attempts have been made to further shorten the exposure time by using two x-ray detectors and x-ray sources instead of one, rotating around the patient. If arranged perpendicular to each other and spinning around the patient three times per second, this system is capable for an imaging acquisition time of 80ms.[4]

It turned out that when imaging the heart with an exposure time as short as 80ms, any motion artifacts may be avoided up a heart rate of 70 beats per minute if reconstructed in the diastole phase of the cardiac cycle. Moreover, 80ms temporal resolution also seems to be short enough to image the heart in the systole phase of the cardiac cycle without major motion artifacts. As the duration of systole slow motion phase changes only to a minor degree in relation to heart rate and rhythm, images with minimal or any artifacts may also be reconstructed in this particular phase of the cardiac cycle, even if patients present with higher heart rates or arrhythmia.[5]

So far, it is not yet clear if CT images reconstructed in the systole phase of the cardiac cycle provide the same kind of information as images reconstructed in the diastole. It is likely that measurements of the degree of stenoses are far more difficult to get from images obtained from the systole rather than from the diastole phase. In the diastole phase, the coronary artery tree is spread out over the myocardium and the coronary arteries are wider due to the increased blood flow.

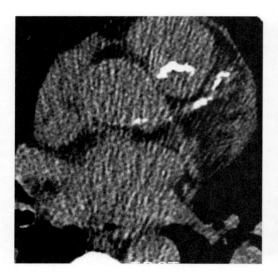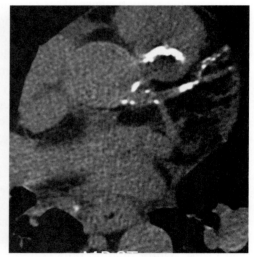

Figure 7.1

As a common standard images with 3mm slice thickness are acquired with electron beam CT as well as with multi-detector row CT. The images are quite comparable in terms of image quality. If evaluated according to guidelines provided by the consortium for standardization of the coronary calcium measurement, the quantities for all different CT scanners are quite well comparable.[11]

The scan mode preferred with multi-detector-row CT scanners with fast gantry rotation and simultaneous acquisition of the electrocardiogram is retrospective ECG gating. For this technique, the data are acquired in the spiral mode of the CT scanner combined with a slow table feed. Image reconstruction is performed by selecting the data during the phase of the least motion during the cardiac cycle. This technique is not very efficient in terms of radiation exposure. With improved spatial and temporal resolution, every new CT scanner generation increased radiation for a cardiac CT examination.[6]

A lot of effort has been invested in order to reduce the radiation exposure by cardiac multidetector-row CT. One of the most effective efforts was to use ECG x-ray-current modulation in conjunction with retrospective ECG gating. For this method, the tube current is reduced during systole and increased during diastole. Radiation exposure may be reduced up to 50% by this technique. Prospective tube current modulation is of limited value in patients with high heart rate and arrhythmia.[7]

Multi-detector CT scanners with increased detector width are now available. These scanners may be capable of imaging the entire heart with one to three heartbeats. The preferred method of image acquisition in these scanners is prospective ECG triggering, which is far more efficient in terms of avoiding redundant radiation. Apparently, cardiac CT examination may be consistently performed with 3mSv, which is almost the same exposure as for an invasive diagnostic cardiac catheter examination.[8]

Various CT protocols exist for coronary calcium screening and plaque imaging, coronary CT angiography, and for the assessment of myocardium and valve function.

CORONARY CALCIUM SCREENING

The prerequisite for screening with CT for coronary calcium is low radiation exposure, no patient preparation, and no contrast media administration. As mentioned previously, image acquisition is performed most of the time with 40 consecutive 3mm slices from the bifurcation to the bottom of the heart. If performed with retrospective ECG gating, overlapping slice reconstruction may improve reproducibility of the coronary calcium quantification. However, in order to keep the radiation exposure to a minimum, prospective ECG triggering is the preferred acquisition mode for CT. The radiation exposure should be in the range of 1mSv and below.

Coronary calcifications are commonly quantified according to the Agatston algorithm. Every pixel in the CT image related to the coronary arteries with a density more than 130 HU is defined as calcium. The area is multiplied by a factor, depending on the peak density of every individual plaque. Plaques with a maximum density between 130 and 199 HU, 200 and 299 HU, 300 and 399 HU, or more than 400 were assigned to a factor of 1, 2, 3, or 4, respectively. The score is calculated as the total sum of all individual plaques.[9]

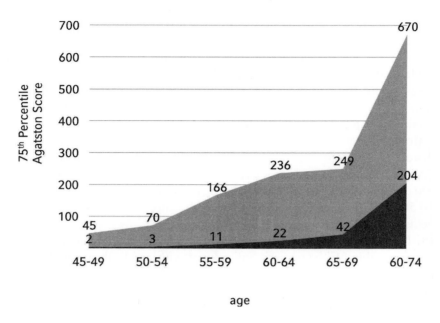

Figure 7.2

Reference values for coronary calcium screening are available from a randomly enrolled cohort of the German population. The 75th percentile that is believed to indicate elevated risk of cardiovascular event in asymptomatic persons is given in the diagram.[23] The reference values may be different for other population cohort and ethnic groups.[24]

One of the major limitations of the Agatston score is the low reproducibility. A method has been proposed that takes the total volume of calcified plaques into account.[10] Because of different acquisition modes and image quality of electron beam CT compared to multidetector-row CT, the Agatston score and volume assessment of the calcified plaque burden are only fairly comparable between these two types of scanners. An international consortium of all CT vendors (Siemens, Toshiba, Philips, and General Electric) and some leading research and clinical institutions agreed upon a standardized measurement for coronary calcium. The consortium provides guidelines for standardized CT scan protocols for any company, as well as guidelines for calibration, quantification, and quality assurance. In addition, the consortium has agreed on the absolute mass quantification as the algorithm with the highest inter-scanner reproducibility.[11] Because the majority of publications are based on the Agatston score, this semiquantitative method still remains the standard of reference.

CORONARY CT ANGIOGRAPHY

Imaging of the coronary arteries by CT requires high spatial resolution and administration of high amounts of contrast media. To avoid motion artifacts with slower CT scanners, patient preparation with beta-blockers may become necessary. This may be done by either oral or intravenous beta-blocker administration.[12] Visualization of stenoses and smaller coronary artery side branches may be improved by the administration of nitroglycerin.[13] Because nitroglycerin may increase the heart rate, it is only advisable to use it in CT scanners with high temporal resolution.

Coronary artery enhancement depends on a variety of factors such as contrast media density, injection rate, patient's blood volume, and cardiac output.[14] Test bolus or bolus-tracking work similarly for the determination of the contrast arrival time.[15]

The use of a dual-head injector for the sequential injection of contrast media and saline is helpful in order to flush the superior vena cava and right atrium where potentially dense contrast media may cause artifacts.[16] Furthermore, cardiac CT examinations are performed in midinspiration to avoid the Valsalva maneuver that potentially may prevent influx of contrast media into the cardiac chambers.

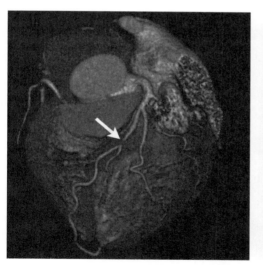 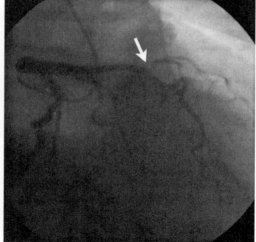

Figure 7.3

With coronary CTA, tight stenosis without calcifications can well be visualized. However, retrograde filling of distal coronary segments remain a pitfall in CTA. (See Color Plate 18.)

One of the limitations to detecting stenoses and plaques by coronary CT angiography is related to calcium or any other dense material, such as stents. These components are overexpressed by CT and prevent assessment of the coronary artery wall and lumen. This blooming artifact depends on spatial resolution and on motion in the CT image. Changing scan and reconstruction parameters to 140kV or a sharper image kernel may reduce these artifacts to a certain degree. However, the blooming artifact remains one of the biggest challenges to perform adequate diagnoses in advanced atherosclerotic disease.

In general, accurate grading of coronary artery stenoses remains a challenge with the spatial resolution available today in CT. Postprocessing workstations may support the diagnoses of a significant stenoses. However, the reliability of any of these workstations depends very much on the algorithm used. The accuracy may vary as much as 25% or more. Therefore, it is advisable to proof the diagnoses of any suspected relevant stenoses with an exercise or stress test.

Coronary CTA is well suited to visualizing the anatomy of patients with coronary anomalies and to identifying patients in whom an aberrant coronary artery, for instance, has its course between the ascending aorta and the pulmonary outflow tract. Coronary CTA may also provide valid and useful information in patients with vasculitis and aneurysms, fistulas, or dissection. In these patients, a CT dataset is best displayed by a 3D volume-rendering technique.

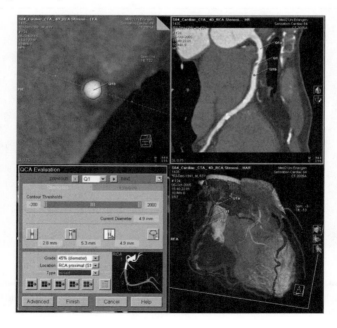

Figure 7.4

Postprocessing software may help in the reporting of a coronary CTA dataset by quantifying the degree of stenosis. (See Color Plate 19.)

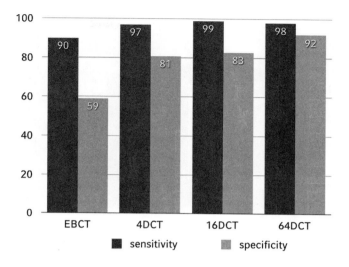

Figure 7.5

Recent meta-analysis from 41 papers provides information about the accuracy of detecting coronary stenoses by CTA as compared to cardiac catheter. Sensitivity and specificity improves with more advanced CT scanners.[25]

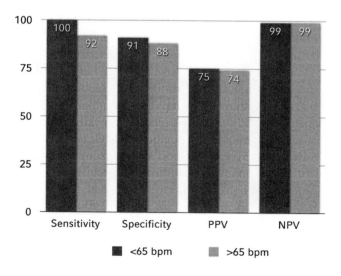

Figure 7.6

The advantage of dual-source CT is the relative independence of the diagnostic accuracy from the heart rate.[26]

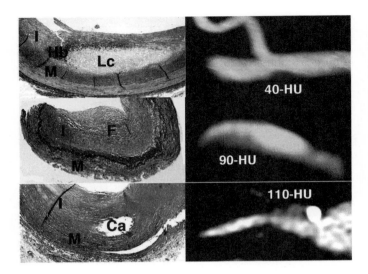

Figure 7.7

The difference in density might give an idea of the component of atherosclerotic plaques in the coronary arteries. Low dense plaques more likely contain lipid or thrombus material, intermediate dense plaques commonly consist of fibrous tissue and calcium. (See Color Plate 20.)

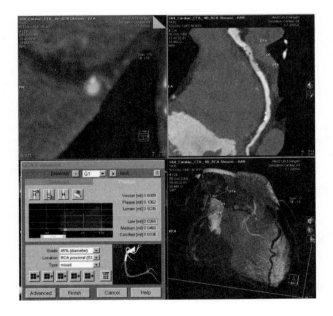

Figure 7.8

Postprocessing software may support in the assessment of atherosclerotic coronary plaques; however, the measurement is often difficult to reproduce. (See Color Plate 21.)

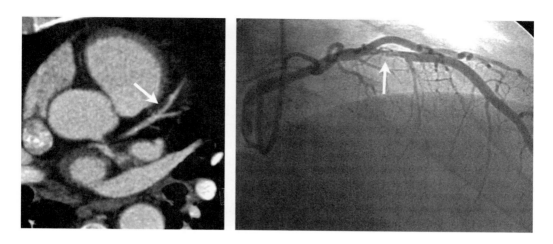

Figure 7.9

Noncalcified plaque that has caused myocardial infarction in a 40-year-old male patient (arrow).

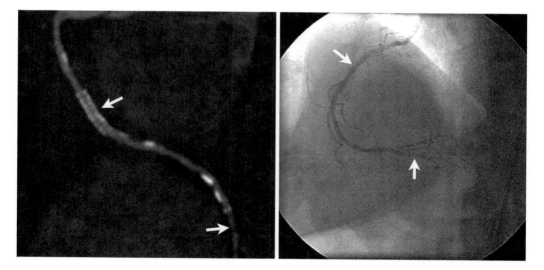

Figure 7.10

The blooming artifact often prevents adequate assessment of the stent lumen (arrow). Extensive atherosclerotic disease is often present beside the stent (arrow).

CT density measurement in carotid and coronary arteries have shown that CT densities of 50 HU and 90 HU within plaques are relatively specific for lipid and fibrous tissue, respectively.[17] However, density measurements of small plaques in CT are often difficult due to partial volume effects.[18]

FUNCTIONAL IMAGING OF THE HEART BY CT

With retrospective ECG gating, data is available for image reconstruction at any point within the cardiac cycle. Putting all images together in a cine loop allows functional assessment of the myocardium and valves. New postprocessing software supports the evaluation of the functional parameters, such as ejection fraction, end-systolic, and end-diastolic left ventricular volumes. For the assessment of the myocardial mass, it is necessary to change the contrast protocol to have some contrast in the right ventricle to delineate the septum. A split bolus technique, with diluted contrast bolus following the main contrast bolus, may be used to achieve an appropriate enhancement of the right ventricle and to avoid a dense contrast in the right cardiac chambers, including the superior vena cava.[19]

Assessment of the cardiac valves is potentially feasible with CT. For preoperative planning, the diameter of the aortic outflow tract can well be measured from CT data. In case of aortic stenosis, the opening area of the valve often is difficult to assess because

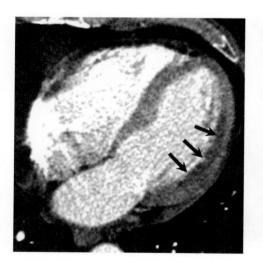 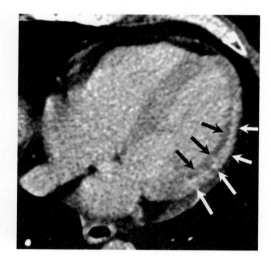

Figure 7.11

Delayed-enhancement CT scanning may allow identification of myocardial infarction (white arrows) and micro-vascular obstruction (black arrows).

of extensive calcifications of the leaflets. Functional assessment of the valve is not possible by CT.[20]

Values obtained from the assessment of the functional parameters of the heart by CT show close correlation to data from MRI.[21] It should be noted that functional assessment of the heart with retrospective ECG gating goes along with higher radiation and more contrast media than imaging the coronary arteries alone with prospective ECG triggering. In particular, assessment of the valves requires the highest quality images at every time point of the cardiac cycle. ECG tube current modulation may not be used if the cardiac valves are to be investigated by CT.

CHALLENGES AND FUTURE POTENTIALS OF CARDIAC CT

By the standardization of the coronary calcium measurements, the results of these studies, originally obtained by EBCT, may also be transferred to MDCT. MDCT scanners are already widely available, and therefore allow for a widespread use of coronary calcium scanning for further risk stratification in subjects with intermediate cardiac event risk.

If the ability of coronary CTA to detect vulnerable plaques in patients with acute coronary syndrome directly holds true, new strategies need to be considered for appropriate treatment of these patients. The noninvasive vulnerable plaque detection may justify intensive medical treatment or may lead to invasive approaches such as plaque sealing.

CTA may soon serve as a tool for complete diagnostic work-up of patients presenting with atypical chest pain. A single CTA investigation will rule in or rule out pulmonary emboli, aortic dissection, or coronary thrombus. Because of the need to administer contrast media and because of the relatively higher radiation exposure for CTA, it currently appears unlikely that coronary CTA may be used as a screening tool for vulnerable plaques in asymptomatic subjects.

Some technical improvements in cardiac CT are foreseeable within the next few years. With wider detectors, prospective ECG triggering will be feasible with a minimal radiation dose if the heart is imaged only at a particular time point of the cardiac cycle. In combination with two or even more x-ray sources, these systems are capable for acquisition times, and will allow image acquisition at any time point of the cardiac cycle, regardless of heart rate and rhythm without any motion. If spatial resolution is improved at the same time, it may result in minor artifacts caused by calcium or stents. By providing a sufficient amount of contrast media, smaller side branches of the coronary artery tree will also become visible.

Myocardial perfusion remains a major challenge for CT. Repeated scanning goes along with high radiation and first pass imaging of the myocardium has frequently been associated with artifacts from dense-contrast media in the cardiac chambers. PET/CT is more likely to provide comprehensive information about morphology and function of the coronary arteries and the myocardium. FDG is a solid tracer commonly used in PET and provides information about viable myocardial comparable to late enhancement MRI. It is a major effort to perform perfusion PET/CT with NH_3, because a cyclotron has to be present next to the scanner. The half time period is in the range of only few minutes. Alternatively, because the tracer can be produced by a generator, rubidium may play an important role for the combined assessment of myocardial ischemia and coronary artery stenoses.

Rotating C-arm CT systems will primarily be used in interventional suites. These systems allow rotation of the C-arm with a flat panel detector around the patient while contrast media is injected through a coronary catheter.[22] The combination of coronary artery imaging by DSA and information about the perfusion of the myocardium provided by CT-like images created from rotating C-arm projections may become of paramount importance in emergency coronary interventions.

In the end, coronary CTA may replace cardiac catheter for the triage of patients for conservative, interventional, or surgical therapy and may reduce the use of an invasive diagnostic procedure to preselected patients in whom coronary interventions are essentially required.

◇◇◇◇◇◇◇◇◇◇◇◇

REFERENCES

1. Sinak, L. J., Hoffman, E. A. & Ritman, E. L. Subtraction gated computed tomography with the dynamic spatial reconstructor: simultaneous evaluation of left and right heart from single right-sided bolus contrast medium injection. *J Comput Assist Tomogr* 8, 1-9 (1984).

2. Boyd, D. P. in *CT of the heart and the great vessels: experimental evaluation and clinical application* (ed Higgins, C. B.) (Futura Publishing Company, Mount Kisco New York, 1983).

3. Flohr, T., Stierstorfer, K., Raupach, R., Ulzheimer, S. & Bruder, H. Performance evaluation of a 64-slice CT system with z-flying focal spot. *Rofo* 176, 1803-1810 (2004).

4. Flohr, T. G. et al. First performance evaluation of a dual-source CT (DSCT) system. *Eur Radiol* 16, 256-268 (2006).

5. Johnson, T. et al. Dual-source CT cardiac imaging: initial expericence. *Eur Radiol* in press, (2006).

6. Einstein, A. J., Henzlova, M. J. & Rajagopalan, S. Estimating risk of cancer associated with radiation exposure from 64-slice computed tomography coronary angiography. *Jama* 298, 317-323 (2007).

7. Jakobs, T. F. et al. Multislice helical CT of the heart with retrospective ECG gating: reduction of radiation exposure by ECG-controlled tube current modulation. *Eur Radiol* 12, 1081-1086 (2002).

8. Hirai, N. et al. Prospective versus retrospective ECG-gated 64-detector coronary CT angiography: assessment of image quality, stenosis, and radiation dose. *Radiology* (2008).

9. Agatston, A. S. et al. Quantification of coronary artery calcium using ultrafast computed tomography. *J Am Coll Cardiol* 15, 827-832 (1990).

10. Callister, T. Q. et al. Coronary artery disease: improved reproducibility of calcium scoring with an electron-beam CT volumetric method. *Radiology* 208, 807-14. (1998).

11. McCollough, C. H. et al. Coronary artery calcium: a multi-institutional, multimanufacturer international standard for quantification at cardiac CT. *Radiology* 243, 527-538 (2007).

12. Shapiro, M. D. et al. Efficacy of pre-scan beta-blockade and impact of heart rate on image quality in patients undergoing coronary multidetector computed tomography angiography. *Eur J Radiol* 66, 37-41 (2008).

13. Dewey, M., Hoffmann, H. & Hamm, B. Multislice CT coronary angiography: effect of sublingual nitroglyc-

erine on the diameter of coronary arteries. *Rofo* 178, 600-604 (2006).

14. Rist, C. et al. Optimization of cardiac MSCT contrast injection protocols dependency of the main bolus contrast density on test bolus parameters and patients' body weight. *Acad Radiol* 15, 49-57 (2008).

15. Cademartiri, F. et al. Intravenous contrast material administration at 16-detector row helical CT coronary angiography: test bolus versus bolus-tracking technique. *Radiology* 233, 817-823 (2004).

16. Cademartiri, F. et al. Non-invasive 16-row multislice CT coronary angiography: usefulness of saline chaser. *Eur Radiol* 14, 178-183 (2004).

17. Becker, C. R. et al. Ex vivo coronary atherosclerotic plaque characterization with multi-detector-row CT. *Eur Radiol* 13, 2094-2098 (2003).

18. Becker, C. R., Knez, A., Ohnesorge, B., Schoepf, U. J. & Reiser, M. F. Imaging of noncalcified coronary plaques using helical CT with retrospective ECG gating. *AJR Am J Roentgenol* 175, 423-44. (2000).

19. Kerl, J. M. et al. Right heart: split-bolus injection of diluted contrast medium for visualization at coronary CT angiography. *Radiology* 247, 356-364 (2008).

20. Saam, T. et al. Assessment of aortic stenosis after aortic valve replacement: comparative evaluation of dual-source CT and echocardiography. *Rofo* 180, 553-560 (2008).

21. Busch, S. et al. Quantitative assessment of left ventricular function with dual-source CT in comparison to cardiac magnetic resonance imaging: initial findings. *Eur Radiol* (2007).

22. Kalender, W. A. & Kyriakou, Y. Flat-detector computed tomography (FD-CT). *Eur Radiol* 17, 2767-2779 (2007).

23. Schmermund, A. et al. Population-based assessment of subclinical coronary atherosclerosis using electron-beam computed tomography. *Atherosclerosis* 185, 177-182 (2006).

24. Schmermund, A. et al. Comparison of subclinical coronary atherosclerosis and risk factors in unselected populations in Germany and US-America. *Atherosclerosis* 195, e207-16 (2007).

25. Janne d'Othée, B. et al. A systematic review on diagnostic accuracy of CT-based detection of significant coronary artery disease. *Eur J Radiol* (2007).

26. Leber, A. W. et al. Diagnostic accuracy of dual-source multi-slice CT-coronary angiography in patients with an intermediate pretest likelihood for coronary artery disease. *Eur Heart J* 28, 2354-2360 (2007).

CHAPTER 8

Magnetic Resonance Imaging

Zahi A. Fayad, PhD, FACC, FAHA*

INTRODUCTION

By 1990, the complications of atherosclerosis had become the leading cause of mortality and morbidity globally. Although death rates in the Western world have been consistently falling since the 1980s, atherosclerosis is now raging throughout the developing world.[1] In 1996, more than 60% of the 15 million worldwide deaths due to circulatory diseases occurred in less-developed nations.

Atherosclerosis is an inflammatory disease affecting medium and large arteries from the first decade of life until death. It has a predilection for certain arterial beds, with the carotid artery and aorta being the most common sites of plaque formation.[2] In the carotid circulation, the end result can be an ischemic cerebral insult causing either temporary (transient ischemic attack—TIA) or permanent (cerebrovascular attack—CVA) symptoms. If unchecked, aortic atherosclerosis can predispose to dissection, intramural hemorrhage, aneurysm formation, and downstream embolus.[3]

PATHOBIOLOGY OF ATHEROSCLEROSIS

Atherosclerosis is characterized by the gradual accumulation of lipid, inflammatory cells, and connective tissue within the arterial wall. It is a chronic, progressive disease with a long asymptomatic phase. The first abnormality is the fatty streak, caused by the collection of lipid and macrophages in the subendothelial space. Fatty streaks develop primarily in regions of endothelial dysfunction. Endothelial cells in these areas have a reduced production of nitric oxide as a result of being exposed to low wall shear stress.[4]

The major atherogenic risk factors, such as smoking, hypertension, and diabetes mellitus, all impair endothelial function.[5] Both the barrier function and secretory capacity of the endothelium become affected. This manifests as an increase in permeability to blood-derived lipids and inflammatory cells.

Once within the subendothelial space, LDL becomes oxidized and attracts monocytes by triggering the release of monocyte chemoattractant protein-1 (MCP-1) from the

*The author of this work is supported by grants from the NIH/NHLBI (R01 HL071021 and R01 HL078667) and the John E. Postley, Jr., MD Fund for the Imaging Science Laboratories.

overlying endothelial cells.[6] Endothelial adhesion molecules, including vascular cell adhesion molecule-1 (VCAM), intercellular adhesion molecule-1, E-selectin, and P-selectin, facilitate the internalization of further monocytes. Once they have escaped the blood pool, monocytes transform into macrophages, and bind and internalize oxLDL via their scavenger receptors.[7, 8] Eventually, the subendothelial accumulation of modified LDL and macrophage-derived foam cells lead to the formation of the atheromatous lipid core.

Under the right conditions (presence of hypertension, diabetes, smoking, and other risk factors), the lipid core may become bound on its luminal side by an endothelialized fibrous cap consisting of vascular smooth muscle cells (VSMC) and connective tissue. VSMCs migrate from the arterial media and synthesize extracellular matrix components such as elastin and collagen, producing the fibrous cap. The cap also contains variable numbers of inflammatory cells, most importantly macrophages.[9] As the plaque enlarges, the affected artery grows outwards by expansion of the external elastic lamina, so that lumen diameter and blood flow is preserved. This process is known as positive remodeling.[10, 11] As the artery's wall stress increases with outward remodeling, further expansion eventually becomes impossible and the plaque starts to encroach into the lumen. This may cause symptoms by compromising blood flow.

Mature plaques may also become calcified, a process that preferentially affects the intima of the artery. Very advanced plaques will also often be perforated by new blood vessels under the influence of angiogenic factors, a process called "neovascularization," is similar to that which occurs within growing tumors. However, these small arteries are structurally fragile, and have a tendency to spontaneously hemorrhage, which can destabilize the plaque, leading to clinical syndromes such as heart attack.[12, 13]

Atherosclerotic plaques may remain quiescent for decades.[14] However, when they initiate clot formation in the vessel lumen, they can become life threatening. This may occur either as a result of fibrous cap rupture, with consequent exposure of the thrombogenic extracellular matrix of the cap and the tissue factor (TF)–rich lipid core to circulating blood. Less commonly, there can be erosion of the endothelial cell layer overlying the fibrous cap, again potentially leading to intravascular thrombosis. Endothelial erosion accounts for around 30% of plaque rupture events.[15] Both forms of plaque disruption invariably lead to local platelet accumulation and activation with subsequent thrombus formation.

It has become clear that the cellular and extracellular composition of the plaque is the primary determinant of plaque stability.[16] Lesions with a large lipid core, thin fibrous cap, preponderance of inflammatory cells, and few VSMCs are at the highest risk of rupture. Inflammatory cells, particularly macrophages, produce metalloproteinase enzymes that break down the matrix proteins in the fibrous cap. In addition, they secrete inflammatory cytokines, in particular interferon γ, which inhibit VSMC proliferation and matrix production. Furthermore, VSMCs in the fibrous cap have a reduced proliferative capacity and a propensity to apoptosis.[17] Consequently, inflammation within the plaques tends towards destruction of the fibrous cap and subsequent thrombosis. There is a dynamic balance within the plaque between macrophages, which promotes erosion and rupture of the fibrous cap, and VSMCs, which nourish and repair it. These processes are independent of plaque size. Consequently, small asymptomatic and angiographically invisible plaques can rupture to precipitate a fatal clinical event, while some large plaques, which obstruct flow to produce symptoms such as angina, may be stable and not life threatening. There is an urgent need to discriminate stable from potentially unstable lesions in clinical practice. This chapter will cover the role of magnetic resonance imaging in this respect.

IMAGING ATHEROSCLEROSIS

The rationale behind the use of imaging in atherosclerosis is that the screening of high-risk patients might allow one to identify dangerous plaques before symptoms and complications develop.[18] Early knowledge of disease might allow the implementation of drug treatment to halt, or even reverse, the process of plaque progression and possibly prevent rupture. The statin drugs have proved efficacious in this regard.[19, 20] Rapid advances in MRI technology, computer software, and a huge array of potential cellular and molecular targets have pushed MRI to the top of the list of potential atherosclerosis imaging modalities.[21]

Multicontrast MRI

Atherosclerotic plaque in the carotid artery is ideally suited for imaging with MRI. Their superficial location, without significant motion, represent less of a technical challenge than imaging of the aorta or the coronary arteries.

Multicontrast MRI of the plaque is based on successive high-resolution black-blood fast-spin echo MR sequences, obtained by nulling the signal of the flowing blood through preparatory pulses. Sequences with several different weightings are generally acquired (T1, T2, and proton density).[22] Analysis of the various signal intensities in each of these sequences allows reasonable differentiation of plaque components (lipid core, fibrous tissue, hemorrhage, fibrous cap, and degree of calcification) by their different relaxation properties on MRI.[23, 24] Yuan et al. demonstrated that multicontrast MRI of human carotid arteries had sensitivity and specificity values of 85% and 92% respectively for the identification of a lipid core.[25, 26]

Recent advances in MRI acquisition protocols have allowed acquisition times to be reduced significantly.[27] Figure 8.1 demonstrates a carotid plaque imaged at 3T, with corresponding T1, T2, and PDW images displayed.

MRI has been validated against transoesophageal echocardiography in the thoracic aorta, with a strong correlation showing mean maximum plaque thickness measured

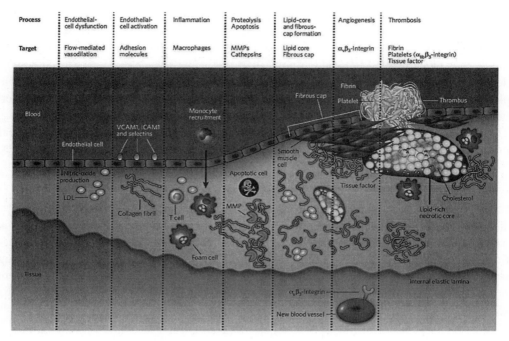

Figure 8.1

Simplified representation of the development and progression of an atherosclerotic lesion. Pathophysiological processes and associated potential targets for molecular imaging of atherothrombosis are indicated. ICAM: intercellular adhesion molecule; LDL: low-density lipoprotein; MMP: matrix metalloproteinase; NO: nitric oxide; VCAM1, vascular cell adhesion molecule-1. (See Color Plate 22.)

Modified from Sanz & Fayad 2008.

by both modalities.[28] Comparison with histology is also favorable, at least in the carotid arteries.[29]

One potential application of MRI is the detection of subclinical atherosclerotic disease.[30, 31] It has proved useful in this respect in several large cohort studies. In asymptomatic subjects enrolled in the Framingham Heart Study (FHS), FHS coronary risk score was strongly associated with asymptomatic aortic atherosclerosis detected by MRI.[32] The prevalence and extent of aortic atherosclerosis significantly increased with age. In a substudy of the Multiethnic Study of Atherosclerosis (MESA), aortic wall thickness measured with MRI also increased as a function of age, but males and black participants had the greatest wall thickness.[33] In a 2004 study of 102 patients undergoing coronary angiography, aortic atherosclerotic plaques were detected with a higher frequency in active smokers and in those with high levels of LDL-cholesterol, but the volume and area of aortic plaques correlated most strongly with age and the presence of high blood pre ssure. Only atherosclerotic plaques located in the thoracic aorta were significantly associated with the presence of coronary artery disease.[34] Taken together, these studies confirm the strong correlation between the presence of cardiovascular risk factors and the incidence of aortic atherosclerosis.[35] It should be noted that there are racial and population differences in the response to individual risk factors, which presumably have a genetic basis.[33]

A benefit readily appreciated by pharmaceutical companies and others wishing to study the effects of drugs on plaque progression (and regression) is the low coefficient of variability of MRI plaque volume measurements.[36] This translates directly into the requirement for low patient numbers for studies investigating the effects of drugs on plaque, because any true drug effect will not be swamped by "noise" within the measuring technique. This was illustrated recently in two separate studies, where high-dose statin regimens were shown to be superior to low in terms of atheroma burden reduction, an effect that could be demonstrated with only 20 patients per group.[37,38]

MRI has sufficient resolution to image the complications of atherosclerosis.[39] A retrospective study imaged the carotid arteries of patients with a recent transient ischemic attack. Ruptured fibrous caps were detected with a much higher frequency in symptomatic patients (70%) than plaques with a fully intact thick fibrous cap (9%), confirming the ability of this technique to illustrate the underlying pathology.[40]

Recent histopathological studies[41,42] suggest that intraplaque hemorrhage may play a role in the triggering of plaque rupture and growth. A first study[43] proved that multi-contrast MRI could accurately image intraplaque hemorrhage in carotid atherosclerotic plaques using T2-weighted sequences. MRI can also distinguish between recent and remote hemorrhage on the basis of its methemoglobin content. In another prospective study,[44] the finding of hemorrhage within carotid atherosclerotic plaques was associated with an accelerated increase in subsequent plaque volume over the next 18 months. This would support the hypothesis that the presence of intraplaque hemorrhage is a potent atherogenic stimulus. These studies show the value of plaque MR imaging for both generating and testing pathological hypotheses about atherosclerosis.

Molecular MRI Imaging of Atherosclerosis

Traditional plaque imaging modalities, such as CT and multicontrast MRI, exploit anatomical variations between tissues to provide images. Molecular (or target-specific) imaging unites molecular and vascular biology with imaging modalities such as MRI, PET, and optical imaging to allow the study of biological processes noninvasively and with high-spatial resolution.[45, 46, 47, 48]

As we have seen, multicontrast MRI can characterize the various plaque components of intermediate to advanced atherosclerosis with a sensitivity in the range of 10^{-3} to 10^{-6} M.[49] But the ability to deliver a larger payload of paramagnetic particles can improve the sensitivity of the technique, especially when trying to image elements of the plaque present at low concentrations (10^{-9} to 10^{-13} M/gram of tissue).[50, 51]

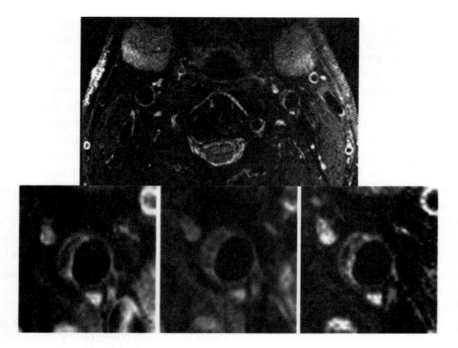

Figure 8.2

An example of multi-contrast plaque imaging at high field stregth (3T). A non-stenotic plaque is well visualized in the left carotid artery. The fibrous cap and lipid core can be seen on the high-magnification images. The T2 TSE images are acquired are a spatial resolution of 0.4 x 0.4 x 2 mm^3.

In the following paragraphs, we will discuss a variety of molecular targets that may provide improved imaging of atherosclerotic plaque using MRI.

Endothelial Dysfunction

Endothelial dysfunction is the first vascular abnormality seen in atherosclerosis and the ability to image the disease at this early stage might allow preemptive lifestyle or drug intervention to slow its progress. However, a great deal of the endothelium is dysfunctional, even in patients with only risk factors for atherosclerosis, as well as those with the established disease. While plaques at risk of rupture may express adhesion molecules, those same molecules will be found throughout the vasculature and will therefore not be a specific marker for high-risk lesions.

The ability to image VCAM has been elegantly demonstrated by Kelly et al.[52] They used a superparamagnetic fluorescent nanoparticle coupled to a payload peptide that was internalized by endothelial cells expressing VCAM. This was tested in ApoE-/- mice fed a high-cholesterol diet and was highly specific for VCAM-expressing cells, with a gold standard of immunohistochemistry.[52] In addition, a recent experimental study demonstrated that microparticles of iron oxide (MPIO) may be used as a functional MRI probe to reveal endothelial adhesion cells in mouse atherosclerosis.[53]

MR imaging of the selectin family of molecules has also been attempted, at least in vitro. Kang et al. showed that a monoclonal antibody fragment tagged with iron oxide nanoparticles was specific for human endothelial cells expressing E-selectin in culture, with an increased binding of 200 times compared to controls.[54] ICAM-1 receptors expressed on the cerebral arterial vascular endothelium have been imaged with MRI, using antibody-conjugated paramagnetic liposomes.[55] MRI provided sufficient signal enhancement to determine the areas of increased expression and binding was verified by fluorescent histopathology.

Angiogenesis

Recent pathological studies have revealed the central role of plaque neovascularization in contributing to atherosclerotic plaque vulnerability.[56, 57, 58] The presence of neovessels is strongly associated with plaque inflammation, macrophage content, and likelihood of rupture,[57] presumably by allowing an alternative route for entry of monocytes into the plaque.

Gadolinium chelates represent the most commonly used MRI contrast agents for imaging plaque new vessels. These paramagnetic agents increase the luminal signal on MRI images after intravenous injection and are therefore good candidates for measuring plaque neovasculature.[59] Such techniques have been used in oncology imaging to quantify new vessels associated with tumors.[60, 61] Although Kerwin and colleagues demonstrated a correlation between the increase in signal intensity in carotid atherosclerotic plaques with gadolinium-enhanced MRI and the extent of neovessels in plaques measured histologically, this imaging modality is not specific for neovascularization and is limited because gadolinium chelates rapidly distribute into the extracellular space.[62] Further improvements in the quantification of plaque neovasculature with these agents will require the development of new compartmental kinetic models of the biodistribution of these contrast agents within atherosclerotic plaques.[63]

Alternatively, MRI contrast agents that remain within the bloodstream, or diffuse more slowly into the extracellular space, are currently being developed.[64] For example, a novel agent targeting the integrin $\alpha_v\beta_3$ (specifically expressed on the endothelial surface of neovasculature) has been developed to identify regions in the vessel wall undergoing neovascularization. Winter et al. demonstrated in a rabbit model of atherosclerosis in which regions of neovascularization in plaques had a 47% increase in signal intensity on MRI after the injection of $\alpha_v\beta_3$-targeted nanoparticles.[65] Another epitope that has been successfully exploited for imaging angiogenesis within plaque (at least in ApoE-/- mice) is fibronectin. The binding of an antifibronectin antibody was confirmed both autoradiographically and by the use of a fluorescent probe, and was specific for the vasovasorum of the atheroscleorisc plaque.[66]

Thrombus

Intraluminal thrombosis represents the final step in the evolution of vulnerable atherosclerotic plaque and is therefore a candidate target for novel specific MRI contrast agents.[67] Histologic studies have demonstrated that superficial thrombus superimposed on a ruptured atherosclerotic plaque characterizes those plaques at high risk of ischemic events,[68] presumably by implying previous asymptomatic rupture.

Several approaches have been taken to image thrombus with MRI. Yu et al. used a gadolinium-loaded nanoparticle coupled to a fibrin antibody and tested this against in vitro thrombus.[69] They were able to demonstrate significant signal enhancement and confirmed tight binding of the antibody with scanning electron microscopy. A similar method, but one using a different nanoparticle construct, was employed successfully by Winter.[70]

A recent paper analyzed the histology of intracoronary thrombus aspirated from 211 patients with acute myocardial infarction. It was shown that more than 50% of the culprit thrombi were at least days or weeks old.[71] Based on this premise, a new fibrin-specific MR contrast agent has recently been designed. With this agent, thrombus resulting from plaque rupture has been identified using MRI in a rabbit model. In the 25 arterial thrombi induced by carotid crush injury, Botnar et al. demonstrated a sensitivity and specificity of 100% for in vivo thrombus detection.[72]

At our own institution, Sirol et al. used the same fibrin-specific MR contrast agent (EP-1242) in 12 guinea pigs to demonstrate that the signal intensity of the thrombus was increased by more than four times compared to noncontrast images. The detection of thrombi improved from 42% pickup precontrast injection compared to 100% detection after injection.[73] The ability to identify different thrombus components with molecular MRI may allow its age to be determined noninvasively. This has important clinical implications because histologic studies have shown that many microplaque rupture events with thrombus formation often predate the catastrophic rupture event that causes the clinical syndrome. The ability to detect these early warnings might allow intense therapy or device placement to avert symptoms.

In this regard, our group has recently tested another experimental fibrin-targeted peptide (EP-2104R) for thrombus detection, and compared it to MRI, both without contrast and with gadolinium contrast MRI.[74] Using this novel agent it was possible to discriminate between occlusive and nonocclusive thrombi and to track thrombus as it aged and became more organized by fibrous tissue infiltration.

Extracellular Matrix

Other novel MRI contrast agents have been found to accumulate within atherosclerotic plaques. For example, gadofluorine M is a lipophilic, macrocyclic, water-soluble, gadolinium chelate complex with a perfluorinated side chain. Both Sirol and Barkhausen separately demonstrated that gadofluorine M significantly increased signal intensity in rabbit aortic plaques compared to controls. A strong correlation was found between the intensity of MRI signal enhancement after the injection of gadofluorine and the presence of lipid-rich plaques on corresponding histological sections.[75, 76] This suggests a high affinity of gadofluorine M for atherosclerotic plaque. There is now emerging data that gadofluorine M is restricted to the extracellular space of plaques and may interact with resident proteins in the extracellular matrix milieu.

Plaque Inflammation

The fibrous cap separates the artery lumen from the thrombogenic core of the plaque and, as such, is the final barrier to thrombus formation. Thus, identifying factors that lead to the disruption of the fibrous cap may aid in targeting therapy to patients at risk of plaque rupture.

Matrix metalloproteinases are responsible for the degradation of proteins in the extracellular matrix causing structural weakening of the cap. The role of MMPs in plaque instability and matrix remodeling in atherosclerotic plaque has been well described.[18] Therefore, the ability to detect MMP activity in the fibrous cap with MRI may not only provide important information regarding risk of possible plaque rupture but may also allow tracking of MMP inhibition with therapy.[77, 78]

Recently, a gadolinium-based MRI constrast agent P947 was evaluated in vivo using ApoE-/- mice and ex vivo in hyperlipidemic rabbits. The agent P947 has affinity and specificity toward matrix metalloproteinase (MMP)-rich plaques. The study showed a showed a preferential accumulation of P947 in atherosclerotic lesions compared with the nontargeted reference compound, Gd-DOTA.[79]

Resident plaque macrophages have been successfully imaged using ultrasmall superparamagnetic particles of iron oxide (USPIO). These are removed from the circulation by the reticuloendothelial system and accumulate in macrophages present in atherosclerotic plaques. Macrophages play a pivotal role in the destabilization of atherosclerotic plaques by secreting large quantities of fibrous cap-degrading MMPs, along with proinflammatory cytokines and tissue factor.[80] Iron oxide contrast agents have superparamagnetic properties, i.e., they decrease T2 relaxation time by generating heterogeneities in the local magnetic field, and can be detected on MRI as signal voids on T2-weighted sequences.

Kooi et al. studied 11 symptomatic patients scheduled for carotid endarterectomy with USPIO-enhanced MRI, and found a 24% decrease in signal intensity on corresponding T2-weighted sequences, and histologically verified uptake of USPIO in 75% of ruptured or rupture-prone lesions.[81] Trivedi et al. expanded on this work and demonstrated that the optimum time for imaging symptomatic carotid plaque was between 24 and 36 hours after injection of USPIO.[82, 83] USPIO plaque imaging with MR has been validated against histopathology at time points out to 8 weeks in an animal model. Iron staining closely matched that of macrophage distribution within the plaque, but interestingly only a subset of smaller-sized macrophages actively accumulated USPIO.[84, 85] New image acquisition methods that render the superparamagnetic signal loss as positive enhancement promises to improve the detection of plaques in vivo.[86] Finally, monocyte/macrophage recruitment into plaques after an inflammatory stimulus has been tracked by USPIO in a mouse model,[87] which might be useful in assessing the antiatherogenic potential of new drugs.

Macrophages within atherosclerotic plaques have also been targeted for imaging by the use of gadolinium-loaded immunomicelles. These agents, with diameters between 20 and 120nm, are composed of phospholipids, a surfactant, and an aliphatic chain with Gd-DTPA attached at the polar head group. The polar head group of the aliphatic chain can be attached to antibodies directly or via a biotin-avidin bridge. Using this model, we have made micelles that have more than 10,000 Gd ions on each micelle surface and the ability to specifically target the macrophage scavenger receptor (MSR). Promising work is currently underway and has demonstrated enhancement of murine atherosclerotic plaque on MRI using immunomicelles that target the MSR-A.[88]

Our group recently developed another type of imaging agent based on a recombinant high-density lipoprotein (rHDL) molecule that incorporates gadolinium-DTPA phospholipids.[89] Natural HDL's role in the body is that of removing lipid from atherosclerotic plaque and returning it to the liver (reverse cholesterol transport). Elevated levels of HDL cholesterol are associated with a reduction in plaque rupture events, presumably because of this protective effect.[90] The rHDL imaging agent has a small diameter (7–12nm) allowing it to diffuse into atherosclerotic plaques, and, by using endogenous transport molecules, it does not trigger any immune reaction. Atherosclerotic plaques had a 35% increase of MRI signal intensity 24 hours after the injection of these rHDL particles in an ApoE knockout mouse model. Furthermore, fluorescent rHDL colocalized with macrophages present in atherosclerotic plaques with confocal microscopy. Figure 8.3 demonstrates the enhancement of atherosclerotic plaques after the injection of rHDL.

CONCLUSIONS AND FUTURE DIRECTIONS

Thanks to the absence of ionizing radiation, MRI represents the imaging technology of choice for the noninvasive high-spatial resolution detection and serial monitoring of atherosclerotic plaques in the carotid arteries and aorta. High image quality and sensitivity to small changes in plaque size mean that there is little variance between measurements, permitting small sample sizes to be used in comparative studies. Thus, multicontrast MRI is ideally suited for use in evaluation of novel antiatheroma drugs.

The development of functional molecular imaging of atherosclerosis may also help to reveal the key pathological steps that lead from a stable atherosclerotic plaque to an acute ischemic event. However, recent clinical studies have underscored the multiple locations of vulnerable and ruptured atherosclerotic plaques and the diffuse inflammation of the arterial tree in patients with acute ischemic events compared to stable patients.[91] Therefore, the concept of detecting infrequent vulnerable atherosclerotic plaques with imaging and treating

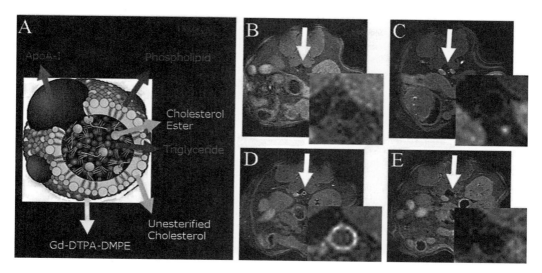

Figure 8.3

(A) This represents the reconstituted HDL-like MRI contrast agent composed of an HDL-like particle and a phospholipid-based contrast agent (Gd-DTPA-DMPE). Transverse in vivo MR images of the abdominal aorta in an 8-week-old mouse at 9.4 Tesla before (B), 1 hour (C), 24 hours (D) and 48 hours (E) after the injection of recombinant HDL-like nanoparticles are displayed. The insets denote the magnification of the aortic region.

Adapted from Frias, Williams, Fisher, & Fayad, 2004.

them individually has started to shift to a more global process of identifying vulnerable patients at high risk of acute clinical events, irrespective of the arterial location.[92]

In the future, atherosclerosis imaging with MRI may help to focus individual evaluation of cardiovascular risk and to optimize anti-atherosclerotic therapies.

◇◇◇◇◇◇◇◇◇◇◇◇

REFERENCES

1. British Heart Foundation Health Promotion Research Group 2005, *Coronary Heart Disease Statistics* London, UK.

2. Svindland, A. & Torvik, A. 1988, Atherosclerotic carotid disease in asymptomatic individuals: An histological study of 53 cases, *Acta Neurol Scand*, vol. 78, no. 6, pp. 506-517.

3. Sanz J, Fayad ZA. Imaging of atherosclerotic cardiovascular disease. *Nature* 2008;451(7181):953-957.

4. Ku, D. N., Giddens, D. P., Zarins, C. K., & Glagov, S. 1985, Pulsatile flow and atherosclerosis in the human carotid bifurcation. Positive correlation between plaque location and low oscillating shear stress, *Arteriosclerosis*, vol. 5, no. 3, pp. 293-302.

5. Cunningham, K. S. & Gotlieb, A. I. 2005, The role of shear stress in the pathogenesis of atherosclerosis, *Lab Invest*, vol. 85, no. 1, pp. 9-23.

6. Cushing, S. D., Berliner, J. A., Valente, A. J., Territo, M. C., Navab, M., Parhami, F., Gerrity, R., Schwartz, C. J., & Fogelman, A. M. 1990, Minimally modified low density lipoprotein induces monocyte chemotactic protein 1 in human endothelial cells and smooth

muscle cells, *Proc Natl Acad Sci U S A*, vol. 87, no. 13, pp. 5134-5138.

7. Hamilton, J. A., Myers, D., Jessup, W., Cochrane, F., Byrne, R., Whitty, G., & Moss, S. 1999, Oxidized LDL can induce macrophage survival, DNA synthesis, and enhanced proliferative response to CSF-1 and GM-CSF, *Arterioscler Thromb Vasc Biol*, vol. 19, no. 1, pp. 98-105.

8. Ross, R. 1999, Atherosclerosis—an inflammatory disease, *N Engl J Med*, vol. 340, no. 2, pp. 115-126.

9. Zernecke A, Bernhagen J, Weber C. 2008 Macrophage Migration Inhibitory Factor in Cardiovascular Disease, *Circulation*, vol. 117, no. 12, pp. 1594-602.

10. Glagov, S., Weisenberg, E., Zarins, C. K., Stankunavicius, R., & Kolettis, G. J. 1987, Compensatory enlargement of human atherosclerotic coronary arteries, *N Engl J Med*, vol. 316, no. 22, pp. 1371-1375.

11. Keenan , N.G., Pennell, D.J., Mohiaddin, R.H. 2008, Glagov remodeling in the atherosclerotic carotid artery by Cardiovascular Magnetic Resonance, *Heart*, vol. 94, no 2, pp. 228.

12. Fuster, V., Moreno, P. R., Fayad, Z. A., Corti, R., & Badimon, J. J. 2005, Atherothrombosis and High-Risk Plaque: Part I: Evolving Concepts, *Journal of the American College of Cardiology*, vol. 46, no. 6, pp. 937-954.

13. Moreno, P.R., Purushothaman, K.R., Sirol, M., Levy, A.P., Fuster, V. 2006, Neovascularization in Human Atherosclerosis, *Circulation*, vol. 113, no. 18, pp. 2245-2252.

14. Juonala, M.,Viikari, J.S., Ronnema, T., Marniemi, J., Jula, A., Loo, B.M., Raitakari, O.T., 2008, Associations of Dyslipidemias From Childhood to Adulthood With Carotid Intima-Media Thickness, Elasticity, and Brachial Flow-Mediated Dilatation in Adulthood. The Cardiovascular Risk in Young Finns Study, *Atherosclerosis Thrombosis Vascular Biology* February 28 (Epub ahead of print).

15. Farb, A., Burke, A. P., Tang, A. L., Liang, T. Y.,Mannan, P., Smialek, J., & Virmani, R. 1996, Coronary plaque erosion without rupture into a lipid core. A frequent cause of coronary thrombosis in sudden coronary death, *Circulation*, vol. 93, no. 7, pp. 1354-1363.

16. Davies, M. J. 1995, Acute coronary thrombosis--the role of plaque disruption and its initiation and prevention, *Eur Heart J*, vol. 16 Suppl L, pp. 3-7.

17. Bennett, M. R., Evan, G. I., & Schwartz, S. M. 1995, Apoptosis of human vascular smooth muscle cells derived from normal vessels and coronary atherosclerotic plaques, *J Clin Invest*, vol. 95, no. 5, pp. 2266-2274.

18. Rudd, J. H., Davies, J. R., & Weissberg, P. L. 2005, Imaging of atherosclerosis—can we predict plaque rupture? *Trends Cardiovasc Med*, vol. 15, no. 1, pp. 17-24.

19. Cannon, C. P., Braunwald, E., McCabe, C. H., Rader, D. J., Rouleau, J. L., Belder, R., Joyal, S. V., Hill, K. A., Pfeffer, M. A., & Skene, A. M. 2004, Intensive versus moderate lipid lowering with statins after acute coronary syndromes, *N Engl J Med*, vol. 350, no. 15, pp. 1495-1504.

20. Schoenhagen, P., Tuzcu, E.M., Apperson-Hansen, C., Wang, C., Wolski, K., Lin, S., Sipahi, I., Nicholls, S.J., Magyar,W.A., Loyd,A., Churchill, T., Crowe, T., Nissen,S.E., 2006, Determinants of arterial wall remodeling during lipid-lowering therapy: serial intravascular ultrasound observations from the Reversal of Atherosclerosis with Aggressive Lipid Lowering Therapy (REVERSAL) trial, *Circulation*, vol.113, no.24, pp. 2826-2834.

21. Ibanez, B., Vilahur, G., Cimmino, G., Speidl, W.S., Pinero, A., Choi, B.G., Zafar, M.U., Santos-Gallego, C.G., Krause, B., Badimon, L., Fuster, V., Badimon, J.J. 2008, Rapid change in plaque size, composition, and molecular footprint after recombinant apolipoprotein A-I Milano (ETC-216) administration: magnetic resonance imaging study in an experimental model of atherosclerosis, *J Am Coll Cardiol*, vol. 15, no. 11, pp. 1104-1109.

22. Saam,T., Hatsukami, T.S., Takaya, N., Chu, B., Underhill, H., Kerwin, W.S., Cai, J., Ferguson, M.S., Yuan, C., 2007, The vulnerable, or high-risk, atherosclerotic plaque: noninvasive MR imaging for characterization and assessment, *Radiology*, vol. 244, no.1,pp.64-77.

23. Fayad, Z. A. & Fuster, V. 2000, Characterization of atherosclerotic plaques by magnetic resonance imaging *Ann NY Acad Sci*, vol. 902, pp. 173-186.

24. Toussaint, J. F., LaMuraglia, G. M., Southern, J. F., Fuster, V., & Kantor, H. L. 1996, Magnetic resonance images lipid, fibrous, calcified, hemorrhagic, and thrombotic components of human atherosclerosis in vivo, *Circulation*, vol. 94, no. 5, pp. 932-938.

25. Yuan, C., Mitsumori, L. M., Beach, K. W., & Maravilla, K. R. 2001a, Carotid atherosclerotic plaque: noninvasive MR characterization and identification of vulnerable lesions, *Radiology*, vol. 221, no. 2, pp. 285-299.

26. Yuan, C., Mitsumori, L. M., Ferguson, M. S., Polissar, N. L., Echelard, D., Ortiz, G., Small, R., Davies, J. W., Kerwin, W. S., & Hatsukami, T. S. 2001b, In vivo accuracy of multispectral magnetic resonance imaging for identifying lipid-rich necrotic cores and

intraplaque hemorrhage in advanced human carotid plaques, *Circulation*, vol. 104, no. 17, pp. 2051-2056.

27. Mani, V., Itskovich, V. V., Szimtenings, M., Aguinaldo, J. G., Samber, D. D., Mizsei, G., & Fayad, Z. A. 2004, Rapid extended coverage simultaneous multisection black-blood vessel wall MR imaging, *Radiology*, vol. 232, no. 1, pp. 281-288.

28. Fayad, Z. A., Nahar, T., Fallon, J. T., Goldman, M., Aguinaldo, J. G., Badimon, J. J., Shinnar, M., Chesebro, J. H., & Fuster, V. 2000, In vivo magnetic resonance evaluation of atherosclerotic plaques in the human thoracic aorta: a comparison with transesophageal echocardiography, *Circulation*, vol. 101, no. 21, pp. 2503-2509.

29. Cai, J. M., Hatsukami, T. S., Ferguson, M. S., Small, R., Polissar, N. L., & Yuan, C. 2002, Classification of human carotid atherosclerotic lesions with in vivo multicontrast magnetic resonance imaging, *Circulation*, vol. 106, no. 11, pp. 1368-1373.

30. Diamond, G.A., Kaul, S., Shah, P.K., 2007, Screen testing cardiovascular prevention in asymptomatic diabetic patients, *J Am Coll Cardiol,* vol.49, no.19, pp.1915-1917.

31. Saam, T., Cai, J., Ma, L., Cai,Y.Q., Ferguson, M.S., Polissar, N.L., Hatsukami, T.S., Yuan, C., 2006,Comparison of symptomatic and asymptomatic atherosclerotic carotid plaque features with in vivo MR imaging, *Radiology,* vol. 240, no. 2, pp.464-472.

32. Jaffer, F. A., O'Donnell, C. J., Larson, M. G., Chan, S. K., Kissinger, K. V., Kupka, M. J., Salton, C., Botnar, R. M., Levy, D., & Manning, W. J. 2002, Age and sex distribution of subclinical aortic atherosclerosis: a magnetic resonance imaging examination of the Framingham Heart Study, *Arterioscler Thromb Vasc Biol,* vol. 22, no. 5, pp. 849-854.

33. Li, A. E., Kamel, I., Rando, F., Anderson, M., Kumbasar, B., Lima, J. A. C., & Bluemke, D. A. 2004, Using MRI to assess aortic wall thickness in the multiethnic study of atherosclerosis: distribution by race, sex, and age, *American Journal of Roentgenology*, vol. 182, no. 3, pp. 593-597.

34. Taniguchi, H., Momiyama, Y., Fayad, Z. A., Ohmori, R., Ashida, K., Kihara, T., Hara, A., Arakawa, K., Kameyama, A., Noya, K., Nagata, M., Nakamura, H., & Ohsuzu, F. 2004, In vivo magnetic resonance evaluation of associations between aortic atherosclerosis and both risk factors and coronary artery disease in patients referred for coronary angiography, *Am Heart J*, vol. 148, no. 1, pp. 137-143.

35. Momiyama, Y., Kato, R., Fayad, Z. A., Tanaka, N., Taniguchi, H., Ohmori, R., Kihara, T., Kameyama, A., Miyazaki, K., Kimura, K., Arakawa, K., Kusuhara, M., Nagata, M., Nakamura, H., & Ohsuzu, F. 2006, A Possible Association Between Coronary Plaque Instability and Complex Plaques in Abdominal Aorta, *Arterioscler Thromb Vasc Biol*

36. Saam, T., Kerwin, W. S., Chu, B., Cai, J., Kampschulte, A., Hatsukami, T. S., Zhao, X. Q., Polissar, N. L., Neradilek, B., Yarnykh, V. L., Flemming, K., Huston, J., III, Insull, W., Jr., Morrisett, J. D., Rand, S. D., DeMarco, K. J., & Yuan, C. 2005, Sample size calculation for clinical trials using magnetic resonance imaging for the quantitative assessment of carotid atherosclerosis, *J Cardiovasc Magn Reson,* vol. 7, no. 5, pp. 799-808.

37. Yonemura, A., Momiyama, Y., Fayad, Z. A., Ayaori, M., Ohmori, R., Higashi, K., Kihara, T., Sawada, S., Iwamoto, N., Ogura, M., Taniguchi, H., Kusuhara, M., Nagata, M., Nakamura, H., Tamai, S., & Ohsuzu, F. 2005, Effect of lipid-lowering therapy with atorvastatin on atherosclerotic aortic plaques detected by noninvasive magnetic resonance imaging, *J Am Coll Cardiol*, vol. 45, no. 5, pp. 733-742.

38. Corti, R., Fuster, V., Fayad, Z. A., Worthley, S. G., Helft, G., Chaplin, W. F., Muntwyler, J., Viles-Gonzalez, J. F., Weinberger, J., Smith, D. A., Mizsei, G., & Badimon, J. J. 2005, Effects of aggressive versus conventional lipid-lowering therapy by simvastatin on human atherosclerotic lesions: a prospective, randomized, double-blind trial with high-resolution magnetic resonance imaging, *J Am Coll Cardiol*, vol. 46, no. 1, pp. 106-112.

39. Briley-Saebo, K.C., Mulder, W.J., Mani, V., Hyafil, F., Amirbekian, V., Aguinaldo, J.G., Fisher, E.A., Fayad, Z.A., 2007, Magnetic resonance imaging of vulnerable atherosclerotic plaques: current imaging strategies and molecular imaging probes, *J Magn Reson Imaging,* vol. 26, no.3, pp.460-479.

40. Yuan, C., Zhang, S. X., Polissar, N. L., Echelard, D., Ortiz, G., Davis, J. W., Ellington, E., Ferguson, M. S., & Hatsukami, T. S. 2002, Identification of fibrous cap rupture with magnetic resonance imaging is highly associated with recent transient ischemic attack or stroke, *Circulation*, vol. 105, no. 2, pp. 181-185.

41. Burke, A. P., Farb, A., Malcom, G. T., Liang, Y., Smialek, J. E., & Virmani, R. 1999, Plaque rupture and sudden death related to exertion in men with coronary artery disease, *JAMA*, vol. 281, no. 10, pp. 921-926.

42. Kolodgie, F. D., Gold, H. K., Burke, A. P., Fowler, D. R., Kruth, H. S., Weber, D. K., Farb, A., Guerrero, L. J., Hayase, M., Kutys, R., Narula, J., Finn, A. V., & Virmani, R. 2003, Intraplaque hemorrhage and progression of coronary atheroma, *N Engl J Med*, vol. 349, no. 24, pp. 2316-2325.

43. Chu, B., Kampschulte, A., Ferguson, M. S., Kerwin, W. S., Yarnykh, V. L., O'Brien, K. D., Polissar, N. L., Hatsukami, T. S., & Yuan, C. 2004, Hemorrhage in the atherosclerotic carotid plaque: a high-resolution MRI study, *Stroke*, vol. 35, no. 5, pp. 1079-1084.

44. Takaya, N., Yuan, C., Chu, B., Saam, T., Polissar, N. L., Jarvik, G. P., Isaac, C., McDonough, J., Natiello, C., Small, R., Ferguson, M. S., & Hatsukami, T. S. 2005, Presence of intraplaque hemorrhage stimulates progression of carotid atherosclerotic plaques: a high-resolution magnetic resonance imaging study, *Circulation*, vol. 111, no. 21, pp. 2768-2775.

45. Wu, J.C., Bengel, F.M., Gambhir, S.S., 2007, Cardiovascular molecular imaging *Radiology*, vol. 244, no.2, pp. 337-355.

46. Jaffer, F.A., Libby, P., Weissleder, R.. 2007, Molecular imaging of cardiovascular disease, *Circulation*, vol.116, no.9, pp.1052-1061.

47. Wickline, S.A., Neubauer, A.M., Winter, P.M., Caruthers, S.D., Lanza, G.M., 2007, Molecular imaging and therapy of atherosclerosis with targeted nanoparticles, *J Magn Reson Imaging*, vol. 25, no.4, pp.667-680.

48. Sosnovik, D.E., Nahrendorf, M., Weissleder, R., 2007, Molecular magnetic resonance imaging in cardiovascular medicine, *Circulation*, vol.115, no.15, pp.2076-2086.

49. Aime, S., Cabella, C., Colombatto, S., Geninatti, C. S., Gianolio, E., & Maggioni, F. 2002, Insights into the use of paramagnetic Gd(III) complexes in MR-molecular imaging investigations, *J Magn Reson Imaging*, vol. 16, no. 4, pp. 394-406.

50. Choudhury, R. P., Fuster, V., & Fayad, Z. A. 2004, Molecular, cellular and functional imaging of atherothrombosis, *Nat Rev Drug Discov*, vol. 3, no. 11, pp. 913-925.

51. Lipinski, M. J., Fuster, V., Fisher, E. A., & Fayad, Z. A. 2004a, Technology insight: targeting of biological molecules for evaluation of high-risk atherosclerotic plaques with magnetic resonance imaging, *Nat Clin Pract Cardiovasc Med*, vol. 1, no. 1, pp. 48-55.

52. Kelly, K. A., Allport, J. R., Tsourkas, A., Shinde-Patil, V. R., Josephson, L., & Weissleder, R. 2005, Detection of vascular adhesion molecule-1 expression using a novel multimodal nanoparticle, *Circ Res*, vol. 96, no. 3, pp. 327-336.

53. McAteer, M.A., Schneider, J.E., Ali, Z.A., Warrick, N., Bursill, C.A., von zur Muhlen, C., Greaves, D.R., Neubauer, S., Channon, K.M., Choudhury, R.P., 2008, Magnetic resonance imaging of endothelial adhesion molecules in mouse atherosclerosis using dual-targeted microparticles of iron oxide, *Arterioscler Thromb Vasc Biol*, vol.28, no. 1, pp.77-83.

54. Kang, H. W., Josephson, L., Petrovsky, A., Weissleder, R., & Bogdanov, A., Jr. 2002, Magnetic resonance imaging of inducible E-selectin expression in human endothelial cell culture, *Bioconjug Chem*, vol. 13, no. 1, pp. 122-127.

55. Sipkins, D. A., Gijbels, K., Tropper, F. D., Bednarski, M., Li, K. C., & Steinman, L. 2000, ICAM-1 expression in autoimmune encephalitis visualized using magnetic resonance imaging, *J Neuroimmunol*, vol. 104, no. 1, pp. 1-9.

56. Kockx, M. M., Cromheeke, K. M., Knaapen, M. W., Bosmans, J. M., De Meyer, G. R., Herman, A. G., & Bult, H. 2003, Phagocytosis and macrophage activation associated with hemorrhagic microvessels in human atherosclerosis, *Arterioscler Thromb Vasc Biol*, vol. 23, no. 3, pp. 440-446.

57. Kumamoto, M., Nakashima, Y., & Sueishi, K. 1995, Intimal neovascularization in human coronary atherosclerosis: its origin and pathophysiological significance, *Hum Pathol*, vol. 26, no. 4, pp. 450-456.

58. Moulton, K. S., Heller, E., Konerding, M. A., Flynn, E., Palinski, W., & Folkman, J. 1999, Angiogenesis inhibitors endostatin or TNP-470 reduce intimal neovascularization and plaque growth in apolipoprotein E-deficient mice, *Circulation*, vol. 99, no. 13, pp. 1726-1732.

59. Mulder WJ, Strijkers GJ, Vucic E, Cormode DP, Nicolay K, Fayad ZA., 2007, Magnetic resonance molecular imaging contrast agents and their application in atherosclerosis, *Top Magn Reson Imaging.*, vol. 18, no.5, pp. 409-417

60. Jacobs, M. A., Barker, P. B., Argani, P., Ouwerkerk, R., Bhujwalla, Z. M., & Bluemke, D. A. 2005, Combined dynamic contrast enhanced breast MR and proton spectroscopic imaging: a feasibility study, *J Magn Reson Imaging*, vol. 21, no. 1, pp. 23-28.

61. Wang, B., Gao, Z. Q., & Yan, X. 2005, Correlative study of angiogenesis and dynamic contrast-enhanced magnetic resonance imaging features of hepatocellular carcinoma, *Acta R adiol*, vol. 46, no. 4, pp. 353-358.

62. Kerwin, W., Hooker, A., Spilker, M., Vicini, P., Ferguson, M., Hatsukami, T., & Yuan, C. 2003, Quantitative magnetic resonance imaging analysis of neovasculature volume in carotid atherosclerotic plaque, *Circulation*, vol. 107, no. 6, pp. 851-856.

63. Lauffer, R. B., Parmelee, D. J., Dunham, S. U., Ouellet, H. S., Dolan, R. P., Witte, S., McMurry, T. J., & Walovitch, R. C. 1998, MS-325: albumin-targeted

contrast agent for MR angiography, *Radiology*, vol. 207, no. 2, pp. 529-538.

64. Port, M., Meyer, D., Bonnemain, B., Corot, C., Schaefer, M., Rousseaux, O., Simonot, C., Bourrinet, P., Benderbous, S., Dencausse, A., & Devoldere, L. 1999, P760 and P775: MRI contrast agents characterized by new pharmacokinetic properties, *MAGMA*, vol. 8, no. 3, pp. 172-176.

65. Winter, P. M., Morawski, A. M., Caruthers, S. D., Fuhrhop, R. W., Zhang, H., Williams, T. A., Allen, J. S., Lacy, E. K., Robertson, J. D., Lanza, G. M., & Wickline, S. A. 2003b, Molecular imaging of angiogenesis in early-stage atherosclerosis with alpha(v) beta3-integrin-targeted nanoparticles, *Circulation*, vol. 108, no. 18, pp. 2270-2274.

66. Matter, C. M., Schuler, P. K., Alessi, P., Meier, P., Ricci, R., Zhang, D., Halin, C., Castellani, P., Zardi, L., Hofer, C. K., Montani, M., Neri, D., & Luscher, T. F. 2004, Molecular imaging of atherosclerotic plaques using a human antibody against the extra-domain B of fibronectin, *Circ Res*, vol. 95, no. 12, pp. 1225-1233.

67. Spuentrup, E., Botnar, R.M., Wiethoff, A.J., Ibrahim, T., Kelle, S., Katoh, M., Ozgun, M., Nagel, E., Vymazal, J., Graham, P.B., Günther, R.W., Maintz, D., 2008, MR imaging of thrombi using EP-2104R, a fibrin-specific contrast agent: initial results in patients *Eur Radiol* Apr 19; [Epub ahead of print]

68. Virmani, R., Kolodgie, F. D., Burke, A. P., Farb, A., & Schwartz, S. M. 2000, Lessons from sudden coronary death: a comprehensive morphological classification scheme for atherosclerotic lesions, *Arterioscler Thromb Vasc Biol*, vol. 20, no. 5, pp. 1262-1275.

69. Yu, X., Song, S. K., Chen, J., Scott, M. J., Fuhrhop, R. J., Hall, C. S., Gaffney, P. J., Wickline, S. A., & Lanza, G. M. 2000, High-resolution MRI characterization of human thrombus using a novel fibrin-targeted paramagnetic nanoparticle contrast agent, *Magn Reson Med*, vol. 44, no. 6, pp. 867-872.

70. Winter, P. M., Caruthers, S. D., Yu, X., Song, S. K., Chen, J., Miller, B., Bulte, J. W., Robertson, J. D., Gaffney, P. J., Wickline, S. A., & Lanza, G. M. 2003a, Improved molecular imaging contrast agent for detection of human thrombus, *Magn Reson Med*, vol. 50, no. 2, pp. 411-416.

71. Rittersma, S. Z., van der Wal, A. C., Koch, K. T., Piek, J. J., Henriques, J. P., Mulder, K. J., Ploegmakers, J. P., Meesterman, M., & de Winter, R. J. 2005, Plaque instability frequently occurs days or weeks before occlusive coronary thrombosis: a pathological thrombectomy study in primary percutaneous coronary intervention, *Circulation*, vol. 111, no. 9, pp. 1160-1165.

72. Botnar, R. M., Perez, A. S., Witte, S., Wiethoff, A. J., Laredo, J., Hamilton, J., Quist, W., Parsons, E. C., Jr., Vaidya, A., Kolodziej, A., Barrett, J. A., Graham, P. B., Weisskoff, R. M., Manning, W. J., & Johnstone, M. T. 2004, In vivo molecular imaging of acute and subacute thrombosis using a fibrin-binding magnetic resonance imaging contrast agent, *Circulation*, vol. 109, no. 16, pp. 2023-2029.

73. Sirol, M., Aguinaldo, J. G., Graham, P. B., Weisskoff, R., Lauffer, R., Mizsei, G., Chereshnev, I., Fallon, J. T., Reis, E., Fuster, V., Toussaint, J. F., & Fayad, Z. A. 2005a, Fibrin-targeted contrast agent for improvement of in vivo acute thrombus detection with magnetic resonance imaging, *Atherosclerosis*, vol. 182, no. 1, pp. 79-85.

74. Sirol, M., Fuster, V., Badimon, J. J., Fallon, J. T., Moreno, P. R., Toussaint, J. F., & Fayad, Z. A. 2005b, Chronic thrombus detection with in vivo magnetic resonance imaging and a fibrin-targeted contrast agent, *Circulation*, vol. 112, no. 11, pp. 1594-1600.

75. Barkhausen, J., Ebert, W., Heyer, C., Debatin, J. F., & Weinmann, H. J. 2003, Detection of atherosclerotic plaque with Gadofluorine-enhanced magnetic resonance imaging, *Circulation*, vol. 108, no. 5, pp. 605-609.

76. Sirol, M., Itskovich, V. V., Mani, V., Aguinaldo, J. G., Fallon, J. T., Misselwitz, B., Weinmann, H. J., Fuster, V., Toussaint, J. F., & Fayad, Z. A. 2004, Lipid-rich atherosclerotic plaques detected by gadofluorine-enhanced in vivo magnetic resonance imaging, *Circulation*, vol. 109, no. 23, pp. 2890-2896.

77. Bremer, C., Tung, C. H., & Weissleder, R. 2001, In vivo molecular target assessment of matrix metalloproteinase inhibition, *Nat Med*, vol. 7, no. 6, pp. 743-748.

78. Nighoghossian, N., Derex, L., & Douek, P. 2005, The vulnerable carotid artery plaque: current imaging methods and new perspectives, *Stroke*, vol. 36, no. 12, pp. 2764-2772.

79. Lancelot, E., Amirbekian, V., Brigger, I., Raynaud, J.S., Ballet, S., David, C., Rousseaux, O., Le Greneur, S., Port, M., Lijnen, H.R., Bruneval, P., Michel, J.B., Ouimet, T., Roques, B., Amirbekian, S., Hyafil, F., Vucic, E., Aguinaldo, J.G., Corot, C., Fayad, Z.A.,2008, Evaluation of matrix metalloproteinases in atherosclerosis using a novel noninvasive imaging approach, *Arterioscler Thromb Vasc Biol*, vol.28, no.3, pp.425-432.

80. Libby, P. 2001, Current concepts of the pathogenesis of the acute coronary syndromes, *Circulation*, vol. 104, no. 3, pp. 365-372.

81. Kooi, M. E., Cappendijk, V. C., Cleutjens, K. B., Kessels, A. G., Kitslaar, P. J., Borgers, M., Frederik, P. M., Daemen, M. J., & van Engelshoven, J. M. 2003, Accumulation of ultrasmall superparamagnetic particles of iron oxide in human atherosclerotic plaques can be detected by in vivo magnetic resonance imaging, *Circulation*, vol. 107, no. 19, pp. 2453-2458.

82. Trivedi, R., King-Im, J., & Gillard, J. 2003, Accumulation of ultrasmall superparamagnetic particles of iron oxide in human atherosclerotic plaque, *Circulation*, vol. 108, no. 19, p. e140.

83. Trivedi, R. A., King-Im, J. M., Graves, M. J., Cross, J. J., Horsley, J., Goddard, M. J., Skepper, J. N., Quartey, G., Warburton, E., Joubert, I., Wang, L., Kirkpatrick, P. J., Brown, J., & Gillard, J. H. 2004, In vivo detection of macrophages in human carotid atheroma: temporal dependence of ultrasmall superparamagnetic particles of iron oxide-enhanced MRI, *Stroke*, vol. 35, no. 7, pp. 1631-1635.

84. Hyafil, F., Laissy, J. P., Mazighi, M., Tchetche, D., Louedec, L., Adle-Biassette, H., Chillon, S., Henin, D., Jacob, M. P., Letourneur, D., & Feldman, L. J. 2006, Ferumoxtran-10-enhanced MRI of the hypercholesterolemic rabbit aorta: relationship between signal loss and macrophage infiltration, *Arterioscler Thromb Vasc Biol,* vol. 26, no. 1, pp. 176-181.

85. Yancy, A. D., Olzinski, A. R., Hu, T. C., Lenhard, S. C., Aravindhan, K., Gruver, S. M., Jacobs, P. M., Willette, R. N., & Jucker, B. M. 2005, Differential uptake of ferumoxtran-10 and ferumoxytol, ultrasmall superparamagnetic iron oxide contrast agents in rabbit: critical determinants of atherosclerotic plaque labeling, *J Magn Reson Imaging*, vol. 21, no. 4, pp. 432-442.

86. Mani, V., Briley-Saebo, K. C., Itskovich, V. V., Samber, D. D., & Fayad, Z. A. 2006, Gradient echo acquisition for superparamagnetic particles with positive contrast (GRASP): Sequence characterization in membrane and glass superparamagnetic iron oxide phantoms at 1.5T and 3T, *Magn Reson Med*, vol. 55, no. 1, pp. 126-135.

87. Litovsky, S., Madjid, M., Zarrabi, A., Casscells, S. W., Willerson, J. T., & Naghavi, M. 2003, Superparamagnetic iron oxide-based method for quantifying recruitment of monocytes to mouse atherosclerotic lesions in vivo: enhancement by tissue necrosis factor-alpha, interleukin-1beta, and interferon-gamma, *Circulation*, vol. 107, no. 11, pp. 1545-1549.

88. Lipinski, M. J., Fuster, V., Fisher, E. A., & Fayad, Z. A. 2004b, Technology insight: targeting of biological molecules for evaluation of high-risk atherosclerotic plaques with magnetic resonance imaging, *Nat Clin Pract Cardiovasc Med*, vol. 1, no. 1, pp. 48-55.

89. Frias, J. C., Williams, K. J., Fisher, E. A., & Fayad, Z. A. 2004, Recombinant HDL-like nanoparticles: a specific contrast agent for MRI of atherosclerotic plaques, *J Am Chem Soc,* vol. 126, no. 50, pp. 16316-16317.

90. Wilson, P. W., D'Agostino, R. B., Parise, H., Sullivan, L., & Meigs, J. B. 2005, Metabolic syndrome as a precursor of cardiovascular disease and type 2 diabetes mellitus, *Circulation*, vol. 112, no. 20, pp. 3066-3072.

91. Rioufol, G., Finet, G., Ginon, I., Andre-Fouet, X., Rossi, R., Vialle, E., Desjoyaux, E., Convert, G., Huret, J. F., & Tabib, A. 2002, Multiple atherosclerotic plaque rupture in acute coronary syndrome: a three-vessel intravascular ultrasound study, *Circulation*, vol. 106, no. 7, pp. 804-808.

92. Naghavi, M., Libby, P., Falk, E., Casscells, S. W., Litovsky, S., Rumberger, J., Badimon, J. J., Stefanadis, C., Moreno, P., Pasterkamp, G., Fayad, Z., Stone, P. H., Waxman, S., Raggi, P., Madjid, M., Zarrabi, A., Burke, A., Yuan, C., Fitzgerald, P. J., Siscovick, D. S., de Korte, C. L., Aikawa, M., Airaksinen, K. E., Assmann, G., Becker, C. R., Chesebro, J. H., Farb, A., Galis, Z. S., Jackson, C., Jang, I. K., Koenig, W., Lodder, R. A., March, K., Demirovic, J., Navab, M., Priori, S. G., Rekhter, M. D., Bahr, R., Grundy, S. M., Mehran, R., Colombo, A., Boerwinkle, E., Ballantyne, C., Insull, W., Jr., Schwartz, R. S., Vogel, R., Serruys, P. W., Hansson, G. K., Faxon, D. P., Kaul, S., Drexler, H., Greenland, P., Muller, J. E., Virmani, R., Ridker, P. M., Zipes, D. P., Shah, P. K., & Willerson, J. T. 2003, From vulnerable plaque to vulnerable patient: a call for new definitions and risk assessment strategies: Part II, *Circulation*, vol. 108, no. 15, pp. 1772-1778.

CHAPTER 9

Nuclear Based Techniques

Louise Thomson, MBChB, FRACP

INTRODUCTION

Nuclear medicine techniques have a well-established role in noninvasive cardiac imaging and have gained wide popularity in the assessment of patients with known or suspected coronary artery disease. The role of nuclear cardiology in daily practice in multiple different applications and clinical questions is supported by a wealth of literature. Although second only to echocardiography in use, most clinicians know very little about the methods underlying cardiac radionuclide imaging.

This chapter aims to provide an overview of these techniques, from the perspective of basic principles through to clinical application. It is the goal of this chapter to familiarize the reader with the basic characteristics of cardiovascular radionuclide imaging, the methods used, and the information provided by these tests.

ISOTOPES AND RADIOPHARMACEUTICALS

Nuclear medicine is the branch of medicine concerned with the use of radioisotopes in the diagnosis, management, and treatment of disease. Nuclear medicine uses small amounts of radioactive materials, or radiopharmaceuticals, which are substances attracted to specific organs, bones, or tissues. By allowing noninvasive visualization of the distribution of the administered radiopharmaceutical, radionuclide imaging provides physiologic and anatomic information that can yield clinically relevant information regarding a number of pathophysiologic processes.

A radioisotope is a version of a chemical element that has an unstable nucleus and emits radiation during its decay to a stable form. When combined with a pharmaceutical for medical imaging, a radiopharmaceutical is produced. Radiopharmaceuticals emit energy that can be detected by gamma or PET cameras, which work in conjunction with computers to generate images of various parts of the body.

Two nuclear medicine imaging approaches used in cardiac imaging are single photon emission computed tomography (SPECT; a gamma camera approach) and positron emission tomography (PET). These approaches are similar in that both can be used for myocardial perfusion or myocardial viability imaging and require the peripheral venous injection of a radiopharmaceutical (that can be taken up by myocardial tissue) in order to generate an image of the left ventricular myocardium. The systems differ in terms of camera design, the type and energy level of the radioactive emission detected by the camera system (thus the radiopharmaceuticals used), and cost and availability.

SPECT is usually performed using radiopharmaceuticals containing either technetium-99m (Tc-99m) or thallium-201 (Tl-201) that are distributed in the myocardium in proportion to coronary blood flow. This imaging approach may also utilize radiopharmaceuticals that demonstrate myocardial metabolism [F18-fluorodeoxyglucose (FDG) SPECT] or the presence and distribution of abnormal tissue within the myocardium (Tc-99m pyrophosphate; see later section on special indications).

The most commonly used isotope in nuclear medicine is Tc-99m. This is produced on site by the molybdenum-99/technetium-99m generator. In this generator, the mother nuclide molybdenum-99 decays into the daughter nuclide Tc-99m, which can be milked from the generator system up to twice a day to provide a laboratory with the raw material required for radiopharmaceutical preparation. The physical half-life of Tc-99m is 6.02 hours (the time taken for the radioactivity of the material to decline to half). With decay, Tc-99m emission is predominantly a gamma ray with an energy level of 140keV.

For myocardial perfusion imaging, available Tc-99m agents include sestamibi (Cardiolite) or tetrafosmin (Myoview), depending on local laboratory preference. These radiopharmaceuticals are distributed throughout the body with a relatively small percentage of the injected dose delivered to the myocardium. The myocardial uptake of these tracers is proportional to coronary artery blood flow at the time of injection and retention of the injected material in the myocardium is due to interaction of the pharmaceutical with the mitochondrial matrix. These radiopharmaceuticals typically clear rapidly from the blood pool and are eliminated from the body via hepatic and renal clearance.

Tl-201 is produced by a cyclotron and has a longer physical half-life (73.1 hours). This material decays sufficiently slowly to permit distribution to laboratories distant from a cyclotron, and it is supplied in the form of an isotonic solution (thallous chloride-201). Tl-201 decays to Mercury Hg-201, and the decay process produces radiation emissions at several different energy levels. The predominant emission utilized for imaging with the gamma camera has an energy level of 68–80.3keV and actually comes from the Mercury Hg-201 daughter product of Tl-201.

For myocardial perfusion imaging, thallium-201 can be considered as an analog of potassium. It is rapidly and efficiently extracted from the blood pool and localizes in the myocardium in proportion to blood flow. Unlike technetium 99m Sestamibi or Tc-99m Tetrafosmin, thallium redistributes in viable myocardium following injection. Imaging must be performed promptly after injection in order to assess the perfusion pattern at the time of injection. This property of Tl-201 has been exploited in its use as an agent to define myocardial viability as the pattern of distribution at 4, 12, and 24 hours has been shown to correlate with presence of viable myocardium.

PET systems are designed to detect high-energy emissions, thus require different isotopes. The most commonly used isotope is F-18 fluorodeoxyglucose (F-18 FDG, physical half-life 110 minutes), which is produced by a cyclotron and is used in oncologic imaging as well as for assessment of myocardial viability. For myocardial perfusion imaging, a variety of different cyclotron produced radioisotopes can be used, such as oxygen-15 water and N-13 ammonia. These agents have very short half-lives (O-15: 110 seconds, N-13: 10 minutes) and this limits their use to institutions with a cyclotron nearby and limits the widespread clinical application of PET myocardial perfusion imaging.

Rubidium-82 is also a high-energy radioisotope that can be used for myocardial perfusion imaging, with a very short half-life of 76 seconds. Unlike O-15 and N-13, this PET agent is available for on-site production by a commercially-available generator system, similar to technetium production described above. The generator contains cyclotron-produced strontium Sr-82 parent isotope and produces approximately a one-month supply of rubidium-82. Rubidium-82 is also an analog of potassium and localizes in the myocardium in proportion to coronary blood flow. Because of its extremely short half-life, it is possible to give large doses (50–60mCi) of rubidium-82 for perfusion imaging and to use the same dose for both rest and stress imaging. The activity required is determined in part by the sensitivity of PET camera being used.

The short-lived radioactive tracers used in PET imaging decay by emission of a positron, which is the antimatter counterpart of an electron. After traveling a few millimeters in tissue, positrons encounter and annihilate with an electron, and produce a pair of annihilation (gamma) photons that move in opposite directions, 180 degrees apart from one another. Fundamental to the PET camera design is the detection of simultaneous (coincident) energy emissions by a ring of detectors around the body, this data is then used to calculate the location of the origin of the energy for images to be reconstructed (see the following section on camera design).

CAMERAS AND CAMERA DESIGN

A gamma camera was first developed in 1957 by Hal Anger[1] and is frequently referred to as an Anger camera. The camera consists of one or more detectors (flat crystal planes) that are optically coupled to numerous photomultiplier tubes, with this detector head system mounted on a gantry. The gantry is connected to a computer system used to control the camera operation and acquire and process image data (see Figure 9.1).

Emitted energy, in the form of gamma rays, is absorbed by the crystal in the camera, which scintillates in response. The photomultiplier tubes detect this incident light event and provide data regarding the timing, location, and summation of events (or counts) detected. The computer reconstructs and displays a two-dimensional (2D) image of the relative spatial count density on a monitor. This reconstructed image reflects the distribution and relative concentration of radioactive tracer elements present in the organs and tissues imaged.

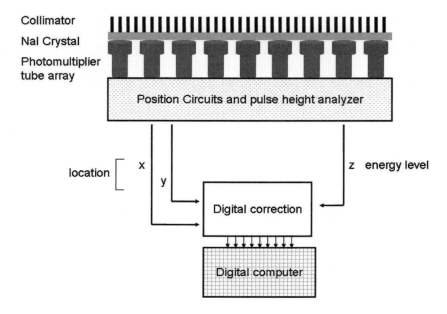

Figure 9.1

Schematic diagram of the Anger camera. NaI: sodium iodide.

A collimator is placed over the camera head in order to obtain spatial information. Collimators, comprised of thick lead containing thousands of adjacent holes, attenuate most (> 99%) incident photons and decrease system sensitivity in the process of gaining spatial information. The best current Anger camera systems can differentiate two separate point sources of gamma photons located a minimum of 1.8cm apart, at 5cm away from the camera face.

Single photon emission computed tomography imaging is performed with one, two, or three detectors (heads) slowly rotated around the patient's torso, in order to produce a three-dimensional (3D) volume of data. This improves detection and localization of abnormalities within the body. Newer generation gamma cameras have recently emerged with novel detector head designs that improve sensitivity, potentially reduce imaging times, and enhance image quality in terms of improved spatial resolution. The newer Spectrum Dynamics D-SPECT Cardiac Imaging System permits data acquisition in only 2 minutes as a result of improved efficiency of count detection. In patients unable to have tomographic imaging (either due to size or inability to transfer to an imaging department), planar (2D) imaging approaches may also be used.

PET cameras were first designed and used for research purposes in the 1970s. There are multiple types of high-density scintillating crystalline materials that have been used for modern PET scanner energy detection. These include Bismuth germinate (BGO), cerium-doped lutetium oxyorthosilicate (Lu2SiO5[Ce] or LSO) and cerium-doped gadolin oxyorthosilicate (Gd2SiO5[Ce]or GSO) and they vary in terms of decay time (determines minimal time of the crystal between detections), light output, and energy resolution. State-of-the-art PET scanners are multidetector full ring systems that axially surround the patient. Attenuation is the loss of detected true energy emissions through the absorption of energy by the body or scattering of energy out of the detector. This is worse with PET than with SPECT and, if uncorrected, causes image noise and artifacts. Attenuation correction is always required for PET images and for cardiac imaging this is performed using a transmission attenuation correction map of the chest. In a PET-only system, the attenuation correction map is generated by detection of an orbiting radioactive source outside the patient (a transmission scan), In a PET/CT scanner, the attenuation map is a CT scan. The latter system provides a more rapid means of attenuation correction, albeit with potential for artifacts predominantly related to differences in diaphragmatic position between the attenuation map and the emission data or CT artifacts.

The development of combined PET/CT and SPECT/CT hybrid systems allows same-scanner acquisition of anatomic and perfusion imaging data. Depending on the capacity of the CT hardware in the system, there is potential to obtain coronary calcium score, CT coronary angiography and myocardial perfusion imaging data at a single imaging session. The clinical utility and cost-effectiveness of a combined anatomic and perfusion imaging approach in the diagnosis and management of coronary artery disease is not clearly defined.

Image Acquisition, Display, and Interpretation

In standard Anger camera systems, the cardiac perfusion image data is acquired over 15–30 minutes with camera detector head(s) moving in an arc of 180 degrees around the patient, spanning from the right anterior oblique to the left posterior oblique views of the chest. Using novel gamma camera technology, the acquisition time may be a low as 2–3 minutes, due to increased sensitivity of the system for detection of emitted radiation. Cardiac gating (scintillation counting timed with the heart contraction relaxation cycle) permits calculation of cardiac volumes and ejection fraction as well as visualization of regional wall motion abnormalities.

Patients are typically positioned supine with arms above the head with ECG electrodes positioned on the torso to permit gated imaging. Images may also be obtained with the patient in the prone position. With some camera systems, the patient is seated or semirecumbent in a chair. PET cameras require patients to lie supine with the arms above the head. Image acquisition time depends on the system but is typically shorter than SPECT.

Prior to display, image data is extensively processed to decrease noise. This is achieved through a complex series of steps that include filtered back projection and smoothing of data, as well as correction for soft tissue attenuation or motion artifact. The 3D image data is then visually inspected to determine the long and short axis of the left ventricle, then images are reconstructed and displayed, typically with rest and stress images alongside one another. Whole imaging field 3D data and gated reformatted images are displayed in a cine loop. Normalization of signal intensity within a dataset (normalized to the brightest pixel of the myocardium) and between rest and stress data also occurs prior to image display.

Standard cardiac axes are inspected: the vertical long axis (2-chamber view), the horizontal long axis (4-chamber view), and the left ventricular short axis. These imaging planes are displayed as a series of slices through the heart, permitting visualization of all regions of the heart in more than one imaging plane. Note is made that the first and last slice of each series of images may underrepresent true image intensity because of partial volume sampling of the myocardium.

The standardized 17-segment model for describing the location of perfusion and wall motion abnormalities within the left ventricle is shown (Figure 9.2). Interpretation of image data includes reporting of left ventricular volumes and ejection fraction, as well as the presence of any ancillary markers of myocardial ischemia or other abnormal findings from the 3D rotating volumetric data.

Interpretation is based on visual and quantitative assessment of the uniformity of left ventricular myocardial signal intensity within each dataset and with comparison of the relative intensity of myocardial signal between rest and stress images. Regional ischemia, as indicated by presence of reduced intensity in a vascular territory at stress as compared to rest (a reversible defect), is described in terms of its location, extent, and severity. Myocardial infarction causes a perfusion defect that is present at rest and stress (a fixed defect) and is associated with regional wall motion abnormality on gated images (Figures 9.3–9.6) Note is made that subendocardial scar, as can be demonstrated by delayed enhancement cardiac MRI, will not be visible by MPS until sufficiently transmural scar is present.[2] Images are typically inspected using a linear scale of signal intensity that may be either in a grey scale or color scale, depending on user preference.

Quantitative analysis of perfusion activity in the myocardium is a software-based approach that compares data obtained in an individual patient to data derived from normal populations of males or females as a means to aid in image interpretation. Quantitative techniques permit rapid evaluation of the extent and severity of perfusion defects and are useful when comparing to a prior study for the same patient.

Stress Testing Protocols and Radiation Dose Estimations

Fundamental to myocardial perfusion imaging is the concept of induced ischemia, indicating presence of impaired coronary flow reserve. Myocardial stress is induced prior to injection of the radiopharmaceutical so that the stress images obtained represent distribution of tracer during a state of maximal coronary blood flow.

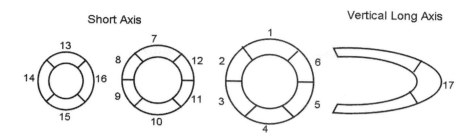

Coronary artery segmentation (varies with anatomic variation)

LAD: 1,2,7,8,13,14,17

RCA: 3,4,9,10,15

LCx: 5,6,11,12,16

Figure 9.2

The 17-segment model of myocardial perfusion. LAD: left anterior descending coronary artery; LCx: left circumflex coronary artery; RCA: right coronary artery.

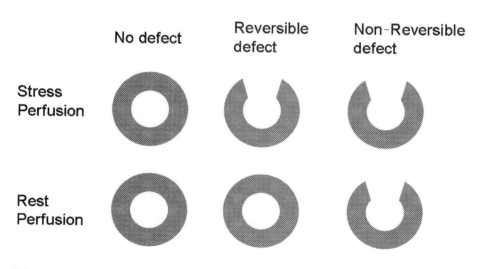

Figure 9.3

Schematic representation of perfusion defect type.

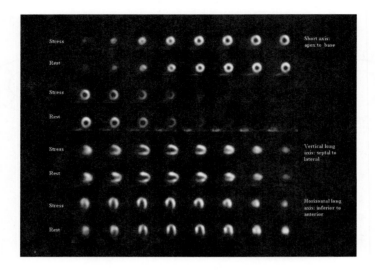

Figure 9.4

Normal stress rest perfusion images in a patient who had Tc-99m Sestamibi for rest and stress imaging. (See Color Plate 23.)

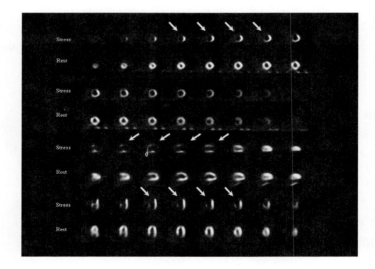

Figure 9.5

Abnormal stress perfusion and normal rest perfusion in a patient who had Tc-99m Sestamibi for rest and stress imaging. The perfusion defect is in the vascular territory of the left anterior descending coronary artery. Additionally, there is a visual impression of dilation of the left ventricular cavity on stress images compared to the rest images. This suggests transient ischemic dilation of the ventricle, and occurs with severe and extensive myocardial ischemia. (See Color Plate 24.)

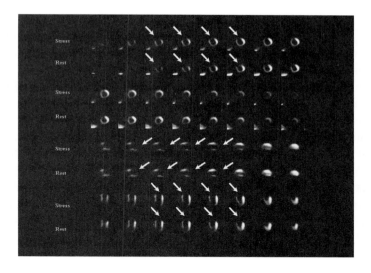

Figure 9.6

Abnormal stress and rest perfusion imaging in a patient with prior left anterior descending coronary artery infarction. The ventricular cavity shape is abnormal, consistent with presence of remodeling of the ventricle, associated with apical thinning and aneurysm. (See Color Plate 25.)

Stress can be induced via exercise (treadmill or bicycle), with peak stress usually defined as achievement of 85% of the maximal age-predicted heart rate. The radiopharmaceutical may also be injected if there is myocardial ischemia prior to achievement of the target heart rate (as defined by ECG changes and/or typical symptoms).

Pharmaceutical stress is also an accurate means of increasing coronary blood flow and is the protocol of choice in patients who are unable to exercise or unable to achieve a target heart rate. The two major pharmaceutical stress types are dobutamine and vasodilator stress. Dobutamine stress testing is performed using protocols similar to those used in dobutamine stress echo with gradually incrementing dose to achieve the desired target heart rate.

Vasodilator stress utilizes agents that act on adenosine receptors to cause coronary vasodilatation and increase in resting coronary blood flow. Dipyridamole was the first such agent available. It is administered as a slow intravenous infusion over 4 minutes, with maximal action at a mean of 6.5 minutes after the commencement of infusion and duration of effect up to 30 minutes. The action of dipyridamole may be reversed by aminophylline. A more direct receptor effect and rapid onset and offset of action occurs with Adenosine, which is administered by intravenous infusion 140mcg/kg/min over 4–6 minutes and has a much shorter half-life (estimated fewer than 10 seconds) so that the effect disappears very soon after discontinuation of the adenosine infusion.

Side effects with vasodilator stress are common but usually mild, with flushing, breathlessness, chest tightness, and nausea being the most common complaints. More troublesome side effects include transient AV nodal block that is typically managed by infusion termination for Adenoscan or agent reversal in the case of dipyridamole. Bronchospasm may also occur, and use of these agents is contraindicated in asthmatics.

More recently, a specific A2A adenosine receptor agonist (Regadenoson, Lexiscan; Astellas Pharma US, Inc.) has become commercially available.[3] This agent is administered as a single, slow intravenous push and causes a rapid increase in intracoronary blood flow that is more than 2.5 times greater than the baseline. Maximal effect is sustained for 2–3 minutes and then coronary blood flow returns to normal over more than 10 minutes. Initial experience with this agent suggests it will decrease time for stress test performance and that it is as efficacious as adenosine for detection of ischemia.[4] Current ASNC guidelines state there is insufficient data to support safety of use of this agent in asthmatics or COPD[5] and the effect of all of these agents is blocked by caffeine or use of medications containing theophylline.

Figure 9.7 outlines typical stress testing SPECT protocols for various myocardial perfusion stress testing protocols. Same-day imaging with rest and stress requires that the emitted signal from the second injection override any background signal in the myocardium from the first injection. This allows you to see the difference between rest and stress perfusion. Thus, there is a requirement that the first injection be a smaller dose or a lower energy isotope than the second injection. Very large patients may require two-day imaging in order to permit injection of sufficient activity to produce interpretable images of the heart. There is an advantage to the use of a high-energy isotope (PET) or camera with increased sensitivity and spatial resolution (PET and newer generation gamma camera) in larger patients. Local experience with the newer gamma camera systems (Cedars Sinai Medical Center, D-SPECT, Spectrum Dynamics) has also been favorable in large patients (130–200kg). Use of thallium 201 permits combined assessment of rest and stress perfusion in addition to myocardial viability. (When using a PET camera, F-18 FDG is the radioisotope of choice for evaluation of myocardial viability.)

The total time duration of protocols vary, with dual isotope protocols (thallium 201 and technetium 99m) being shorter than single isotope protocols. The dual isotope protocol has a higher estimated radiation exposure to the patient than single isotope protocol, but has the advantage of permitting assessment of viability by obtaining late Tl-201 redistribution images. Imaging protocols designed specifically for viability imaging with thallium 201 are discussed later in the section on special applications. Imaging protocols with PET cameras permit acquisition of rest and stress images within a 30-minute table time on the camera, by virtue of the short half-life of the radioisotope being administered. Duration of a protocol may also be shortened by use of newer gamma camera technology, when image acquisition is reduced from 15–20 minutes to 2–3 minutes as a function of increased sensitivity of the crystal array for detection of the emitted energy.[6]

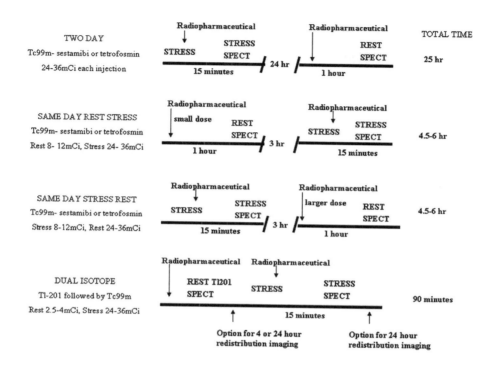

Figure 9.7

Example protocols for myocardial perfusion imaging utilizing a single-isotope or dual-isotope technique.

Image Artifacts (Attenuation, Motion, Camera-Related Image Artifacts)

Optimization of nuclear imaging accuracy demands attention to potential sources of error. Image artifacts diminish accuracy and confidence for reader interpretation, but can be minimized.

The Association of Electrical and Medical Imaging Equipment Manufacturers (NEMA) has defined standards for manufacture of nuclear medicine imaging equipment. Gamma camera performance is assessed on a regular basis by use of a variety of acceptance tests to confirm intrinsic and extrinsic (system) function. These tests are classified as NEMA and non-NEMA standards and include checks of energy resolution, spatial resolution, and field uniformity for planar imaging. For SPECT systems, the tests include checking for angular linearity errors, field uniformity, tomographic slice uniformity, rotational uniformity, system volume sensitivity, and tomographic resolution.

The reader is referred to the Nuclear Medicine Resources Manual published by the International Atomic Energy Agency, Austria, in 2006 (available at www-pub.iaea.org) for a detailed account of the recommended procedures to check imaging instrumentation.

The imaging physician should always inspect raw projection data prior to interpretation of the processed data in order to confirm quality of the image acquisition. This allows the evaluation of the extent of soft tissue, motion artifact, and any abnormal tracer uptake (e.g., in pulmonary or breast malignancy, parathyroid adenoma). Raw data can be motion corrected by software algorithms, but this is generally most effective when the motion is in the craniocaudal direction and is not excessive.

The use of prone imaging as an adjunct to supine imaging has the advantage of being associated with less patient motion. Prone imaging also alters the cardiac position relative to the diaphragm and shifts breast and chest wall soft tissues. This may result in improvement in the visualization of the inferior wall (frequently attenuated in men or large patients) and decrease artifacts related to motion. Reliance on presence of normal wall motion to define a segment with diminished activity as artifact rather than real is suboptimal, due to the potential for preserved wall motion in the setting of mild ischemia and subendocardial infarction. However, it is recognized that the routine use of gated SPECT and interrogation of wall motion helps to differentiate presence of infarction from attenuation.

Attenuation correction is available on many SPECT camera systems, utilizing an internal source of energy (transmission source) within the camera to generate a patient-specific estimate of attenuation coefficients. This data is then used to correct the SPECT data (emission data) prior to reconstruction of images. Although this concept appears at first to be the ideal solution to image attenuation artifact, correction of the data is difficult. SPECT photons originating from different depths within the patient will experience different levels of attenuation depending on their position relative to the surface of the patient. Even with gamma cameras that have the ability to acquire transmission data, the advantage of current attenuation correction implementations has not been consistently demonstrated. Thus, correction may not be complete in all patients and it is recommended that nonattenuation correction and attenuation correction data be inspected and integrated in the interpretation of studies. It is noted, however, that the use of attenuation correction software has been shown to decrease the number of equivocal studies, as has the use of prone imaging.[7] Similarly, the use of gated SPECT improved test specificity in women by permitting differentiation of fixed defects caused by infarction (abnormal wall motion) from fixed defects due to attenuation artifact (normal wall motion).

PET system specifications are defined in a NEMA publication (Performance Measurements of Positron Emission Tomographs; NEMA NU 2 Revision/Edition: 07) and performance quality control tests are also required on a regular basis as detailed in the IAEA Nuclear Medicine Resources Manual.

PET camera systems have an inherent advantage with regard to attenuation, which is fundamental to the improvement in image quality compared to gamma camera systems. In PET, the total attenuation factor is the same along any given line of response, irrespective of where the annihilation event took place, because both photons (180 degrees apart) have to escape the body. Attenuation correction is performed using either a transmission source or by use of a CT attenuation correction map, with correction data acquired for each emission scan.

For spatial resolution and myocardial perfusion imaging, PET systems have superior spatial resolution to SPECT camera systems. The observed spatial resolution of PET is dependent on the distance traveled by a positron between its point of initial delivery to myocardium and its interaction with tissue (annihilation). This distance is a function of the isotope concerned and is one of the reasons why Rb-82 (PET myocardial blood flow tracer) images do not usually exhibit significantly higher resolution than corresponding SPECT images.

Information Provided by Stress Radionuclide Myocardial Perfusion Imaging

Compared to modalities such as echocardiography and CMR, myocardial perfusion imaging (MPI) techniques yield a limited range of data. Several parameters are considered a standard part of routine reporting. Stress versus rest myocardial perfusion should be reported, both globally and regionally. If performed, results of viability imaging using a validated protocol should be reported as well. Use of gated SPECT techniques allows reporting of LV ejection fraction, end systolic and end diastolic volumes, regional wall motion, and ventricular shape. Of note, gated SPECT may be reported for either rest images or poststress images or both. Gated SPECT techniques do not currently permit routine peak stress imaging; hence, poststress data is reported. The calculation of cardiac volumes and ejection fraction by gated SPECT or PET is based on ventricular myocardial contour detection algorithms and volumetric model assumptions.

The data potentially acquired from stress PET studies differ slightly from that acquired from SPECT. First, in light of the shorter half-lives of PET tracers, peak pharmacologic stress LV ejection fraction, volumes, and wall motion are reported. Recent reports indicate that the failure to increase LV ejection fraction during pharmacologic stress PET compared to rest ejection fraction suggests the presence of multivessel CAD.[8] Further, studies indicate that rest and peak stress flow, thus coronary flow reserve, can be determined using Rb-82 with an accuracy similar to that for NH_3-13 PET.[9] The ability to determine flow reserve as a part of routine testing may extend the applications of PET MPI to include detection of small vessel disease and, possibly, noninvasive assessment of the hemodynamic significance of nonobstructive coronary lesions.

Gated Equilibrium Blood Pool Scan

The terms gated equilibrium blood pool scan (GBPS), radioventriculography, blood pool scan, or multiple gated acquisition (MUGA) are synonymous and describe the nuclear medicine technique for inspection of ventricular function by visualizing the blood pool within the ventricles. Radiopharmaceuticals for this purpose include Tc-99m–human serum albumin, Tc-99m–labeled red blood cells, and O-15–labeled carbon monoxide. This technique is an accurate and reproducible method for calculation of both right and left ventricular ejection fraction, and is considered the gold standard to which performance of alternative imaging methods is compared.

Red cell labeling is achieved by addition of technetium pertechnetate to cells that have been exposed to the reducing agent, stannous pyrophosphate. This can be achieved in vivo (injecting tracer after stannous pyrophosphate) or in vitro (removing 50ml of blood, adding stannous pyrophosphate followed by technetium pertechnetate, and then reinjecting the labeled red cells). The in vitro method has superior labeling efficiency but an in vivo approach allows the acquisition of dynamic first pass radionuclide angiography during the bolus injection of technetium pertechnetate (advantageous for right ventricular ejection fraction measurement and the demonstration of shunts).

Imaging of the patient is by planar and/or tomographic data acquisition. Postprocessing of data involves selection of a region for analysis and the calculation of cardiac volumes is based on the detection of counts within this region in systole and diastole. The use of this counts-based method avoids errors that occur when ventricular shape must be mathematically assumed. Potential errors with radioventriculography may result from failure to label red cells, failure to gate for identification of end systole/end diastole, or from the incorporation of nonventricular overlying structures in the region of interest. The use of tomographic imaging (gated blood pool SPECT) is more accurate than planar imaging in terms of being able to accurately identify the ventricular volume of interest, separate from adjacent structures and with 3D visualization of regional wall motion. When comparing ejection fraction calculated by gated blood pool SPECT as opposed to myocardial perfusion SPECT (MPS), it is important to recognize the differences in technique will result in a small difference in the measured ejection fraction. The presence of marked cardiac enlargement with a large prior infarction or a very small ventricle may result in a greater observed differences between techniques.[10, 11] The type of software used to process MPS data will also influence the result obtained and, ideally, follow up studies looking for interval changes in ventricular volumes and ejection fraction should be performed using the same technique and same software.

Radioventriculography is a valuable tool for serial measurement of ventricular function in patients being monitored for adverse effects of chemotherapy and in management of heart failure. An application of gated blood pool SPECT is its use in evaluation of ventricular dyssynchony, where phase analysis profiles may help predict risk of ventricular arrhythmia in dilated cardiomyopathy and demonstrate effectiveness of resynchronization therapy for heart failure.[12]

Diastolic function may be evaluated using radioventriculography. By using commercially available software packages for RNA, the rate of change of counts in diastole can be analyzed to calculate indices of diastolic filling, including the peak LV filling rate, time to peak filling, and atrial contribution to filling.[13]

APPLICATIONS OF STRESS MYOCARDIAL PERFUSION IMAGING AND SELECTION OF CANDIDATES FOR TESTING

Myocardial perfusion imaging has been used in numerous populations to address many different clinical questions. There is a wealth of literature validating use of MPI in patients with known or suspected coronary artery disease, including the identification of obstructive lesions, patient risk stratification on the basis of test results, and the management of patients based on results of these tests. However, with the increased emphasis on evidence-based care, it can now be appreciated that the role of MPI is best limited to specific situations and populations.

1. **Identification of obstructive CAD.** In the United States, the identification of obstructive CAD is considered an appropriate indication for MPI in symptomatic patients with intermediate or high pretest probability of CAD.[14] This indication includes those patients able to exercise to their age-predicted target heart rate (and without left bundle branch block or permanent pacemaker), as well as those unable to do so who will require pharmacologic stress. Additionally, the use of MPI in patients with intermediate Duke Treadmill score, repeat testing in patients with changing symptoms, and exercise MPI to assess the significance of intermediate lesions (25–75% stenosis) are also included this category.

   MPI diagnostic accuracy is good, with sensitivity and specificity for detection of significant CAD, as defined by catheterization, expected to be approximately 85%. The observed test performance is influenced by the prevalence of disease in the population studied and the number of patients referred on to a gold standard test. The sensitivities and specificities for exercise and adenosine stress SPECT, based on pooled data from the ACC/AHA radionuclide guidelines, are shown in Table 9.1. However, published estimates of diagnostic test accuracy, are limited by partial verification bias (also known as posttest referral bias), that results from patients being frequently referred to a gold standard (catheterization) after an abnormal test result, but infrequently referred after a normal test result. Thus, estimates of test sensitivity are overestimated (resulting from the few false negative studies), while estimates of specificity are underestimated (resulting from the relatively low number of documented true negative studies as compared to number of false positives). Methods to correct for partial verification bias exist, and aid in the understanding of observed test performance, with the adjusted values of sensitivity and specificity also shown

Table 9.1   Myocardial Perfusion Test Performance Before and After Adjustment for Referral Bias

Year	Author	Modality	Total Number	Sensitivity % Raw	Sensitivity % Adjusted	Specificity % Raw	Specificity % Adjusted
1986	Diamond[28]	Ex. Planar T1-201	2269	91	68	34	71
1993	Schwartz[29]	T1-201	845	67	45	59	78
1996	Cecil et al.[26]	Ex. MPS T1-201	2688	98	82	14	59
1998	Santana-Boado et al.[27]	Ex./Dip.MPS Tc-99m	Men 100	93	88	89	96
			Women 63	85	87	91	91
2002	Miller et al.[25]	Ex.MPS Tc-99m/T1-201	1853	98	65	13	67

in Table 9.1. The methods discussed earlier regarding minimization of image artifacts (section on image artifacts) result in improved test specificity by reducing the frequency of false positive studies due to artifacts.

2. **Risk assessment/risk stratification.** This application by far has the most extensive support for the use of MPI. To date, outcomes in thousands of patients followed after exercise or pharmacologic stress have been reported, suggesting that *in general* patients after normal MPI are at very low risk (defined as < 1% rate of cardiac death per year of follow-up).[15] Risk after an abnormal MPI increases in proportion to the extent and severity of perfusion defects, thus, risk stratification relative to normal or lower risk MPI is achieved. Further, even after initial risk stratification of a patient population by clinical parameters, MPI will further enhance risk stratification in each of these patient subsets.[16]

Nonetheless, it must be noted that the risk of patients after MPI, as the case with all testing, is a function of their baseline risk. Thus, for the same extent and severity of perfusion defect, observed risk will vary with the patient's baseline risk, demographics, cardiac risk factors, and history of prior CAD.

While it is commonly stated that MPI is best applied for risk stratification in patients with a clinically intermediate risk of a subsequent cardiac event (analogous to the optimal diagnostic application of nuclear testing to patients with an intermediate likelihood of CAD),[17] studies support the concept that even in high-risk patients, a normal MPS is associated with low risk. Indeed, a study of MPI in patients with high pre-MPI likelihood of CAD (> 85%) reported that a majority of patients had normal MPI, and these studies were low risk.[18]

3. **Pre-operative assessment.** MPI has long been used in the assessment of patients prior to noncardiac surgery. While this modality is unquestionably capable of identifying the presence of jeopardized myocardium, therefore identifying the high-risk patient, the yield of this testing has been called into question and the role of MPI has been reduced to a relatively minor one in recent years. This can be attributed to large, multicenter trials demonstrating the value of aggressive medical manage-

ment in the prevention of perioperative events. Hence, in large part, the role of MPI is likely limited to the assessment of patients with intermediate (mild angina, prior MI, compensated or prior heart failure, diabetes, and renal insufficiency) or minor clinical risk predictors (advanced age, abnormal ECG, rhythm other than sinus, low functional capacity, history of CVA, and uncontrolled hypertension) and poor functional capacity (less than 4 METS) who require high-risk noncardiac surgery (defined as emergent operations [particularly in the elderly], aortic and other major vascular surgery, peripheral vascular surgery, and other prolonged operations during which major fluid shifts are anticipated [i.e., reported cardiac risk often more than 5%]) when used in conjunction with pharmacologic stress. Similarly, patients with intermediate clinical risk predictors, abnormal baseline ECGs, and moderate or excellent functional capacity (greater than 4 METS) being evaluated prior to high-risk noncardiac surgery are also MPI candidates.[17]

4. **Acute emergency department use of MPI.** Based on the growing body of literature on the use of emergency department imaging of patients with chest pain, it appears that the sensitivity and specificity of acute rest imaging for MI appears very high, especially at the onset of acute MI. A strategy of initial triage based on symptoms, ECG, and history, rest SPECT imaging in the emergency department appears to identify high-risk patients (in need of admission) versus low-risk patients able to be discharged. In the United States, the use of MPI in an emergency department setting has a class I indication in two circumstances. First, the use of rest MPI for risk assessment in patients with possible ACS but nondiagnostic ECG and initial serum markers and enzymes. Also, the use of same day stress/rest perfusion imaging for CAD diagnosis in possible ACS patients with chest pain, nondiagnostic ECG, and negative serum markers and enzymes.[17]

5. **Post-MI risk stratification.** In the United States, post-MI risk stratification is considered a class I indication for MPI in these settings: First, for the assessment of LV function. Further, for the detection of inducible ischemia and jeopardized myocardium in patients treated with thrombolytic therapy without catheterization. Finally, for the assessment of infarct size and residual viable myocardium in patients with acute STEMI.[17]

6. **Patients with heart failure.** Nuclear techniques potentially play several roles in patients presenting with heart failure. First, either gated MPS or gated equilibrium blood pool scan techniques can be used to assess and follow LV and RV function and volumes, (class I indication for testing). Further, MPI can assess for the presence of viable myocardium, therefore suitability for revascularization, in patients with CAD and LV systolic dysfunction who do not have angina (also a class I indication). Several other clinical applications are feasible in this population. In patients with heart failure, gated blood pool and MPS techniques are particularly well suited for

differentiating systolic versus diastolic function as the etiology of symptoms. Also, MPS can be used to distinguish ischemic versus nonischemic etiologies for heart failure in patients with new presentations.[17]

Identification of Optimal MPI Candidates

The cost-effectiveness of stress MPI has been extensively studied in a number of populations. First, the use of stress MPI has been found to be a superior strategy to direct referral to catheterization in stable patients with chest pain.[19] While intermediate-term outcomes are similar for the two strategies, the use of noninvasive testing results in 30–45% reduced cost compared to the invasive strategy, as well as a reduced frequency of normal catheterization results.[20] With respect to the optimal cost-effective selection of patients, several studies have shown that, although MPI results can risk stratify patients in all clinical risk subsets, this stratification attains cost-effectiveness only in patients with intermediate or high risk.[21-23] Although low-risk patients are risk stratified, this stratification is associated with unacceptable cost levels. Further, while earlier studies claimed that radionuclide techniques were not cost-effective for the identification of high-risk anatomic CAD (left main or three vessel CAD) in patients with normal rest ECG, they were cost-effective in the risk stratification of patients with normal rest ECG. Hence, it appears that MPI is cost-effective in the setting of intermediate to high risk or likelihood of CAD and with respect to outcomes, rather than an anatomic endpoint.

TESTING FOR SPECIAL INDICATIONS

Viability

As already mentioned above, myocardial viability may be assessed using nuclear imaging techniques. Thallium-201 redistribution MPS and F-18 FDG PET may be used to predict global or segmental recovery of left ventricular function in patients who have resting perfusion abnormalities associated with dysfunctional myocardium and occlusive coronary artery disease. MPS and PET viability imaging has been shown to correlate with delayed enhancement CMR. Nitrate enhanced rest perfusion MPS using technetium Sestamibi has also been shown to be useful in the demonstration of myocardial viability, although with sensitivity less than thallium-201 redistribution MPS.

There are inherent differences between thallium-201 redistribution MPS and F-18 FDG PET that may influence results obtained. Thallium-201 is a potassium analog and presence of uptake in myocardium depends upon intact cell membranes. Thallium-201 has a lower energy emission than F-18 FDG and is more likely to be attenuated by soft tissues or pleural/ pericardial fluid. Imaging is also fundamentally different between the gamma camera and PET systems. The presence of radioactive glucose uptake in the myocardium requires glucose metabolism to occur at the time

Table 9.2   Radionuclide Imaging Agents Commonly Used to Assess Myocardial Viability

Agent	Mechanism	Causes of Underestimation of Viability
Tl-201 (rest-redistribution imaging)	Myocyte cell membrane integrity for uptake	Attenuation Thin wall
Tc-99m-sestamibi (nitrate enhanced rest perfusion)	Requires myocyte cell membrane integrity for uptake and binds to mitochondria	Decreased mitochondrial content of hibernating myocytes Thin wall
F-18-FDG in combination with a rest perfusion image)	Requires preserved myocyte glucose uptake and phosphorylation; insulin drives cell uptake.	Suboptimal uptake in chronic (read hyperglycemia

of FDG injection. Hibernating myocardium metabolizes glucose is preferable to free fatty acid, but whole heart radioactive glucose uptake is promoted by careful patient preparation prior to F-18 FDG injection. This requires fasting followed by administration of an oral glucose load or a euglycemic hyperinsulinemic metabolic clamp technique prior to injection of radioactive glucose. It may be challenging to achieve this myocardial preparation in diabetic patients, leading to potential for underestimation of viability by PET (Table 9.2).

Myocardial Infiltrative Diseases

Technetium pyrophosphate is a radiopharmaceutical that is used in detection of myocardial involvement in systemic amyloidosis. Pyrophosphate was historically an agent used in bone imaging and is not normally retained in myocardium. The demonstration of pyrophosphate activity in the myocardium represents an abnormal appearance and is highly suggestive of the presence of abnormal protein deposition. More recently, enhancement patterns with delayed gadolinium-enhanced MRI have been shown to be valuable in identification of cardiac amyloidosis. The accuracy of these methods in comparison to each other has not been established, however it is likely that both approaches will vary depending upon the extent and type of abnormal protein deposition within the myocardium.[24]

CONCLUSION

Nuclear medicine techniques have a well-established role in noninvasive cardiac imaging for the diagnosis and management of coronary artery disease, both in terms of detection of impaired coronary flow reserve and in detection of myocardial viability.

The radiation emitted from the intravenously injected tracer is converted to light energy via a process of crystal scintillation within the gamma or PET camera, converted to digital data and then displayed in standardized form for interpretation. Relative change in regional activity comparing rest and stress perfusion is the basis for detection of fixed or reversible defects, suggesting presence of infarction or ischemia respectively. Gated imaging utilizing a myocardial perfusion tracer or blood pool labeling permits assessment of ventricular function. This adds incrementally to perfusion data for detection of ischemia and prediction of risk. Gated blood pool SPECT is also an accurate and reproducible means of assessing ventricular volumes and function, with application in serial measurements to monitor response to treatment.

Technical developments have been made in gamma camera and PET camera technology, offering promise of improved specificity and sensitivity for detection of CAD and ongoing clinical utility of nuclear imaging techniques in cardiac disease.

Nuclear medicine techniques permit the noninvasive evaluation of coronary artery disease, detection of myocardial ischemia and viability, accurate assessment of ventricular wall motion volumes and LVEF, and evaluation of diastolic filling and ventricular dyssynchony. Newer techniques improve accuracy through more sensitive and specific imaging, and facilitate more rapid evaluation of myocardial perfusion and function.

◇◇◇◇◇◇◇◇◇◇◇◇

REFERENCES

1. Anger HO. Scintillation camera with multichannel collimators. *J Nucl Med* 1964 65:515-31.
2. Wagner A, Mahrholdt H, Holly TA, et al. Contrast-enhanced MRI and routine single photon emission computed tomography (SPECT) perfusion imaging for detection of subendocardial myocardial infarcts: an imaging study. *Lancet* 2003 361:374-9.
3. Hendel RC, Bateman TM, Cerqueira MD, et al. Initial clinical experience with Regadenoson, a novel selective A2A agonist for pharmacologic stress single-photon emission computed tomography myocardial perfusion imaging. *J Am Coll Cardiol* 2005;46:2069-75.
4. Iskandrian AE, Bateman TM, Belardinelli L, et al. Adenosine versus regadenoson comparative evaluation in myocardial perfusion imaging: results of the ADVANCE phase 3 multicenter international trial. *J Nucl Cardiol* 2007;14:645-658.
5. Henzlova MJ, Cerqueira MD, Hansen CL, Taillefer R, Yao SS. ASNC imaging guidelines for nuclear cardiology procedures. Stress protocols and tracers. *J Nucl Cardiol.* 2009;16:331.

6. Gambhir SS, Berman DS. A Novel High-Sensitivity Rapid-Acquisition Single-Photon Cardiac Imaging Camera. *J Nucl Med* 2009;50:635-643.
7. Malkerneker D, Brenner R, Martin WH, et al. CT-based attenuation correction versus prone imaging to decrease equivocal interpretations of rest/stress Tc-99m tetrofosmin SPECT MPI. *J Nucl Cardiol* 2007;14:314-23.
8. Dorbala S, Vangala D, Sampson U, Limaye A, Kwong R, Di Carli MF. Value of vasodilator left ventricular ejection fraction reserve in evaluating the magnitude of myocardium at risk and the extent of angiographic coronary artery disease: a 82Rb PET/CT study. *J Nucl Med* 2007 48:349-58.
9. Anagnostopoulos C, Almonacid A, El Fakhri G, et al. Quantitative relationship between coronary vasodilator reserve assessed by 82Rb PET imaging and coronary artery stenosis severity. *Eur J Nucl Med Mol Imaging* 2008 35:1593-601.
10. Chua T, Yin LC, Thiang TH, Choo TB, Ping DZ, Leng LY. Accuracy of the automated assessment of left ventricular function with gated perfusion SPECT

in the presence of perfusion defects and left ventricular dysfunction: correlation with equilibrium radionuclide ventriculography and echocardiography. *J Nucl Cardiol* 2000 7:301-11.

11. Daou D, Vilain D, Colin P, et al. Comparative value of ECG-gated blood pool SPET and ECG-gated myocardial perfusion SPET in the assessment of global systolic left ventricular function. *Eur J Nucl Med Mol Imaging* 2003 30:859-67.

12. Fauchier L, Marie O, Casset-Senon D, Babuty D, Cosnay P, Fauchier JP. Ventricular dyssynchrony and risk markers of ventricular arrhythmias in nonischemic dilated cardiomyopathy: a study with phase analysis of angioscintigraphy. *Pacing Clin Electrophysiol.* 2003 26:352-6.

13. Muntinga HJ, van den Berg F, Knol HR, et al. Normal values and reproducibility of left ventricular filling parameters by radionuclide angiography. *Int J Card Imaging* 1997;13:165-71.

14. Hendel RC, Berman DS, Di Carli MF, et al. ACCF/ASNC/ACR/AHA/ASE/SCCT/SCMR/SNM 2009 Appropriate Use Criteria for Cardiac Radionuclide Imaging. *J. Am. Coll. Cardiol* 2009;53:inpress.

15. Fraker TD, Jr, Fihn SD, Gibbons RJ, et al. American College of Cardiology; American Heart Association; American College of Cardiology/American Heart Association Task Force on Practice Guidelines Writing Group. 2007 chronic angina focused update of the ACC/AHA 2002 guidelines for the management of patients with chronic stable angina: a report of the American College of Cardiology/American Heart Association Task Force on Practice Guidelines Writing Group to develop the focused update of the 2002 guidelines for the management of patients with chronic stable angina. *Circulation* 2007 116:2762-72.

16. Hachamovitch R, Berman DS, Kiat H, et al. Exercise myocardial perfusion SPECT in patients without known coronary artery disease: incremental prognostic value and use in risk stratification. *Circulation* 1996;93:905-14.

17. Klocke FJ, Baird MG, Bateman TM, et al. ACC/AHA/ASNC guidelines for the clinical use of cardiac radionuclide imaging: a report of the American 1995 guidelines for the clinical use of radionuclide imaging. *Circulation* 2003;108:1404-18.

18. Hachamovitch R, Hayes SW, Friedman JD, Cohen I, Berman DS. Stress myocardial perfusion SPECT is clinically effective and cost-effective in risk-stratification of patients with a high likelihood of CAD but no known CAD. *J Am Coll Cardiol* 2004;43:200-8.

19. Marwick TH, Shaw LJ, Lauer MS, et al. The noninvasive prediction of cardiac mortality in men and women with known or suspected coronary artery disease. *. Am J Med* 1999;106:172-178.

20. Shaw LJ, Hachamovitch R, Berman DS, et al. The economic consequences of available diagnostic and prognostic strategies for the evaluation of stable angina patients: an observational assessment of the value of precatheterization ischemia. Economics of Noninvasive Diagnosis (END) Multicenter Study Group. *J Am Coll Cardiol* 1999 33:661-9.

21. Berman DS, Hachamovitch R, Kiat H, et al. Incremental value of prognostic testing in patients with known or suspected ischemic heart disease: a basis for optimal utilization of exercise technetium-99m sestamibi myocardial perfusion single-photon emission computed tomography. *J Am Coll Cardiol* 1995;26:639-47.

22. Hachamovitch R, Berman DS, Kiat H, Cohen I, Friedman JD, Shaw LJ. Value of stress myocardial perfusion single photon emission computed tomography in patients with normal resting electrocardiograms: an evaluation of incremental prognostic value and cost-effectiveness. *Circulation* 2002;105:823-9.

23. Hachamovitch R, Hayes SW, Friedman JD, Cohen I, Berman D. Stress Myocardial Perfusion SPECT is Clinically Effective and Cost-effective in Risk-stratification of Patients with a High Likelihood of CAD but No Known CAD. *J Am Coll Cardiol* 2004;43:200-8.

24. Thomson LE. Cardiovascular magnetic resonance in clinically suspected cardiac amyloidosis: diagnostic value of a typical pattern of late gadolinium enhancement. *J Am Coll Cardiol* 2008; 51:1031-2.

25. Miller TD, Hodge DO, Christian TF, Milavetz JJ, Bailey KR, Gibbons RJ. Effects of adjustment for referral bias on the sensitivity and specificity of single photon emission computed tomography for the diagnosis of coronary artery disease. *Am J Med* 2002;112:290-7.

26. Cecil MP, Kosinski AS, Jones MT, et al. The importance of work-up (verification) bias correction in assessing the accuracy of SPECT thallium-201 testing for the diagnosis of coronary artery disease. 49 1996.

27. Santana-Boado C, Candell-Riera J, Castell-Conesa J, et al. Diagnostic accuracy of technetium-99m -MIBI myocardial SPECT in women and men. *J Nucl Med* 1998;39:751-5.

28. Diamond GA, Rozanski A, Forrester JS, et al. A model for assessing the sensitivity and specificity of tests subject to selection bias. Application to exercise radionuclide ventriculography for diagnosis of coronary artery disease. *J Chronic Dis.* 1986;39:343-55.

29. Schwartz RS, Jackson WG, Celio PV, Richardson LA, Hickman JR, Jr. Accuracy of exercise 201Tl myocardial scintigraphy in asymptomatic young men. *Circulation* 1993;87:165-72.

CHAPTER 10

Novel Intravascular Imaging Technologies

Hector M. Garcia-Garcia, MD, MSc
Nieves Gonzalo, MD
Peter Barlis, MBBS, MPH, FRACP
Patrick W. Serruys, MD, PhD

INTRODUCTION

The ability to detect vulnerable plaques in vivo is essential to study their natural history and to evaluate potential therapeutic interventions that may ultimately favorably impact on acute coronary syndrome (ACS) and death. Coronary angiography offers valuable information on the long-term behavior of complex coronary lesions but does have several limitations. Goldstein et al.[1] reported that patients with ST-segment elevation myocardial infarction (STEMI) and multiple complex lesions had an increased incidence of recurrent ACS during the year following STEMI when compared to patients with a single complex lesion (19.0% vs 2.6%, p < 0.001, respectively). Taking this into consideration, angiography only permits a two-dimensional view of the arteries and is unable to give precise detail about the vessel wall. As a result, a number of invasive imaging modalities are being tested or used, specifically geared toward the evaluation of vulnerable plaque.[2] These techniques are capable of providing unique detail on the vessel wall, lumen, plaque tissue composition, and the status of inflammation, and therefore circumvent many of the limitations of coronary angiography. This chapter will provide a contemporary review of these technologies with particular reference to their use in the assessment of vulnerable plaque and coronary stents.

HISTOPATHOLOGIC VULNERABLE PLAQUE DEFINITIONS

The classical, most-described phenotype of vulnerable plaque is a thin-capped fibroatheroma (TCFA),[3] characterized by a large necrotic core with an overlying thin cap infiltrated by macrophages. Smooth muscle cells within the cap are absent or few. The thickness of the fibrous cap near the rupture site measures 23 ± 19μm, with 95% of caps measuring < 65μm.[4, 5] Rupture of a TCFA with exposure of the thrombogenic necrotic core to circulating platelets is thought to be responsible for 60% of all acute coronary syndromes.[5]

Macrophage infiltration of the thin cap with release of matrix metalloproteinases and local inflammation can cause extracellular matrix degradation and subsequent plaque rupture.[6, 7] Excessive mechanical strain, particularly at the junction of the TCFA and the normal vessel wall is another factor predisposing to rupture.[8, 9]

Chevuru et al.[10] reported new pathological evidence on TCFA characterization. The prevalence of TCFA and rupture is low (0.46 ± 0.95 and 0.38 ± 0.70 per heart, respectively), focal in nature, and located in the proximal segments of coronary arteries. In earlier studies, up to three TCFA were found per heart.[11] Necrotic core size was relatively small for both, TCFA ($1.6 ± 1.8mm^2$; length 2.7 ± 2.0mm) and ruptured plaques ($2.2 ± 1.9mm^2$; length 1.9 ± 3.6mm). In previous studies, the size of necrotic core in TCFAs was $1.7 ± 1.1mm^2$ with a length of 8mm (range 2–17mm), and in ruptured plaques $3.8 ± 5.5mm^2$, with a length of 9mm (range 2.5–22mm).[12]

The second recognized phenotype of vulnerable plaque, accounting for approximately 40% of coronary thromboses in pathology series is plaque erosion in lesions consisting of either pathologic intimal thickening or thick-capped fibroatheroma.[13] These lesions typically have a high smooth muscle cell content, are rich in proteoglycans and are more common in young women and smokers, but are not associated with other conventional risk factors such as hypercholesterolemia.[14, 15]

Thirdly, there are calcified nodules, which may protrude into the vessel lumen and comprise up to 5% of lesions in pathological series. These lesions are characterized by an absence of endothelial and inflammatory cells.[15] In addition, intraplaque hemorrhage secondary to leakage from the vasa vasorum may also a pathologic role.[16]

IMAGING OF VULNERABLE PLAQUES

Angioscopy

Coronary angioscopy (CAS) is a well-established technique that allows direct visualization of the plaque surface and intraluminal structures. It enables assessment of the plaque color (white, red, yellow), and can illuminate plaque complications such as rupture, intimal tears, and thrombosis with a higher sensitivity compared to angiography.[17-20] On angioscopy, normal artery segments appear as glistening white, whereas atherosclerotic plaques can be categorized based on their angioscopic color as yellow. Platelet-rich thrombus at the site of plaque rupture is characterized as white granular material, and fibrin/erythrocyte-rich thrombus as an irregular, red structure protruding into the lumen. Yellow plaques are associated with ACS[21] and thrombosis.[22] They have also been correlated with other features of vulnerability such as positive remodeling and increased distensibility.[23] Quantitative colorimetric angioscopic analysis provides objective and highly reproducible measurements of angioscopic color. This technique can correct for important chromatic distortions present in modern angioscopic systems. It can also help overcome current limitations in angioscopy research and clinical use imposed by the reliance on visual perception of color.[24]

The major limitation of angioscopy is that it is a rather specialized technique that requires a blood-free field during image acquisition, which can be obtained either by complete vessel occlusion or by continuous saline flushing distal to the angioscope. Presently, coronary angioscopy (Vecmova®, Clinical Supply Co., Gifu, Japan) can be performed while blood is cleared from the field of view by injection of 5–10ml normal saline. Nevertheless, angioscope only allows limited assessment of the coronary tree (i.e., vessels > 2mm diameter) and assessment of stenotic lesions may prove technically difficult. Furthermore, imaging is only of the luminal surface and, although changes in the vessel wall are reflected on the surface, this might not be sufficiently sensitive to detect subtle alterations in plaque composition or plaque burden in the presence of positive remodeling.[25]

Kubo et al.[20] used CAS, optical coherence tomography (OCT) and IVUS to assess culprit lesion morphology in acute myocardial infarction (AMI). The incidence of plaque rupture observed by OCT was 73%, by CAS 47% (p = 0.035), and by IVUS 40%, (p = 0.009). Furthermore, OCT (23%) was superior to CAS (3%, p = 0.022) and IVUS (0%, p = 0.005) in the detection of fibrous cap erosion. The intracoronary thrombus was observed in all cases by OCT and CAS, but was identified in 33% by IVUS (vs OCT, p = 0.001).

Intravascular Ultrasound Radiofrequency Analysis: Virtual Histology

Description of the Technique

Grayscale IVUS imaging is formed by the envelope (amplitude) of the radiofrequency signal, discarding a considerable amount of information lying beneath and between the peaks of the signal. The frequency and power of the signal commonly differ between tissues, regardless of similarities in the amplitude. IVUS-Virtual Histology (IVUS-VH, Volcano Corp., Rancho Cordoba, USA) involves spectral analysis of the data and evaluates different spectral parameters (Y-intercept, minimum power, maximum power, midband power, frequency at minimum power, frequency at maximum power, slope, etc.) to construct tissue maps that classify plaque into four major components (fibrous, fibrolipidic, necrotic core, and calcium). Different plaque components are assigned different color codes: calcified (white), fibrous (green), fibrolipidic (greenish-yellow), and necrotic core (red).[26] Although this classification was initially evaluated in vitro, more recently IVUS-VH pre- and postprocedure have also been correlated with pathological atherectomy specimens showing good correlation for all four tissue types.[27] As assessed by IVUS-VH, the sensitivity and specificity for fibrous tissue was 86% and 90.5%, fibro-fatty 79.3% and 100%, necrotic core 67.3% and 92.9%, and dense calcium 50% and 98.9%, respectively. More recently, these tissue maps have been validated ex vivo by comparison with histology via 899 selected regions (n = 94 plaques) that comprised 471 fibrous tissue, 130 fibro-fatty, 132 necrotic core, and 156 dense calcium regions. The overall predictive accuracies were 93.5% for fibrous, 94.1% for fibro-fatty, 95.8% for necrotic core, and

96.7% for dense calcium with sensitivities and specificities ranging from 72 to 99%. The kappa statistic was calculated to be 0.845 indicating very high agreement with histology.[28]

IVUS-VH data is currently acquired using a commercially available 64-element phased-array catheter (Eagle Eye™ 20MHz catheter, Volcano Corporation, Rancho Cordova, USA). Using an automated pullback device, the transducer is withdrawn at a continuous speed of 0.5mm/s up to the ostium. IVUS-VH acquisition is ECG-gated at the R-wave peaks using a dedicated console.

IVUS B-mode images are reconstructed by customized software and contour detection is performed using cross-sectional views with semiautomatic contour detection software to provide quantitative geometrical and compositional measurements. Because of the limitations of manual calibration,[29] the radiofrequency data is normalized using a technique known as blind deconvolution, an iterative algorithm that deconvolves the catheter transfer function from the backscatter, thus accounting for catheter-to-catheter variability.[30, 31]

It has been our observation that in the near field, an excessive amount of necrotic core is present. The developers have accounted for this with a corrected version introduced in the latest release of the classification tree.

Virtual Histology and Plaque Characterization

Lesion classification is based on static images obtained from autopsy specimens. In brief, some believe that atherosclerotic lesion progression starts with pathologic intimal thickening in which lipid accumulates in areas rich in proteoglycans (lipid pools), but no trace of necrotic core. Others believe that the earliest change of atherosclerosis is the fatty streak, also called as intimal xanthoma. The earliest lesion with a necrotic core is the fibroatheroma (FA), and this is the precursor lesion that may give rise to symptomatic heart disease. Thin-capped fibroatheroma (TCFA) is a lesion characterized by a large necrotic core containing numerous cholesterol clefts. The overlying cap is thin and rich in inflammatory cells, macrophages, and T-lymphocytes with few smooth muscle cells. Plaques prone to rupture are those with decrease cap thickness, large lipid-necrotic core, and severe inflammatory infiltrate. A study done by Burke et al.[4] identified a cut-off value for cap thickness of < 65 microns for vulnerable coronary plaque definition.

Virtual Histology can potentially identify detect thin-capped fibroatheromas (TCFAs). In addition, the progression of the disease can also be followed up. Table 10.1 outlines the Virtual Histology plaque and lesion types that are proposed based on the above pathologic data (Figure 10.1).

Our group evaluated the incidence of IVUS-derived thin-cap fibroatheroma (IDTCFA) using IVUS-VH.[32] Two independent IVUS analysts defined IDTCFA as a lesion fulfilling the following criteria in at least three consecutive cross-sectional areas: (1) necrotic core $\geq$ 10% without evident overlying fibrous tissue; (2) lumen obstruction $\geq$ 40 %. In this study, 62% of patients had at least one IDTCFA in the interrogated vessels. ACS patients had a significantly higher incidence of IDTCFA than stable patients < 3.0 (interquartile range 0.0, 5.0) IDTCFA/coronary vs 1.0 (interquartile range 0.0, 2.8) IDTCFA/coronary,

Table 10.1   VH-IVUS Proposed Lesion Types

Lesion Type	Brief Description
Adaptative Intimal Thickening (AIT)	< 600µm of intima thickness
Pathological Intimal Thickening (PIT)	≥ 600µm thickness for > 20% of the circumference with FF > 15%, and no confluent NC or DC
Fibrotic Plaque (FT)	Dominant FT and no confluent NC or DC
Fibrocalcific Plaque (FC)	Confluent DC with no confluent NC
Fibroatheroma (FA)	Confluent NC not at the lumen on three consecutive frames
Thin Cap Fibroatheroma (TCFA)	Confluent NC at the lumen on three consecutive frames

FT: fibrous tissue; FF: fibro-fatty tissue; NC: necrotic core; and DC: dense calcium.

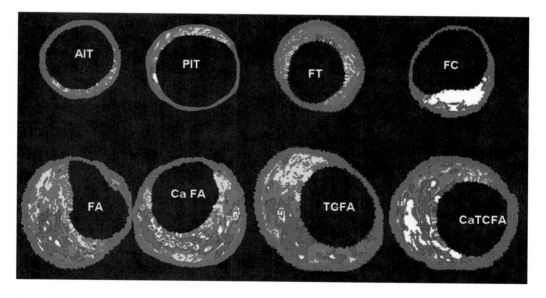

Figure 10.1

IVUS-Virtual Histology proposed lesion types. AIT: adaptative intimal thickening; PIT: pathological intimal thickening; FT: fibrotic plaque; FC: fibrocalcific; FA: fibroatheroma; CaFA: calcified fibroatheroma; TCFA: thin-capped fibroatheroma. (See Color Plate 26.)

p = 0.018; (3) Finally, a clear clustering pattern was seen along the coronaries, with 66.7% of all IDTCFAs located in the first 20mm whereas further along the vessels the incidence was significantly lower (33.3%, p = 0.008). This distribution of IDTCFAs is consistent with previous ex vivo and clinical studies, with a clear clustering pattern from the ostium demonstrating a nonuniform distribution of vulnerable plaques along the coronary tree.[33]

Patients presenting with ACS had a significantly higher prevalence of IDTCFA even in nonculprit vessels, supporting the concept of a multifocal process.[34] Of note, the lesion percent area stenosis and the mean necrotic core areas of the IDTCFAs detected by IVUS-VH were also similar to previously reported histopathological data (55.9% vs 59.6% and 19% vs 23%, respectively).[12]

It is worth mentioning that, although the most accepted threshold to define a cap as "thin" has previously been set at $< 65\mu m$, this was based on postmortem studies of ruptured plaques.[35] Extrapolation of such criteria to in vivo studies therefore requires caution. It is well established that tissue shrinkage occurs during tissue fixation.[36] Shrinkage (particularly of collagen, the main component of fibrous caps) of up to 60%, 15%, and 80% can occur during critical-point-drying, free-drying, and air-drying respectively.[37] Furthermore, postmortem contraction of arteries is an additional confounding factor.[38, 39] Since the axial resolution of IVUS-VH is $246\mu m$, we assumed that the absence of visible fibrous tissue overlying a necrotic core suggested a cap thickness of below $246\mu m$ and used the absence of such tissue to define a thin fibrous cap.[40]

We have developed software to quantify the amount of necrotic core in contact with the lumen, enabling refinement of our analysis. Our current definition of an IVUS-derived TCFA (IDTCFA) is a lesion fulfilling the following criteria in at least three consecutive cross-sectional areas (CSAs): (1) plaque burden $\geq 40\%$; (2) confluent necrotic core $\geq 10\%$ in direct contact with the lumen (i.e., no visible overlying tissue) in the investigated CSA; (3) all consecutive CSAs having the same morphologic characteristics are considered as part of the same IDTCFA lesion.[41] In a study, using this refined definition of TCFA as assessed by IVUS-VH, in patients with ACS who underwent IVUS of all three epicardial coronaries, on average, there were two IVUS-derived thin cap fibroatheroma (IDTCFA) per patient with half of them showing outward remodeling.[41]

The potential value of IVUS-VH in the prediction of adverse coronary events is currently under evaluation in two international multicenter prospective studies (PROSPECT and IBIS 2 trials). In the IBIS 2 trial administration of the lipoprotein-associated phospholipase A2 inhibitor, darapladib, was demonstrated to slow progression of the necrotic core on IVUS-VH on serial evaluation. The impact of this therapy on clinical outcome is currently being investigated in a large event-based trial. Initial review of the PROSPECT review revealed that patients with evidence of an IDTCFA are much more likely to have a subsequent cardiovascular event in the 3 years following an acute coronary syndrome when compared with subjects with no evidence of IDTCFA. These observations further underscore the potential utility of IVUS-VH in the ability to characterize serial changes within the coronary arteries.

Virtual Histology and Coronary Embolization

Identification of subclinical high-risk plaques is potentially important because they may have greater likelihood of rupture and subsequent thrombosis. In 55 patients, a nonculprit vessel with $< 50\%$ diameter stenosis was studied with IVUS-VH. Mean necrotic core percentage was significantly larger in patients with acute coronary syndrome when compared with stable patients (12.26% ± 7.0% vs 7.40% ± 5.5%, p = .006). In addition, stable patients showed more fibrotic vessels (70.97% ± 9.3% vs 63.96% ± 9.1%, p = .007).[42] However, not only the is amount of necrotic larger in patients with ACS, but it appears that NC is also unevenly distributed. In 51 consecutive patients, a nonculprit vessel was investigated through IVUS-VH. The overall length of the region of interest, subsequently divided into 10mm segments, was 41.5 ± 13mm long. No significant change was observed in terms of relative plaque composition along the vessel with respect to fibrous, fibro-fatty, and calcified tissue, whereas the percentage of necrotic core turned out to be increased in the first (median: 8.75%; IQR: 5.7–18) vs the third (median: 6.1%; IQR: 3.2–12) (p = 0.036) and fourth (median: 4.5%; IQR: 2.4–7.9) (p = 0.006) segment. At multivariable regression analysis, distance from the ostium resulted in an independent predictor of relative necrotic content [beta = -0.28 (95%CI: -0.15, -0.41)], together with older age, unstable presentation, no use of statin, and presence of diabetes mellitus.[43]

Two studies evaluated the usefulness of IVUS-VH plaque composition to predict the risk of embolization during stenting.[44, 45] In one of them, 71 patients with STEMI who underwent primary PCI within 12 hours of the beginning of the symptoms were included. After crossing the lesion with a guidewire and performing thrombectomy with an aspiration catheter, IVUS-VH of the infarct-related vessel was performed. The stent was then deployed without embolic protection. ST segment reelevation was used as a marker of distal embolization during stenting. Eleven patients presented with ST segment reelevation after stenting. Total plaque volume was similar in both groups, but the NC volume was significantly higher in the group of patients with ST segment reelevation (32.9 ± 14.1mm^3 vs 20.4 ± 19.1mm^3, p < 0.05). On receiver-operating characteristic curves, NC volume was the best predictor of ST reelevation after stent deployment as compared with fibrous, fibro-lipid, dense calcium, and total plaque volumes. The cut-off point for NC volume that was best predictive for ST reelevation was 33.4mm^3, with a sensitivity of 81.7% and a specificity of 63.6%. The second study included 44 patients who underwent elective coronary stenting. Plaque composition was assessed with IVUS-VH, and small embolic particles liberated during stenting were detected as high-intensity transient signals (HITS) with a Doppler guidewire. Patients were divided into the tertiles according to the HITS counts. Dense calcium and NC area were significantly larger in the highest tertile. In the multivariate logistic regression analysis, only necrotic core area was an independent predictor of high HITS counts (odds ratio 4.41, p = 0.045).

Intravascular Ultrasound Radiofrequency Analysis: Palpography

This technique allows the assessment of local mechanical tissue properties. For a defined pressure difference, soft tissue (e.g., lipid-rich) components will deform more than hard tissue components (e.g., fibrous, calcified).[46, 47] Radiofrequency data obtained at different pressure levels are compared to determine the local tissue deformation.

Each palpogram represents the strain information for a certain cross-section over the full cardiac cycle. The longitudinal resolution of the acquisitions depends on heart rate and pullback speed. With a heart rate of 60bpm and a pullback speed of 1.0mm/s, the longitudinal resolution is 1.0mm. Palpograms are acquired using a 20MHz phased array IVUS catheter (Eagle Eye™ 20MHz catheter, Volcano Therapeutics, Rancho Cordova, USA). Digital radiofrequency data are acquired using a custom-designed workstation.

The local strain is calculated from the gated radiofrequency traces using cross-correlation analysis and displayed, color-coded, from blue (for 0% strain) to red to yellow (for 2% strain).[48] Plaque strain values are assigned a Rotterdam Classification (ROC) score ranging from 1 to 4 (ROC I = 0–< 0.6%; ROC II = 0.6–< 0.9%; ROC III = 0.9–< 1.2%; ROC IV = > 1.2%)[49] (Figure 10.2). Our group has demonstrated that palpography has a high sensitivity (88%) and specificity (89%) to detect vulnerable plaques in vitro.[46] Postmortem coronary arteries were investigated with intravascular elastography and subsequently processed for histology. There was a positive correlation between the presence of high strain and the degree of macrophage infiltration ($p < 0.006$) and an inverse relation between the amount of smooth muscle cells and strain ($p < 0.0001$). Vulnerable plaques identified by palpography had a thinner cap than nonvulnerable plaques ($p < 0.0001$). In a subsequent study, 55 patients with either stable or unstable angina, or acute MI were analyzed. Among patients with stable angina, the prevalence of deformable plaques was significantly lower per vessel (0.6 ± 0.6) than in patients presenting with unstable angina (1.6 ± 0.7, $p = 0.0019$) or with acute MI (2.0 ± 0.7, $p < 0.0001$). In the IBIS I study, on palpography, both the absolute number of high-strain spots (grade 3/4) in the ROI ($p = 0.009$) and their density per cm ($p = 0.012$) decreased significantly between baseline and follow-up. This decrease in the overall population was largely driven by changes in the subgroup of patients with STEMI; this group had both the highest number of high-strain spots at baseline and the most marked relative decrease during follow-up compared to patients with other clinical presentations. At 6-month follow-up, the density of high-strain spots (1.2 ± 1.4/cm) was comparable among clinical subgroups.[50]

The potential value of IVUS-palpography is currently under evaluation in two international multicenter prospective studies, PROSPECT and IBIS 2 trials. These two studies have also obtained IVUS-VH during the same IVUS pullback, allowing for the assessment of both morphologic and biomechanic properties of a particular plaque. Assessing several characteristics of a given plaque could potentially enhance invasive risk stratification by identifying very high-risk plaques, thereby lowering the number of vulnerable plaques that deserve to be serially followed and ultimately treated (see Figure 10.2).

Optical Coherence Tomography

Optical coherence tomography (OCT) is an optical analog of ultrasound; however, it uses light instead of sound to create an image.[51, 52] For OCT imaging, low-coherence, near infrared light with a wavelength around 1300nm is used because it minimizes the energy

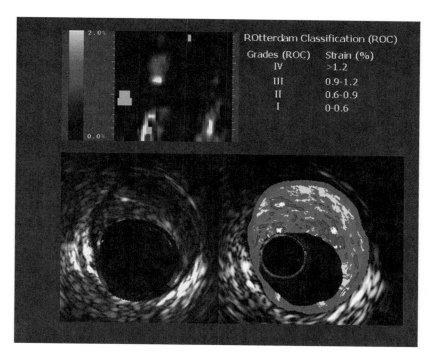

Figure 10.2

IVUS-palpography. In the upper left side the palpography strain map is opened up. The local strain is calculated from the gated radiofrequency traces using cross-correlation analysis and displayed, color-coded (see Color Plate 27), from 0% strain to 2% strain. Plaque strain values are assigned a Rotterdam Classification (ROC) score ranging from 1 to 4 (ROC I = 0–< 0.6%; ROC II = 0.6–< 0.9%; ROC III = 0.9–< 1.2%; ROC IV = > 1.2%). At the bottom, in the same cross-sectional area a high-strain spot (ROC III) is shown (left); in the Virtual Histology (VH) image (right) a confluent necrotic core area in contact with the lumen is seen, suggesting an IVUS-derived thin capped fibroatheroma.

absorption in the light beam caused by protein, water, hemoglobin, and lipid. The light waves are reflected by the internal microstructures within biologic tissues as a result of their differing optical indices.

This technique provides a resolution of 10–20μm in vivo;[53] this level of detail is well beyond the level of resolution of IVUS (100–150μm).[54] OCT has been demonstrated to be highly sensitive and specific for characterizing atherosclerotic plaques in vitro when compared with histological analysis[55-57] with a sensitivity and specificity of 71–79% and 97–98% for fibrous plaques, 95–96% and 97% for fibrocalcific plaques, and 90–94% and 90%–92% for lipid-rich plaques. In addition, the inter- and intraobserver reliabilities of OCT assessment were high (kappa values of 0.88 and 0.91, respectively).[57] In vitro comparison of OCT with IVUS have demonstrated superior delineation by OCT of structural details such as thin caps, lipid pools, or tissue proliferation.[58] An in vitro comparison of OCT, integrated backscatter IVUS (similar methodology to IVUS-VH), and conventional IVUS found that OCT had the best potential for tissue characterization of coronary plaques, with higher sensitivity and specificity compared to the other imaging modalities.[59] However, a recent study comparing OCT to histopathology reported a lower sensitivity for plaque components. Misclassification occurred in 41% of lesions, predominantly resulting from a combination of incomplete penetration depth into the vessel wall and the inability to distinguish calcium deposits from lipid pools.[60]

In a pilot clinical study, our group performed in vivo OCT analysis of the coronary arterial wall in patients who were undergoing percutaneous coronary intervention. Imaging was possible in all patients and the entire vessel circumference was visualized at all times. A wide spectrum of different plaque morphologies was observed. OCT allowed for differentiation of the normal artery wall and inhomogeneous, mixed plaques, as well as thin cap fibroatheromas with inhomogeneous, low-reflecting necrotic cores, covered by highly reflecting thin fibrous caps.[54]

As a result of its high axial resolution, there is no doubt that OCT is the in vivo gold standard for identifying and measuring the thickness of the fibrous cap (Figure 10.3); an in vivo study found a significant difference in minimal cap thickness between acute MI and stable angina patients, with median (interquartile range) values of 47.0 (25.3–184.3) μm and 102.6 (22.0–291.1) μm, respectively (p = 0.02).[61] In addition to its reliability as a tool to measure the thickness of the cap in vivo, recent postmortem and in vivo studies have shown that OCT is capable of evaluating the macrophage content of infiltrated fibrous caps.[62, 63]

Kubo et al.[20] evaluated the ability of intracoronary OCT to assess culprit lesions during primary PCI in patients with acute MI. The thickness of the remnants of the fibrous cap after symptomatic rupture measured was 49 ± 21 μm. The main limitation of OCT is the shallow tissue penetration depth (1.5–2mm), which hampers imaging of the entire vessel wall in large vessels and light absorbance by blood that currently needs to be overcome by saline infusion and balloon occlusion, thereby precluding interrogation of long and proximal segments of the coronary tree. This has been partly overcome with the use of nonocclusive techniques whereby contrast is flushed through the guiding catheter during simultaneous image acquisition at 3.0mm/seconds (M3, LightLab Imaging Inc., Westford, MA, USA). Furthermore, even more encouraging is the use of optical frequency domain imaging (OFDI) that enables even faster pullback speeds without compromise of image quality and resolution.

Thermography

Atherosclerosis is accompanied by inflammation, and vulnerable plaques have been associated with increased macrophage activity, metabolism, and inflammation.[64] Activated macrophages produce thermal energy, which might be detected on the surface of these atherosclerotic lesions using specially designed catheters equipped with thermistor

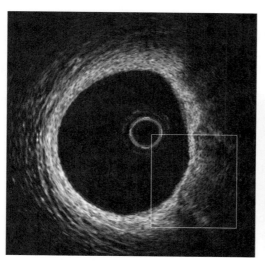
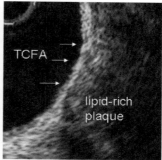

Figure 10.3

The optical coherence tomography image shows thin cap fibrous atheroma (TCFA). The cross-section demonstrates a region of low reflectivity with diffuse borders between the 3 and 5 o'clock positions consistent with a lipid-rich plaque. This is covered by a thin, highly reflective fibrous cap (TCFA) that measures between 10–30 microns in thickness.

sensors at the distal tip.[65] A rise in temperature can be found in atherosclerotic plaques as compared to disease-free coronary segments. Temperature differences between an atherosclerotic plaque and normal vessel wall increase progressively from patients with stable angina to patients with acute MI with a maximum temperature difference to the background temperature of $1.5 \pm 0.7°C$.[66] In a prospective study, Stefanadis et al. reported an association between temperature heterogeneity and the incidence of adverse events at follow-up in patients with coronary artery disease undergoing successful PCI.[67] In addition, treatment with statins seemed to affect the thermographic results: in nonculprit lesions the temperature difference was lower in the group treated with statins compared with the untreated group $(0.06 \pm 0.05°C$ vs $0.11 \pm 0.10°C; p = 0.05)$.[68]

More recently, a correlation between morphologic and functional characteristics of culprit lesions (CL) in patients with acute coronary syndromes and chronic stable angina (CSA) has been reported.[69] In 81 consecutive patients (48 with ACS and 33 with CSA), remodeling index (Ri) by IVUS and temperature difference (DeltaT) by angioscopy between the CL and the proximal vessel wall were measured. Patients with ACS had greater remodeling index than patients with CSA $(1.15 \pm 0.18$ vs $0.90 \pm 0.12; p < 0.01)$, as well as increased DeltaT $(0.08 \pm 0.03$ degrees C vs 0.04 ± 0.02 degrees C; $p < 0.01)$. Patients with positive Ri had higher DeltaT than patients with negative Ri $(0.07 \pm 0.03$ degrees C vs 0.04 ± 0.02 degrees C; $p < 0.001)$. Patients with rupture plaque had increased

DeltaT compared with patients without rupture plaques ($0.09 \pm 0.03°C$ vs $0.05 \pm 0.02°C$; $p < 0.01$). Multivariate analysis showed that DeltaT was independently correlated with the presence of rupture plaque, positive Ri, and ACS.

However, there are several different aspects that deserve further investigation. The prevalence and distribution of inflammatory cells in stable and unstable atherosclerotic plaque is unclear, and the predictive value of warm lesions remains elusive. Furthermore, the impact of different coronary flow conditions on plaque temperature (cooling effect) is still not completely understood.[70, 71] Simulations have revealed that the correct interpretation of intravascular thermographic measurements requires data on the flow and on the morphologic characteristics of the atherosclerotic plaque.[72]

There are a few limitations to the routine use of thermography in the catheterization laboratory: (a) most of the catheters used still comprise over-the-wire systems; (b) accurate temperature assessment requires direct contact of the thermistors with the vessel wall, with the associated potential risk of endothelial damage;[73] and (c) as the temperature within the vessel changes rapidly with fluid application, any intracoronary injection of contrast, flush, or medication has to be avoided before and during measurements.[74]

Intravascular Magnetic Resonance

Magnetic resonance (MR) is a nonionizing diagnostic tool exploiting the spins of the nuclear protons in a strong magnetic field. For intravascular diagnosis, two different approaches have been introduced.

The first, conventional approach visualizes the anatomic structure by using a coil placed in a catheter or wire in combination with an external magnet (MR imaging). While this approach has been shown to provide detailed information on structure and composition of the arterial wall and plaque,[75] the procedure has to be performed in a MR magnet, not in a cardiac catheterization laboratory. The accuracy for MRI differentiation of plaque components has been validated in vitro and feasibility demonstrated in vivo.[76] The 0.030-inch IVMRI coil had a sensitivity and specificity of 73% and 85% respectively for lipid, 83% and 81% respectively for fibrous tissue, and 100% and 97% respectively for calcification. Subsequently, the same system was applied in human iliac arteries in vivo using a 1.5T magnet with a resolution of 312μm. Complete vessel wall analysis was possible in all 25 patients and required 20 minutes for an arterial segment of 20mm length. Compared to IVUS, mean lumen diameters were similar, but the outer wall area was overestimated by IVMRI (mean $116.4 \pm 4.7mm^2$ vs $86.6 \pm 5.8mm^2$, $p = 0.0001$). However, interobserver agreements for IVMRI were much higher (kappa 0.68–0.79) than for IVUS (kappa 0.21).

The other novel approach analyzes the chemical composition by placing both the coils and miniaturized magnets on the tip of a catheter, without the need of external magnets (MR spectroscopy) and can be performed in the cardiac catheterization laboratory.[77]

MR spectroscopy can identify fibrous and lipid-rich tissue by measuring differential water diffusion in a field of view. Acquired data is displayed as color-coded sectors based on the lipid fraction index (LFI) for each zone of the FOV. Blue indicates no lipid, gray corresponds to intermediate lipid content and yellow indicates high lipid content (Figure 10.4). Clinical feasibility of catheter-based, self-contained IV MR spectroscopy has been recently demonstrated in patients scheduled for coronary catheterization.[78]

Preclinical trials employing this technology demonstrated its capacity to differentiate plaque components of human aortas, coronary and carotid arteries in vitro: IVMR spectroscopy was able to accurately detect different components (fibrous cap, smooth muscle cells, organizing thrombus, fresh thrombus, edema, lipid, and calcium) with sensitivities and specificities ranging from 84–100%. Agreement with histology for grading

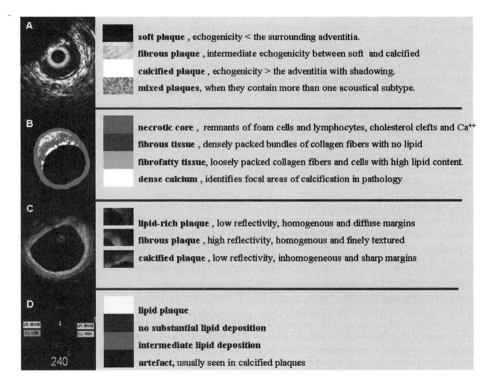

Figure 10.4

Multi-imaging in the coronary arteries. The same coronary segment (represented by one frame) has been imaged by 4 different imaging techniques: grayscale IVUS (panel A), IVUS-Virtual Histology (panel B), optical coherence tomography (panel C) and intravascular magnetic resonance spectroscopy (IVMR). Of note, in the upper left quadrant of the plaque, a calcified area is seen in three imaging modalities, but not in IVMR where an artifact is observed. On the right hand side, the different plaque and tissues types across the coronary imaging techniques is shown. (See Color Plate 28.)

the extent of intraplaque lipid accumulation was 74% and 80% for grading intimal thickness. Further analysis revealed high correlation to histologic analysis of a wide spectrum of plaque types in 15 of 16 (94%) aortic lesions and 16 of 18 (89%) coronary lesions (sensitivity 100%, specificity 89%), including one plaque rupture, three TFCAs, seven thick-cap fibrous atheroma, four fibrocalcific plaques, two intimal xanthomas, and one adaptive intimal thickening.[79]

Current limitations include the limited field of view, the size of the catheter, the need for direct vessel wall contact, and the time required for acquisition. In the past, the use of an autoperfusion balloon during data acquisition has been proposed to limit ischemia.[80]

Clearly IVMR diagnostics remain an exciting area still under development. Catheter-based system will further increase the user friendliness, their sample volume and allow for scanning of longer arterial segments. Upcoming developments include the improvement MR plaque differentiation by the use of contrast agents, such as paramagnetic gadolinium-based contrast[81] or supraparamagnetic contrast agents (iron oxide nanoparticles), that can accumulate in macrophages.[82] There are still a few unanswered questions, including the effect of the thermal energy generated on small arteries and on coronary artery stents, although conventional MRI appears safe in this setting.[83]

A study has been started in our center to explore a multimodality imaging approach of atherosclerotic plaque in vivo. The same coronary segment is assessed by greyscale IVUS, IVUS-VH, and OCT and IVMR (see Figure 10.4). This has been a challenging process, because we are dealing with the different imaging resolutions and the lack of common nomenclature and classification across these imaging techniques.

Raman and Near Infrared Spectroscopy

A number of spectroscopic intravascular imaging techniques have been developed recently and are still under investigation.[84] Spectroscopy can provide qualitative and quantitative information about chemical plaque composition. The Raman effect is created when incident laser light (typically 750–850nm wavelength) excites molecules in a tissue sample, which scatter light at a different wavelength. This change in wavelength, called the Raman effect, is dependent on the chemical components of the tissue sample[85, 85] and can therefore provide quantitative information about molecular composition.[87-89] Raman spectroscopy has shown acceptable correlation compared with histology (r = 0.68 for cholesterol and r = 0.71 calcification)[89] and with IVUS in vitro.[88]

Raman spectroscopy technology collects scattered light with optical fibers and routes the collected signal to spectrometer systems for analysis. Previously optical fiber probes utilized a region of the Raman spectrum called the fingerprint (FP) region (< ~1800 cm^{-1} shifted light) to conduct remote assays, but because of technical problems with this approach, it has been recently replaced by using another region of the Raman spectrum, called high wave number (HW) Raman shifted light (> ~2500 cm^{-1} shifted light). This allows us to collect Raman spectra via a single optical fiber, simplifying the size and

Table 10.2   Plaque/Vessel Components Detectable by Raman Spectroscopy

Demonstrated:	Collagen
	Elastin
	Myosin
	Triglycerides
	Beta-carotene
	Foam cells
	Cholesterol/esters
	Hemoglobin
	Fibrin
Possible:	Metalloproteinases
	Low density lipoprotein (LDL)
	Oxidized LDL
	Proteoglycans
	Glycosaminoglycans
	Plasmin
	Nucleic acids
	Nitrotyrosine

complexity of the catheter and making it clinically feasible (Eurointervention 2008, in press). Thus, the optical catheter system (OCS) (vPredict™) has been introduced as a tool for measuring the chemical composition of coronary vessels in vivo using Raman spectroscopy and the subsequent mapping and quantification of the vessel and plaque components for evaluating plaque progression. In a xenograft model, lipid-laden plaque were identified with the collected Raman spectra by utilizing the overall cholesterol content, i.e., the sum of the free cholesterol and cholesterol esters contents, and setting a decision threshold at 12%, as determined in previous studies. As expected, the lipid-laden plaques exhibit an increased content of free cholesterol and cholesterol esters, while the nonatherosclerotic samples are mainly protein and triglycerides (Table 10.2).

The vPredict OCS delivers infrared light to the vessel wall through optical fibers contained within a small flexible catheter and captures a portion of the reflected light for spectral analysis. This analysis provides information about the composition of the underlying tissue (Figure 10.5).

Alternatively, near infrared (NIR) molecular vibrational transitions can be measured in the NIR region (750–2500nm)[90] and laser spectroscopy using wavelengths of 360–510nm has been evaluated in vitro.[91]

Near-infrared spectroscopy observes how different substances absorb and scatter NIR light to different degrees at various wavelengths. A NIR spectrometer emits light into a sample and measures the proportion of light that is returned over a wide range of optical wavelengths. The return signal is then plotted as a graph of absorbance (y-axis) at different wavelengths (x-axis) called a spectrum.

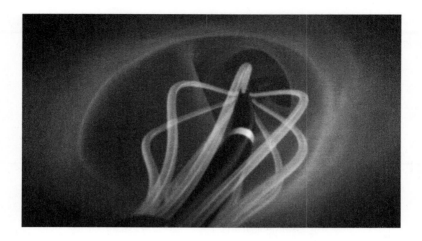

Figure 10.5

vPredict™ optical catheter system (OCS). This catheter has 8 optical fibers that deliver infrared light to the vessel wall and captures a portion of the reflected light for spectral analysis.

Image courtesy of Prescient Medical, Inc.

In aortic and coronary artery autopsy specimens, the ability of the technique to identify lipid-rich TCFA through blood has been confirmed.[92] A catheter-based system has been developed to address the challenges that must be overcome for use in patients—access to the coronary artery, blood, motion, and the need to scan. Initial clinical experience in six patients with stable angina demonstrates that high-quality NIR spectra can be safely obtained.[93] Additional studies are planned to validate the ability of the technique to identify lipid-rich coronary artery plaques and ultimately link chemical characterization with subsequent occurrence of an ACS.[94, 95]

IMAGING OF CORONARY STENTS

Intravascular Ultrasound Radiofrequency Analysis: Virtual Histology

Intravascular ultrasound–Virtual Histology classifies stent struts as dense calcium (DC) and necrotic core (NC). We applied this property to follow-up the degradation of a bioabsorbable stent by measuring the temporal changes in IVUS-VH characteristics. Twenty-seven consecutive patients treated with a single bioabsorbable everolimus-eluting stent (BVS, Abbott Laboratories, IL USA) in simple lesions were imaged with IVUS-VH after predilation (presenting cohort of 13 patients), poststenting, and again in 6 months. There was an increase in absolute dense calcium and necrotic core by 297% and 256% respectively from pre- to poststenting. Overall, patients (n = 27) with poststent-

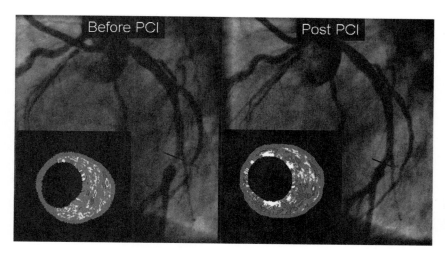

Figure 10.6

IVUS-Virtual Histology in stented segments. In the left-hand side, a coronary angiogram of the left coronary system shows on the distal segment of the left circumflex artery an eccentric lesion. A presenting Virtual Histology (VH) frame showed a fibrotic type of plaque (location of VH frame is indicated by a black line). On the right hand side, the post-stenting VH frame is depicted. Of note, at the lumen and surrounding areas an increase in the amount of "dense calcium" and "necrotic core" is observed. This is due to the presence of stent struts that are misclassified by VH. PCI, percutaneous coronary intervention. (See Color Plate 29.)

ing and follow-up VH showed a significant decrease in dense calcium (28.3% vs 20.9, p = 0.001). Individually, in 21 out of 27 patients, there was a regression in the calcified pattern. Although not significantly, necrotic core content also decreased (22.4% vs 20.3, p = 0.227). In turn, both fibro-fatty and fibrous tissue increased (5.0% vs 7.4, p = 0.024 and 44.3% vs 51.4%, p = 0.006 respectively). In conclusion, the quantitative assessment of the IVUS-VH changes at 6 months suggests a reduction of the DC compatible with early struts alteration of the BVS (Figure 10.6).

Optical Coherence Tomography

OCT permits the detailed assessment of stents and their relation to the vessel wall, both immediately following implantation and at follow-up. Furthermore, OCT also allows the quantification of neointimal tissue surrounding each individual stent strut. Unlike bare metal stents (BMS), which develop circumferential coverage with an average thickness of 500mm or more well visualized with IVUS and angiography,[96] drug-eluting stents (DES) delay and prevent this hyperplastic response so that the average late lumen loss can be as low as 0.1 or 0.2mm,[97, 98] which means the amount of intimal tissue will not be detectable with IVUS.[96]

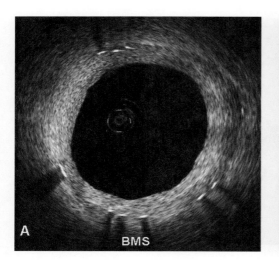
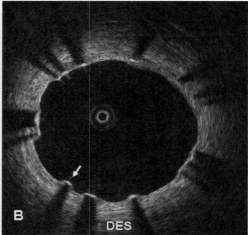

Figure 10.7

OCT and stent. Panel A: Demonstrates the optical coherence tomography (OCT) imaging of a bare metal stent 4 months following implantation. The circumferential tissue struts are visible with shadowing induced by the metal. The neointimal tissue measured between 140 and 220 microns in thickness. Panel B: OCT imaging of a drug-eluting stent (DES) at 4 months follow-up showing the circumferential struts with a very thin neointimal layer (10–40 microns thick). The arrow indicates a strut with no visible tissue coverage. (See Color Plate 30.)

Several small studies have recently been published highlighting the application of OCT in the detection of stent tissue coverage at follow-up. Matsumoto et al.[99] studied 34 patients following sirolimus-eluting stent (SES) implantation. The mean neointima thickness was 52.5 microns, and the prevalence of struts covered by thin neointima undetectable by IVUS was 64%. The average rate of neointima-covered struts in an individual SES was 89%. Nine SES (16%) showed full coverage by neointima, whereas the remaining stents had partially uncovered struts.[99] Similarly, Takano et al.[100] studied 21 patients (4,516 struts) 3 months following SES implantation. Rates of exposed struts and exposed struts with malapposition were 15% and 6%, respectively. These were more frequent in patients with ACS than in those with non-ACS (18% vs 13%, p < 0.0001; 8% vs 5%, p < 0.005, respectively). The ability of OCT to image at high resolution is the major advantage over IVUS and it also affords the potential to quantify the amount of neointimal tissue formed over struts, an application that remains elusive for a technique like angioscopy. OCT is now also being incorporated in more and more clinical stent trials with the goal of assessing neointimal tissue coverage, an important potential surrogate marker for late thrombosis[101, 102] (Figure 10.7).

CONCLUSION

Several invasive imaging techniques are currently under development to detect vulnerable coronary plaques in human coronary arteries in vivo. To date, however, none of the techniques described above have been sufficiently validated and, more importantly, they have not demonstrated a sound and reproducible ability to predict future adverse cardiac events. Intravascular palpography and Virtual Histology, based on conventional IVUS catheters, appear to be very promising and their predictive role is presently under investigation in a large international trial.

Very rigorous and well-designed studies are compelling for defining the role of each imaging modality. Noninvasive techniques and the assessment of humoral and genetic factors comprise complementary and important tools in this direction.

At present, the main purpose of all these evolving techniques is to improve our understanding of atherosclerotic disease and to define its natural history. Ultimately, the aim is to identify patients at high risk for future cardiovascular events and to evaluate the benefits from either local or systemic therapeutic interventions.

◇◇◇◇◇◇◇◇◇◇◇◇

REFERENCES

1. Goldstein JA, Demetriou D, Grines CL, Pica M, Shoukfeh M, O'Neill WW. Multiple complex coronary plaques in patients with acute myocardial infarction. *N Engl J Med* 2000;343:915-22.

2. Waxman S, Ishibashi F, Muller JE. Detection and treatment of vulnerable plaques and vulnerable patients: novel approaches to prevention of coronary events. *Circulation* 2006;114:2390-411.

3. Kolodgie FD, Burke AP, Farb A, et al. The thin-cap fibroatheroma: a type of vulnerable plaque: the major precursor lesion to acute coronary syndromes. *Curr Opin Cardiol.* 2001;16:285-92.

4. Burke AP, Farb A, Malcom GT, Liang YH, Smialek J, Virmani R. Coronary risk factors and plaque morphology in men with coronary disease who died suddenly. *N Engl J Med* 1997;336:1276-82.

5. Virmani R, Kolodgie FD, Burke AP, Farb A, Schwartz SM. Lessons from sudden coronary death: a comprehensive morphological classification scheme for atherosclerotic lesions. *Arterioscler Thromb Vasc Biol* 2000;20:1262-75.

6. Moreno PR, Falk E, Palacios IF, Newell JB, Fuster V, JT. F. Macrophage infiltration in acute coronary syndromes. Implications for plaque rupture. *Circulation* 1994;90:775-8.

7. Ross R. Atherosclerosis—An Inflammatory Disease. *N Engl J Med* 1999;340:115-126.

8. Loree HM, Kamm RD, Stringfellow RG, RT. L. Effects of fibrous cap thickness on peak circumferential stress in model atherosclerotic vessels. *Circ Res* 1992;71:850-8.

9. Richardson PD, Davies MJ, GV. B. Influence of plaque configuration and stress distribution on fissuring of coronary atherosclerotic plaques. *Lancet* 1989;2:941-4.

10. Cheruvu PK, Finn AV, Gardner C, et al. Frequency and distribution of thin-cap fibroatheroma and ruptured plaques in human coronary arteries: a pathologic study. *J Am Coll Cardiol* 2007;50:940-9.

11. Kolodgie FD, Virmani R, Burke AP, et al. Pathologic assessment of the vulnerable human coronary plaque. *Heart* 2004;90:1385-91.

12. Virmani R, Burke AP, Kolodgie FD, Farb A. Vulnerable plaque: the pathology of unstable coronary lesions. *J Interv Cardiol* 2002;15:439-46.

13. Farb A, Burke AP, Tang AL, et al. Coronary plaque erosion without rupture into a lipid core: a frequent cause of coronary thrombosis in sudden coronary death. *Circulation* 1996;93:1354-1363.

14. Arbustini E, Dal Bello B, Morbini P, et al. Plaque erosion is a major substrate for coronary thrombosis in acute myocardial infarction. *Heart* 1999;82:269-272.

15. Virmani R, Kolodgie FD, Burke AP, Farb A, Schwartz SM. Lessons from sudden coronary death: a comprehensive morphological classification scheme for atherosclerotic lesions. *Arterioscler Thromb Vasc Biol* 2000;20:1262-1275.

16. Kolodgie FD, Gold HK, Burke AP, et al. Intraplaque Hemorrhage and Progression of Coronary Atheroma. *N Engl J Med* 2003;349:2316-2325.

17. Mizuno K, Satomura K, Miyamoto A, et al. Angioscopic evaluation of coronary-artery thrombi in acute coronary syndromes. *N Engl J Med* 1992;326:287-291.

18. Sherman CT, Litvack F, Grundfest W, et al. Coronary angioscopy in patients with unstable angina pectoris. *N Engl J Med* 1986;315:913-919.

19. de Feyter PJ, Ozaki Y, Baptista J, et al. Ischemia-related lesion characteristics in patients with stable or unstable angina: a study with intracoronary angioscopy and ultrasound. *Circulation* 1995;92:1408-1413.

20. Kubo T, Imanishi T, Takarada S, et al. Assessment of culprit lesion morphology in acute myocardial infarction: ability of optical coherence tomography compared with intravascular ultrasound and coronary angioscopy. *J Am Coll Cardiol* 2007;50:933-9.

21. Thieme T, Wernecke KD, Meyer R, et al. Angioscopic evaluation of atherosclerotic plaques: validation by histomorphologic analysis and association with stable and unstable coronary syndromes. *J Am Coll Cardiol* 1996;28:1-6.

22. Ueda Y, Ohtani T, Shimizu M, Hirayama A, Kodama K. Assessment of plaque vulnerability by angioscopic classification of plaque color. *Am Heart J* 2004;148:333-5.

23. Takano M, Mizuno K, Okamatsu K, Yokoyama S, Ohba T, Sakai S. Mechanical and structural characteristics of vulnerable plaques: analysis by coronary angioscopy and intravascular ultrasound. *J Am Coll Cardiol* 2001;38:99-104.

24. Lehmann KG, Oomen JA, Slager CJ, deFeyter PJ, Serruys PW. Chromatic distortion during angioscopy: assessment and correction by quantitative colorimetric angioscopic analysis. *Cathet Cardiovasc Diagn* 1998;45:191-201.

25. Smits PC, Pasterkamp G, de Jaegere PP, de Feyter PJ, Borst C. Angioscopic complex lesions are predominantly compensatory enlarged: an angioscopy and intracoronary ultrasound study. *Cardiovasc Res* 1999;41:458-64.

26. Nair A, Kuban BD, Tuzcu EM, Schoenhagen P, Nissen SE, Vince DG. Coronary plaque classification with intravascular ultrasound radiofrequency data analysis. *Circulation* 2002;106:2200-2206.

27. Nasu K, Tsuchikane E, Katoh O, et al. Accuracy of in vivo coronary plaque morphology assessment: a validation study of in vivo virtual histology compared with in vitro histopathology. *Journal of the American College of Cardiology* 2006;47:2405-2412.

28. Nair A MP, Kuban BD, Vince DG. Automated coronary plaque characterization with intravascular ultrasound backscatter: ex vivo validation. *Eurointervention* 2007;3:113-130.

29. Rodriguez-Granillo GA, Aoki J, Ong AT, et al. Methodological considerations and approach to cross-technique comparisons using in vivo coronary plaque characterization based on intravascular ultrasound radiofrequency data analysis: insights from the Integrated Biomarker and Imaging Study (IBIS). *Int J Cardiovasc Intervent* 2005;7:52-8.

30. Kaaresen K. Deconvolution of sparse spike trains by iterated window maximization. *IEEE Trans Signal Process* 1997;45:1173-1183.

31. Kaaresen K, Bolviken E. Blind deconvolution of ultrasonic traces accounting for pulse variance. *IEEE Trans Ultrason Ferroelectr Freq Control* 1999;46:564-573.

32. Rodriguez-Granillo GA, Garcia-Garcia HM, Mc Fadden EP, et al. In vivo intravascular ultrasound-derived thin-cap fibroatheroma detection using ultrasound radiofrequency data analysis. *Journal of the American College of Cardiology* 2005;46:2038-2042.

33. Wang JC, Normand SL, Mauri L, Kuntz RE. Coronary artery spatial distribution of acute myocardial infarction occlusions. *Circulation* 2004;110:278-84.

34. Rioufol G, Finet G, Ginon I, et al. Multiple atherosclerotic plaque rupture in acute coronary syndrome: a three-vessel intravascular ultrasound study 10.1161/01.CIR.0000025609.13806.31. *Circulation* 2002;106:804-808.

35. Burke AP, Farb A, Malcom GT, Liang Y, Smialek J, R V. Coronary risk factors and plaque morphology in men with coronary disease who died suddenly. *N Engl J Med* 1997;336:1276-1282.

36. Lowder ML, Li S, Carnell PH, RP. V. Correction of distortion of histologic sections of arteries. *Journal of Biomechanics*;In Press, Corrected Proof.

37. Boyde A, Jones SJ, Tamarin A. Dimensional changes during specimen preparation for scanning electron microscopy. *Scanning Electron Microsc* 1977;1:507-18.

38. Fishbein MC, Siegel RJ. How big are coronary atherosclerotic plaques that rupture? *Circulation* 1996;94:2662-6.

39. Siegel RJ, Swan K, Edwalds G, Fishbein MC. Limitations of postmortem assessment of human coronary artery size and luminal narrowing: differential effects of tissue fixation and processing on vessels with different degrees of atherosclerosis. *J Am Coll Cardiol* 1985;5:342-6.

40. Nair A, Calvetti D, DG V. Regularized autoregressive analysis of intravascular ultrasound data: improvement in spatial accuracy of plaque tissue maps. *IEEE Trans Ultrason Ferroelectr Freq Control* 2004;51:420-431.

41. Garcia-Garcia HM, Goedhart D, Schuurbiers JC, et al. Virtual histology and remodeling index allow in vivo identification of allegedly high risk coronary plaques in patients with acute coronary syndromes: a three vessel intravascular ultrasound radiofrequency data analysis. *Eurointervention* 2006;2:338-344.

42. Rodriguez-Granillo GA, McFadden EP, Valgimigli M, et al. Coronary plaque composition of nonculprit lesions, assessed by in vivo intracoronary ultrasound radio frequency data analysis, is related to clinical presentation. *Am Heart J* 2006;151:1020-24.

43. Valgimigli M, Rodriguez-Granillo GA, Garcia-Garcia HM, et al. Distance from the ostium as an independent determinant of coronary plaque composition in vivo: an intravascular ultrasound study based radiofrequency data analysis in humans. *Eur Heart J* 2006;27:655-63.

44. Kawaguchi R, Oshima S, Jingu M, et al. Usefulness of virtual histology intravascular ultrasound to predict distal embolization for ST-segment elevation myocardial infarction. *J Am Coll Cardiol* 2007;50:1641-6.

45. Kawamoto T, Okura H, Koyama Y, et al. The relationship between coronary plaque characteristics and small embolic particles during coronary stent implantation. *J Am Coll Cardiol* 2007;50:1635-40.

46. Schaar JA, de Korte CL, Mastik F, et al. Characterizing vulnerable plaque features with intravascular elastography. *Circulation* 2003;108:2636-2641.

47. Schaar JA, Regar E, Mastik F, et al. Incidence of high-strain patterns in human coronary arteries: assessment with three-dimensional intravascular palpography and correlation with clinical presentation. *Circulation* 2004;109:2716-2719.

48. de Korte CL, Carlier SG, Mastik F, et al. Morphological and mechanical information of coronary arteries obtained with intravascular elastography; feasibility study in vivo. *Eur Heart J* 2002;23:405-13.

49. van Mieghem CAG, Bruining N, Schaar JA, et al. Rationale and methods of the integrated biomarker and imaging study (IBIS): combining invasive and noninvasive imaging with biomarkers to detect subclinical atherosclerosis and assess coronary lesion biology.

The International Journal of Cardiovascular Imaging (formerly Cardiac Imaging) 2005;21:425-441.

50. Van Mieghem CA, McFadden EP, de Feyter PJ, et al. Noninvasive detection of subclinical coronary atherosclerosis coupled with assessment of changes in plaque characteristics using novel invasive imaging modalities: the Integrated Biomarker and Imaging Study (IBIS). *J Am Coll Cardiol* 2006;47:1134-42.

51. Regar E vLA, Serruys PW. Optical coherence tomography in cardiovascular research. London: *Informa Healthcare* 2007;ISBN 1841846112.

52. Huang D, Swanson EA, Lin CP, et al. Optical coherence tomography. *Science* 1991;254:1178-81.

53. Brezinski ME, Tearney GJ, Bouma BE, et al. Imaging of coronary artery microstructure (in vitro) with optical coherence tomography. *Am J Cardiol* 1996;77:92-3.

54. Regar E, Schaar JA, Mont E, Virmani R, Serruys PW. Optical coherence tomography. *Cardiovascular Radiation Medicine* 2003;4:198-204.

55. Jang IK, Bouma BE, Kang DH, et al. Visualization of coronary atherosclerotic plaques in patients using optical coherence tomography: comparison with intravascular ultrasound. *J Am Coll Cardiol* 2002;39:604-9.

56. Patwari P, Weissman NJ, Boppart SA, et al. Assessment of coronary plaque with optical coherence tomography and high-frequency ultrasound. *Am J Cardiol* 2000;85:641-4.

57. Yabushita H, Bouma BE, Houser SL, et al. Characterization of human atherosclerosis by optical coherence tomography. *Circulation* 2002;106:1640-1645.

58. Brezinski ME, Tearney GJ, Weissman NJ, et al. Assessing atherosclerotic plaque morphology: comparison of optical coherence tomography and high frequency intravascular ultrasound. *Heart* 1997;77:397-403.

59. Kawasaki M, Bouma BE, Bressner J, et al. Diagnostic Accuracy of Optical Coherence Tomography and Integrated Backscatter Intravascular Ultrasound Images for Tissue Characterization of Human Coronary Plaques. *Journal of the American College of Cardiology* 2006;48:81-88.

60. Manfrini O, Mont E, Leone O, et al. Sources of Error and Interpretation of Plaque Morphology by Optical Coherence Tomography. *The American Journal of Cardiology* 2006;98:156-159.

61. Jang IK, Tearney GJ, MacNeill B, et al. In Vivo Characterization of Coronary Atherosclerotic Plaque by Use of Optical Coherence Tomography. *Circulation* 2005;111:1551-1555.

62. Tearney GJ, Yabushita H, Houser SL, et al. Quantification of macrophage content in atherosclerotic plaques by optical coherence tomography. *Circulation* 2003;107:113-119.

63. MacNeill BD, Jang IK, Bouma BE, et al. Focal and multi-focal plaque macrophage distributions in patients with acute and stable presentations of coronary artery disease. *Journal of the American College of Cardiology* 2004;44:972-979.

64. Fuster V. Human lesion studies. *Ann N Y Acad Sci* 1997;811:207-24; discussion 224-5.

65. Casscells W, Hathorn B, David M, et al. Thermal detection of cellular infiltrates in living atherosclerotic plaques: possible implications for plaque rupture and thrombosis. *Lancet* 1996;347:1447-51.

66. Stefanadis C, Diamantopoulos L, Vlachopoulos C, et al. Thermal heterogeneity within human atherosclerotic coronary arteries detected in vivo: A new method of detection by application of a special thermography catheter. *Circulation* 1999;99:1965-71.

67. Stefanadis C, Toutouzas K, Tsiamis E, et al. Increased local temperature in human coronary atherosclerotic plaques: an independent predictor of clinical outcome in patients undergoing a percutaneous coronary intervention. *J Am Coll Cardiol* 2001;37:1277-83.

68. Toutouzas K, Drakopoulou M, Mitropoulos J, et al. Elevated plaque temperature in non-culprit de novo atheromatous lesions of patients with acute coronary syndromes. *J Am Coll Cardiol* 2006;47:301-6.

69. Toutouzas K, Synetos A, Stefanadi E, et al. Correlation between morphologic characteristics and local temperature differences in culprit lesions of patients with symptomatic coronary artery disease. *J Am Coll Cardiol* 2007;49:2264-71.

70. Stefanadis C, Toutouzas K, Tsiamis E, et al. Thermal heterogeneity in stable human coronary atherosclerotic plaques is underestimated in vivo: the "cooling effect" of blood flow. *J Am Coll Cardiol* 2003;41:403-8.

71. Diamantopoulos L, Liu X, De Scheerder I, et al. The effect of reduced blood-flow on the coronary wall temperature: Are significant lesions suitable for intravascular thermography? 10.1016/S0195-668X(03)00440-8. *Eur Heart J* 2003;24:1788-1795.

72. ten Have AG, Gijsen FJ, Wentzel JJ, Slager CJ, van der Steen AF. Temperature distribution in atherosclerotic coronary arteries: influence of plaque geometry and flow (a numerical study). *Phys Med Biol* 2004;49:4447-62.

73. Verheye S, De Meyer GRY, Krams R, et al. Intravascular thermography: Immediate functional and morphological vascular findings. *Eur Heart J* 2004;25:158-165.

74. ten Have AG GF, Wentzel JJ, Slager CJ, Serruys PW, van der Steen AFW. Intracoronary thermography: heat generation, transfer and detection. *Eurointervention* 2005;1:105-114.

75. Correia LC, Atalar E, Kelemen MD, et al. Intravascular magnetic resonance imaging of aortic atherosclerotic plaque composition. *Arterioscler Thromb Vasc Biol* 1997;17:3626-32.

76. Larose E, Yeghiazarians Y, Libby P, et al. Characterization of human atherosclerotic plaques by intravascular magnetic resonance imaging. *Circulation* 2005;112:2324-31.

77. Blank A, Alexandrowicz G, Muchnik L, et al. Miniature self-contained intravascular magnetic resonance (IVMI) probe for clinical applications. *Magn Reson Med* 2005;54:105-12.

78. Regar E HB, Grube E, Halon D, Wilensky R.L, Virmani R, Schneiderman J, Sax S, Friedmann H, Serruys PW, Wijns W. First-In-Man application of a miniature self-contained intracoronary magnetic resonance probe. A multi-centre safety and feasibility trial. *Eurointervention* 2006;2:77-83.

79. Schneiderman J, Wilensky RL, Weiss A, et al. Diagnosis of thin-cap fibroatheromas by a self-contained intravascular magnetic resonance imaging probe in ex vivo human aortas and in situ coronary arteries. *J Am Coll Cardiol* 2005;45:1961-9.

80. Quick HH, Ladd ME, Hilfiker PR, Paul GG, Ha SW, Debatin JF. Autoperfused balloon catheter for intravascular MR imaging. *J Magn Reson Imaging* 1999;9:428-34.

81. Barkhausen J, Ebert W, Heyer C, Debatin JF, Weinmann HJ. Detection of atherosclerotic plaque with Gadofluorine-enhanced magnetic resonance imaging. *Circulation* 2003;108:605-9.

82. Kooi ME, Cappendijk VC, Cleutjens KB, et al. Accumulation of ultrasmall superparamagnetic particles of iron oxide in human atherosclerotic plaques can be detected by in vivo magnetic resonance imaging. *Circulation* 2003;107:2453-8.

83. Porto I, Selvanayagam J, Ashar V, Neubauer S, Banning AP. Safety of magnetic resonance imaging one to three days after bare metal and drug-eluting stent implantation. *Am J Cardiol* 2005;96:366-8.

84. Moreno PR, Muller JE. Identification of high-risk atherosclerotic plaques: a survey of spectroscopic methods. *Current Opinion in Cardiology* 2002;17:638-647.

85. Brennan JF, 3rd, Romer TJ, Lees RS, Tercyak AM, Kramer JR, Jr., Feld MS. Determination of human coronary artery composition by Raman spectroscopy. *Circulation* 1997;96:99-105.

86. Baraga JJ, Feld MS, Rava RP. In situ: optical histochemistry of human artery using near infrared fourier transform Raman spectroscopy. *PNAS* 1992;89:3473-3477.

87. Romer TJ, Brennan JF, Fitzmaurice M, et al. Histopathology of human coronary atherosclerosis by quantifying its chemical composition with Raman spectroscopy. *Circulation* 1998;97:878-885.

88. Romer TJ, Brennan JF, Puppels GJ, et al. Intravascular Ultrasound Combined With Raman Spectroscopy to Localize and Quantify Cholesterol and Calcium Salts in Atherosclerotic Coronary Arteries. *Arterioscler Thromb Vasc Biol* 2000;20:478-483.

89. van de Poll SWE, Kastelijn K, Schut TCB, et al. On-line detection of cholesterol and calcification by catheter based Raman spectroscopy in human atherosclerotic plaque ex vivo. *Heart* 2003;89:1078-1082.

90. Wang J, Geng YJ, Guo B, et al. Near-infrared spectroscopic characterization of human advanced atherosclerotic plaques. *J Am Coll Cardiol* 2002;39:1305-13.

91. Marcu L, Fishbein MC, Maarek JM, Grundfest WS. Discrimination of human coronary artery atherosclerotic lipid-rich lesions by time-resolved laser-induced fluorescence spectroscopy. *Arterioscler Thromb Vasc Biol* 2001;21:1244-1250.

92. Moreno PR, Lodder RA, Purushothaman KR, Charash WE, O'Connor WN, Muller JE. Detection of lipid pool, thin fibrous cap, and inflammatory cells in human aortic atherosclerotic plaques by near-infrared spectroscopy. *Circulation* 2002;105:923-7.

93. Moreno PR, Muller JE. Identification of high-risk atherosclerotic plaques: a survey of spectroscopic methods. *Curr Opin Cardiol* 2002;17:638-47.

94. Caplan JD, Waxman S, Nesto RW, Muller JE. Near-infrared spectroscopy for the detection of vulnerable coronary artery plaques. *J Am Coll Cardiol* 2006;47:C92-6.

95. Waxman S, Ishibashi F, Caplan JD. Rationale and use of near-infrared spectroscopy for detection of lipid-rich and vulnerable plaques. *J Nucl Cardiol* 2007;14:719-28.

96. Tanigawa J, Barlis P, Di Mario C. Intravascular Optical Coherence Tomography: Optimisation of image acquisition and quantitative assessment of stent strut apposition. *Eurointervention* 2007;3:128-136.

97. Morice MC, Serruys PW, Sousa JE, et al. A randomized comparison of a sirolimus-eluting stent with a standard stent for coronary revascularization. *N Engl J Med* 2002;346:1773-80.

98. Fujii K, Mintz GS, Kobayashi Y, et al. Contribution of stent underexpansion to recurrence after sirolimus-eluting stent implantation for in-stent restenosis. *Circulation* 2004;109:1085-8.

99. Matsumoto D, Shite J, Shinke T, et al. Neointimal coverage of sirolimus-eluting stents at 6-month follow-up: evaluated by optical coherence tomography. *Eur Heart J* 2006.

100. Takano M, Inami S, Jang IK, et al. Evaluation by optical coherence tomography of neointimal coverage of sirolimus-eluting stent three months after implantation. *Am J Cardiol* 2007;99:1033-8.

101. Finn AV, Joner M, Nakazawa G, et al. Pathological correlates of late drug-eluting stent thrombosis: strut coverage as a marker of endothelialization. *Circulation* 2007;115:2435-41.

102. Finn AV, Nakazawa G, Joner M, et al. Vascular responses to drug eluting stents: importance of delayed healing. *Arterioscler Thromb Vasc Biol* 2007;27:1500-10.

Part III

Imaging and Cardiovascular Research

CHAPTER 11

Monitoring Regression and Progression of Atherosclerosis

Stephen J. Nicholls, MBBS, PhD, FRACP, FACC
Pia Lundman, MD, PhD, FESC

INTRODUCTION

Technological advances in arterial wall imaging permit the opportunity to visualize the disease process at all stages of its development. This has provided important insights into the relationship between clinical factors and the natural history of atherosclerosis. Serial imaging of atherosclerosis has also enabled a unique opportunity to evaluate the impact of a range of medical therapies on plaque progression. This has provided further characterization of the mechanism that underlies the clinical benefit observed with medical therapies in randomized controlled trials.

More recently, arterial wall imaging has been incorporated into clinical development programs of novel antiatherosclerotic therapies. In the setting of increased rates of concomitant use of proven medical therapies, declining placebo event rates create a scenario in which large numbers of patients (greater than 10,000) need to be followed for longer periods (more than 7 years) to demonstrate clinical efficacy. Given that this proposition is largely prohibitive for the development of new compounds, increasing interest has focused on the use of surrogate markers of efficacy to triage therapies with the greatest likelihood of clinical benefit through to later stages of drug development. This provides a unique opportunity for vascular imaging in the development of novel antiatherosclerotic agents.

MODALITIES FOR IMAGING PLAQUE PROGRESSION

Since its inception in 1958, coronary angiography has been the clinical gold standard for the detection and quantitation of obstructive coronary artery disease. This has guided the use of medical and revascularization strategies in millions of patients worldwide. Standardized techniques for quantitation of lumen stenoses has been incorporated in a serial fashion in clinical trials that assess the impact of medical therapies. The relationship between the extent of angiographic disease and clinical outcome has supported the use of QCA to evaluate new agents (see Figure 11.1). However, given that angiography generates a two-dimensional silhouette of the arterial lumen and does not visualize the vessel wall, it does not directly image the full extent of atherosclerotic plaque.[1] As a result, imaging modalities that visualize the entire vessel wall are required to investigate the effect of therapies on the full extent of disease.

Noninvasive B-mode ultrasonic imaging can detect and quantify early thickening of the intimal-medial layer of the carotid and femoral arteries. Increasing carotid intimal-medial thickness (CIMT) has been reported to be associated with the presence of cardiovascular risk factors, atherosclerotic disease in other vascular territories, and the prospective risk of clinical events.[2-4] Accordingly, this technique permits assessment of the impact of medical therapies on the development and progression of very early changes in the artery wall (see Figure 11.2). However, this generates a two-dimensional evaluation and does not quantify the volumetric extent of disease. Similarly, CIMT analysis provides no characterization of the arterial wall components that contribute to arterial wall thickening.

While initially proposed in the 1970s, a number of advances in catheter and transducer technology were required to enable the clinical application of intravascular ultrasound (IVUS). Placement of a high-frequency ultrasound transducer (20–45MHz) within close proximity to the endothelial surface generates high-resolution cross-sectional tomographic images of the entire vessel wall. As a result, IVUS visualizes a greater burden of atherosclerosis than suggested by conventional angiography. In fact, the presence of substantial plaque in regions that appear normal or minimally diseased on angiography[5] reflects the

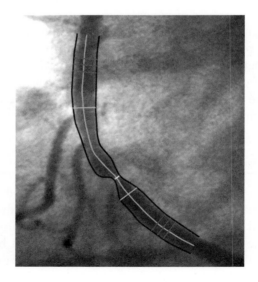

Figure 11.1

Illustrative example of measurements obtained during quantitative coronary angiography. (See Color Plate 31.)

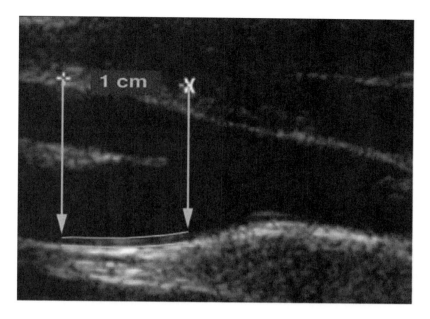

Figure 11.2

Illustrative example of measurements obtained of carotid intimal-medial thickness.

ability of the vessel wall to remodel in response to plaque accumulation.[6] Expansion of the artery wall in the early stages of atherosclerosis tends to preserve lumen dimensions, giving a normal angiographic appearance despite the presence of extensive disease.[6] As a result IVUS imaging provides an accurate determination of the extent of disease within a defined arterial segment, which can be evaluated at different time points to assess the effect of therapies on disease progression (see Figures 11.3–11.5).[7] Emerging developments in backscatter analysis provide a tissue map of radiofrequency spectra, which correlate with histology findings.[8] This enables additional assessment of the effect of therapies on disease composition (see Figure 11.6).

Advances in computed tomography (CT) and magnetic resonance (MR) permit non-invasive arterial imaging in vivo. Detection and quantitation of coronary calcification by CT has been associated with the extent of atherosclerotic disease and prospective risk of cardiovascular events.[9, 10] It remains to be determined to what degree coronary calcification enhances risk stratification in an incremental fashion beyond traditional risk factor assessment. Improving resolution has enabled the visualization of atherosclerotic plaque within the coronary artery wall.[11] While this may permit its use clinically in the assessment of the intermediate-risk patient, the imaging resolution currently lacks the precision

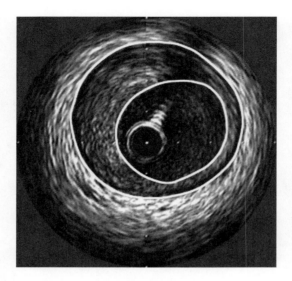

Figure 11.3

Illustrative example of measurements obtained of intravascular ultrasound imaging. The leading edge of the intima (inner circle) and adventitial border (outer circle) are defined.

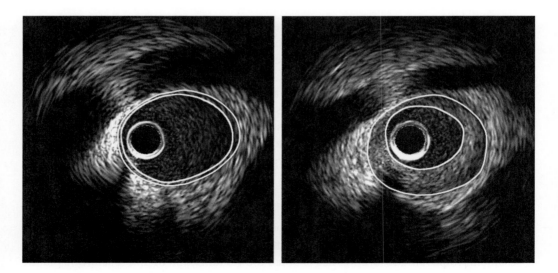

Figure 11.4

Illustrative example of progression of coronary atherosclerosis on serial evaluation with intravascular ultrasound.

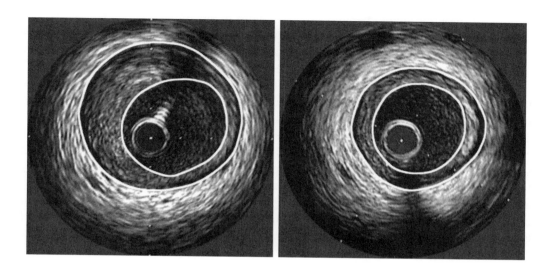

Figure 11.5

Illustrative example of regression of coronary atherosclerosis on serial evaluation with intravascular ultrasound.

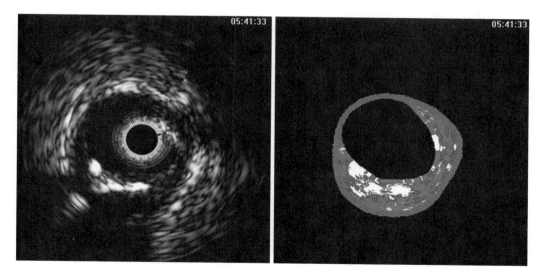

Figure 11.6

Illustrative example of plaque composition derived from radiofrequency analysis of intravascular ultrasound imaging. (See Color Plate 32.)

required to monitor small changes in disease with medical therapies. MR imaging has been used to characterize the extent and composition of plaque within the carotid arteries and aorta, with suitable resolution for evaluation of medical therapies.[12-14] The ability to visualize disease within the coronary tree is currently suboptimal for clinical trials.

A number of additional imaging modalities are currently in development, with view to further characterize atherosclerotic plaque. Optical coherence tomography (OCT) is an invasive technique, which involves analysis of light, in contrast with sound with IVUS. This generates high-resolution images of the artery wall, enabling visualization of fibrous cap thickness, neointimal hyperplasia, inflammatory components of plaque, and stent struts. The greater resolution comes at the expense of tissue penetration, limiting its ability to quantify the extent of disease.[15] Invasive assessment of distensibility,[16] temperature,[17] and chemical composition using spectroscopy[18] have each been proposed as methods to evaluate plaque vulnerability. Administration of contrast labeled with chemicals that bind to specific molecular components of plaque enables imaging of inflammatory, metabolic, apoptotic, angiogenic, and thrombotic activity within plaque.[19, 20] This may provide the opportunity to assess the impact of therapies on the extent, composition, and functional activity of coronary atherosclerosis.

LESSONS LEARNED FROM MEDICAL THERAPIES

Lowering LDL Cholesterol

For more than 100 years the role of cholesterol in the pathogenesis of plaque formation has been well established. Lowering low-density lipoprotein (LDL) cholesterol levels is associated with reductions in clinical event rates in randomized controlled trials.[21-26] As a result, LDL cholesterol has become a major target for therapeutic intervention in guidelines for cardiovascular prevention. The impact of therapies that lower LDL cholesterol on disease progression has been widely studied.

Serial QCA was applied in early studies that evaluated the impact of lowering LDL cholesterol on disease progression. Lowering LDL cholesterol by 26% with cholestyramine resulted in a lower percentage of patients who demonstrated disease progression (32% vs 49%) in the National Heart, Lung and Blood Institute Type II Coronary Intervention Study.[27] When combined with dietary intervention in the St. Thomas' Atherosclerosis Regression Study (STARS), cholestyramine therapy was associated with attenuation of disease progression and a greater proportion of subjects with evidence of regression.[28] The benefit of lowering LDL cholesterol was extended beyond use of medical therapies in the Program on the Surgical Control of the Hyperlipidemias (POSCH), in which lowering LDL cholesterol by 38% with partial ileal bypass surgery was associated with a reduction in cardiovascular events and less disease progression on evaluation of angiograms over 10 years of follow-up.[29]

Poorly controlled lipid levels in patients with familial hypercholesterolemia contributes to accelerated disease progression and early incidence of cardiovascular events. LDL-apheresis has been employed in patients whose lipid levels remain substantially elevated, despite the use of medical therapies. It is therefore interesting that, despite anecdotal reports of regression with LDL-apheresis,[30, 31] clinical trials were only able to demonstrate attenuation of angiographic disease progression. In the Familial Hypercholesterolemia Regression Study addition of either LDL-apheresis or colestipol with simvastatin halted progression.[32] Similarly, addition of LDL-apheresis had no incremental benefit in slowing disease progression in statin-treated patients in the LDL-apheresis Atherosclerosis Regression Study (LAARS).[33] More recently, the application of IVUS did permit a greater benefit of LDL-apheresis on disease progression. In the Low-Density Lipoprotein-Apheresis Coronary Morphology and Reserve Trial (LACMART), addition of LDL-apheresis to medical therapy resulted in greater LDL cholesterol lowering, in association with a reduction in plaque area and increase in minimum lumen diameter, consistent with regression of atherosclerotic plaque.[34]

A large number of studies employed CIMT and QCA to demonstrate a benefit of lowering LDL cholesterol with statins on disease progression. In clinical trials of CIMT, this benefit was observed in the setting of primary and secondary prevention. In asymptomatic patients, lovastatin was associated with regression at the most-diseased site in the Asymptomatic Carotid Artery Progression Study (ACAPS),[35] while pravastatin slowed progression in the Kuopio Atherosclerosis Prevention Study.[36] In the setting of established coronary disease, CIMT progression was attenuated with lovastatin in the Monitored Atherosclerosis Regression Study (MARS)[37] and pravastatin in the Regression Growth Evaluation Statin Substudy (REGRESS).[38] More recently, the benefit of statin therapy was extended to hypercholesterolemic patients at low risk in the Measuring Effects on Intima-Media Thickness: an Evaluation of Rosuvastatin (METEOR) study, a cohort who would not normally meet the criteria for lipid lowering treatment.[39] Similar benefits were observed with regard to the impact of statin therapy on progression of obstructive coronary artery disease. The Monitored Atherosclerosis Regression Study (MARS),[40] Pravastatin Limitation Atherosclerosis in the Coronary Arteries (PLAC-1)[41] and Multicentre Anti-Atherosclerosis Study (MAAS)[42] each demonstrated that statin therapy slowed disease progression and was associated with a greater proportion of patients with evidence of regression. Accordingly, meta-analyses of both CIMT[43] and angiographic[44] studies revealed a direct relationship between the degree of LDL cholesterol lowering with statins and the rate of disease progression. The report that incremental LDL cholesterol lowering with addition of ezetimibe to simvastatin in patients with familial hypercholesterolemia does not slow CIMT progression in the Ezetimibe and Simvastatin in Hypercholesterolemia Enhances Atherosclerosis Regression (ENHANCE) study suggests that the benefit of LDL cholesterol lowering may depend on the therapy employed.[45]

Arterial wall imaging has played an important role in supporting the concept that intensive lowering of LDL cholesterol is associated with clinical benefit. In the Atorvastatin versus Simvastatin Atherosclerosis Progression (ASAP) study of heterozygous familial hypercholesterolemia, intensive lipid lowering with atorvastatin 80mg daily resulted in CIMT regression, compared with evidence of progression in moderately treated patients, who received simvastatin 40mg daily.[46] A similar finding was observed in middle-aged hypercholesterolemic males in the Arterial Biology for the Investigation of Treatment Effects of Reducing Cholesterol (ARBITER) study, in which CIMT regression was observed with atorvastatin 80mg daily and progression with pravastatin 40mg daily.[47] Collectively, these findings suggested that intensive lipid lowering with statin therapy had an incremental benefit on progression of very early changes in the carotid artery.

The German Atorvastatin Investigation (GAIN) was the first clinical trial to employ IVUS to evaluate the impact of intensive lipid lowering on coronary atheroma volume. Despite achieving lower LDL cholesterol levels, open-label use of atorvastatin did not slow disease progression, although increased plaque echogenicity, suggesting a beneficial effect on plaque composition.[48] Subsequent randomized clinical trials did demonstrate that intensive lipid lowering had a favorable impact on plaque progression. In the Reversal of Atherosclerosis with Aggressive Lipid Lowering (REVERSAL) study intensive lipid lowering with atorvastatin 80mg daily halted the progression of disease observed in moderately treated patients who received pravastatin 40mg daily. A direct relationship was observed between the degree of LDL cholesterol lowering and changes in atheroma volume.[49] Interestingly, pravastatin-treated patients required incremental lowering of LDL cholesterol to achieve the same impact on plaque progression as observed in atorvastatin-treated patients. This suggested that differences in factors, in addition to LDL cholesterol, were likely to have contributed to the benefit of atorvastatin. Greater CRP lowering with atorvastatin, and the finding of a direct relationship between CRP lowering and changes in atheroma volume, supported the concept that anti-inflammatory properties are likely to contribute to the benefit of statins.[50]

The benefit of very intensive LDL cholesterol lowering was further investigated in A Study to Evaluate the Effect of Rosuvastatin on Intravascular Ultrasound-Derived Coronary Atheroma Burden (ASTEROID), in which lowering LDL cholesterol by 53% to 60.8mg/dL and raising HDL cholesterol by 14.7% to 49mg/dL was associated with plaque regression.[51] This is supported by reports of regression with atorvastatin in patients with an acute coronary syndrome in the ESTABLISH study and in a cohort of middle-aged males treated with simvastatin.[52] The contribution of HDL cholesterol elevation with statins was investigated in a pooled analysis of four clinical trials that employed IVUS evaluations of 1455 statin-treated patients. Although modest, raising HDL cholesterol independently predicted a beneficial effect of statins on plaque progression.[53] The finding that the change in the apolipoprotein B/A-I ratio was the strongest predictor of plaque progression highlights the importance of lowering levels of atherogenic lipids and promoting protective lipids.[53] Subsequent analysis from ASTEROID demonstrated evidence of angiographic regression with rosuvastatin.[44] Extending pooled analysis of angiographic studies involving statin therapy, changes in obstructive coronary artery disease correlated directly with achieved levels of LDL cholesterol and inversely with HDL cholesterol.[44]

More recently, noninvasive atherosclerosis imaging has been employed to assess the impact of intensive lipid lowering. Despite an initial report that cerivastatin slowed progression of coronary calcification,[54] two subsequent studies failed to demonstrate an impact of using an intensive versus moderate lipid lowering strategy.[55, 56] These observations contrast with the finding that intensive lipid lowering has a favorable influence on plaque volume and clinical events and question whether this is a useful tool for the assessment of antiatherosclerotic therapies. Magnetic resonance imaging of the carotid artery and aorta has demonstrated evidence of regression in statin-treated patients.[57, 58] While a small study failed to demonstrate an incremental benefit of high-dose statin therapy, the finding that patients with LDL cholesterol levels less than 100mg/dL demonstrated the greatest degree of regression supports the benefit of intensive lipid lowering.[59] More recently, the Outcome of Rosuvastatin Treatment on Carotid Artery Atheroma: a Magnetic Resonance Imaging Observation (ORION) demonstrated that rosuvastatin slowed disease progression and had a beneficial impact on the size of the lipid-rich necrotic core.[60] This impact of statins on necrotic core size is consistent with reports of a beneficial influence on plaque composition in studies that investigated the radiofrequency backscatter of IVUS[61] and histopathology.[62]

Promoting HDL Function

Niacin is the most effective HDL-cholesterol-raising agent available in clinical practice. In ARBITER-2, serial changes in CIMT were evaluated in patients with established coronary disease and low HDL-cholesterol levels, who were treated with extended release niacin or placebo, in addition to background statin therapy. Raising HDL cholesterol with niacin was associated with slowing CIMT progression at 12 months and regression on extended follow-up.[63] This suggested that promoting HDL, in addition to LDL-cholesterol lowering, could have an incremental benefit on very early changes in the artery wall. A similar benefit was observed with regard to progression of coronary atherosclerosis. In the HDL-Atherosclerosis Treatment Study (HATS) the combination of simvastatin and niacin promoted angiographic regression, a benefit associated with a reduction in clinical events. This benefit was no longer observed when patients also received a cocktail of potentially antioxidant vitamins.[64] The benefit of niacin on both early and advanced stages of disease is compatible with the report of clinical efficacy in the Coronary Drug Project.[65] The impact of niacin-based therapies, which aim to reduce flushing on disease progression has yet to be evaluated.

While fibric acid derivatives have a number of effects on plasma lipid levels, raising HDL cholesterol predicts their ability to reduce event rates in clinical trials. This benefit was extended to slowing angiographic disease progression. In the Bezafibrate Coronary Atherosclerosis Intervention Trial (BECAIT) administration of bezafibrate attenuated the reduction in minimum lumen diameter in dyslipidemic male survivors of myocardial infarction.[66] Similarly, micronised fenofibrate slowed progression in diabetic subjects with diffuse coronary disease in the Diabetes Atherosclerosis Intervention Study (DAIS).[67] More recently, magnetic resonance has been employed to demonstrate evidence of plaque regression and stabilization by treatment with fenofibrate in a rabbit model of atherosclerosis.[68]

Considerable interest has been focused on the potential efficacy of infusional therapy with reconstituted HDL or apolipoprotein A-I. Early reports that infusional therapy improves endothelial function[69] and enhances fecal sterol excretion,[70] a surrogate marker of reverse cholesterol transport, provide optimism that this approach will have a favorable impact on coronary atherosclerosis. Two preliminary studies suggest that infusing HDL has a rapid influence on coronary atheroma burden. In the first study of 57 patients within 2 weeks of an acute coronary syndrome, infusion of reconstituted HDL containing recombinant human apolipoprotein A-I$_{Milano}$ weekly for 5 weeks promoted rapid plaque regression.[71] More profound regression was observed in the 10mm segments containing the greatest amount of plaque at baseline, consistent with mobilization of lipid from the artery wall.[72] The finding of no change in lumen dimensions with regression further supported the need to image the entire vessel wall to evaluate the impact of medical therapies.[72] More recently, infusions of reconstituted HDL containing wild-type apolipoprotein A-I weekly for 4 weeks were associated with a trend toward regression and an improvement in plaque echogenicity, consistent with stabilization.[73] The potential benefit of infusing lipid-deplete forms of HDL has stimulated interest in delipidating a patient's HDL for use as infusional therapy. An early study in a small cohort of patients demonstrated disease regression following treatment with delipidated HDL infusions.[74] The impact of infusional therapy on clinical outcome remains to be elucidated.

Substantial elevation of HDL cholesterol with cholesteryl ester transfer protein (CETP) inhibitors has been proposed to be of potential use in cardiovascular prevention. At the time that development of the CETP inhibitor torcetrapib was ceased because of excessive mortality, three imaging trials had been completed. The impact of torcetrapib on CIMT progression was assessed in subjects with familial hypercholesterolemia and atherogenic dyslipidemia in the Rating Atherosclerotic Disease Changes by Imaging with a New Cholesteryl-Ester-Transfer Protein Inhibitor (RADIANCE) 1 and 2 studies.[75, 76] Raising HDL cholesterol by more than 50% and incremental lowering of LDL cholesterol with torcetrapib in combination with atorvastatin did not slow CIMT progression, compared with atorvastatin alone. A similar lack of efficacy on progression of coronary atherosclerosis was observed in the Investigation of Lipid Level Management Using Coronary Ultrasound to Assess Reduction of Atherosclerosis by CETP Inhibition and HDL Elevation (ILLUSTRATE) study.[77] More recent analysis revealed an inverse relationship between achieved levels of HDL cholesterol with torcetrapib and the rate of coronary atherosclerosis progression, with evidence of regression in patients achieving very high levels of HDL cholesterol. This benefit was not observed in subjects with reductions in potassium levels, consistent with the concept that activation of the renin-angiotensin-aldosterone axis with torcetrapib may be associated with vascular toxicity and mitigate any potential benefit of raising HDL cholesterol.[78] Accordingly, development of CETP inhibitors, which lack such off-target toxicities, may have a beneficial influence on cardiovascular risk.

Antihypertensive Therapy

Hypertension is associated with accelerated progression of carotid intimal-medial thickness and is the major clinical risk factor for cerebrovascular events.[79] A number of small clinical trials have demonstrated that administration of calcium channel antagonists,[80, 81] ACE inhibitors,[82, 83] and beta-blockers[84-86] have a beneficial influence on progression of both CIMT and established atherosclerotic plaque in the carotid arteries in hypertensive subjects. It is therefore of interest that administration of ACE inhibitors has not been demonstrated to have a beneficial impact on progression of obstructive disease in the coronary arteries. Treatment with quinapril in the Quinapril Ischemic Event Trial (QUIET)[87] and enalapril in the Simvastatin/Enalapril Coronary Atherosclerosis Trial (SCAT)[88] had no influence on angiographic progression.

In the Prospective Randomized Evaluation of the Vascular Effects of Norvasc Trial (PREVENT), patients with established coronary artery disease and well-controlled blood pressures were treated with amlodipine or a placebo. While amlodipine administration was not associated with a beneficial impact on progression of angiographic disease, slowing of carotid CIMT was observed. This benefit was associated with a lower clinical event rate and suggested that use of antihypertensive therapies might continue to be of clinical utility in patients with CAD, whose blood pressure is below the current treatment target.[89]

The Comparison of Amlodipine Versus Enalapril to Limit Occurrences of Thrombosis (CAMELOT) trial randomized patients with angiographic coronary artery disease and normal blood pressure levels to treatment with amlodipine, enalapril, or placebo. A subset of patients underwent serial evaluation by coronary IVUS, which demonstrated that amlodipine therapy was associated with halting of disease progression, a finding consistent with a significant reduction in cardiovascular endpoints in the main study. A direct relationship was observed between achieved levels of systolic blood pressure and changes in atheroma volume.[90] More recent observations that progression rates were less in patients who were normotensive (systolic blood pressure < 120mmHg) and lower than those deemed to be prehypertensive (systolic blood pressure 120–140mmHg) or hypertensive (systolic blood pressure > 140mmHg) with therapy suggests that blood pressure should be lowered more intensively than proposed by current guidelines.[91] It was therefore of interest to note that in a substudy of the European Trial on Reduction of Cardiac Events with Perindopril in Stable Coronary Artery Disease (EUROPA), that treatment with the antihypertensive perindopril did not slow disease progression on angiography or IVUS, although the small number of subjects studied provided limited power to detect a therapeutic effect.[92]

Antidiabetic Therapies

Diabetes is characterized by the presence of diffuse angiographic abnormalities with accelerated disease progression and an adverse clinical prognosis. The accelerated disease progression provides an ideal scenario to test the impact of antidiabetic therapies. In early studies of small cohorts, targeting glycemic control with a number of therapies, including the oral hypoglycemics metformin or gliclazide,[93] mitiglinides,[94] or the a-glucosidase inhibitor acarbose in patients with impaired glucose homeostasis,[95, 96] the greatest impact has been observed with the use of peroxisome proliferator-activated receptor (PPAR) agonists. In the Diabetes Atherosclerosis Intervention Study (DAIS) the PPAR-a agonist fenofibrate slowed angiographic progression.[67] Using serial assessment of CIMT, the PPAR-g agonist, pioglitazone, which has a beneficial influence on both insulin sensitivity and lipid levels was associated with halting of disease progression in the Carotid Intima-Media Thickness in Atherosclerosis Using Pioglitazone (CHICAGO) study.[97] A recent post hoc analysis revealed that the strongest predictor of benefit of pioglitazone was the 15% rise in HDL-cholesterol levels.[98]

Subgroup analysis of clinical trials demonstrating the benefit of therapeutic approaches targeting LDL-cholesterol and systolic blood pressure on progression of coronary atherosclerosis with intravascular ultrasound revealed similar effects in patients with and without diabetes.[49, 51, 90] In a pooled analysis of studies that employed IVUS to evaluate medical therapies, residual disease progression was observed, despite the benefit of intensive LDL-cholesterol lowering.[99] This suggests that additional therapies will be required to complement the impact of targeting LDL cholesterol and blood pressure on disease progression in diabetes. The metabolic benefits of pioglitazone were recently demonstrated to contribute to halting progression of coronary disease in the Pioglitazone Effect on Regression of Intravascular Sonographic Coronary Obstruction Prospective Evaluation (PERISCOPE) study. In a similar study design to the CHICAGO study, accelerated disease progression was observed in patients treated with the sulphonylurea glimepiride, while plaque growth was arrested in patients treated with pioglitazone.[100] These results suggest that targeting the lipid and inflammatory factors that are commonly encountered in patients with diabetes are likely to result in an incremental benefit.

Novel Antiatherosclerotic Therapies

Elucidation of the molecular events that drive the accumulation of lipid, inflammatory, and necrotic material within the artery wall provides the opportunity to develop novel therapeutic agents that directly target these pathologic cascades. The factor acyl:cholesterol acyltransferase (ACAT) promotes the esterification of cholesterol, which is taken up by macrophages to become foam cells, the cellular hallmark of atherosclerotic plaque.[101] Inhibition of ACAT has been proposed to be of potential therapeutic value, given consistent beneficial effects in animal models of atherosclerosis.[102] However, two studies have failed to demonstrate that ACAT inhibitors slow disease progression in humans. The lack of an effect of the ACAT inhibitor avasimibe in the Avasimibe and Progression of coronary Lesions assessed by intravascular Ultrasound (A-PLUS) was attributed to its ability to induce statin metabolism and therefore result in higher LDL-cholesterol levels.[103] In the ACAT Intravascular Atherosclerosis Treatment Evaluation (ACTIVATE) study, despite having no effect on LDL-cholesterol levels pactimibe administration was associated with greater progression than observed in placebo-treated patients.[104] The potential proathero-genic effect of ACAT inhibition in humans may result from an increase in cytotoxicity caused by elevated cellular levels of free cholesterol.[105]

AGI-1067 is a vascular protectant with antioxidant and anti-inflammatory activities. In a preliminary study of patients who underwent percutaneous coronary intervention, a trend to regression was observed with AGI-1067, although this was not statistically significant from placebo.[106] However, it does raise the potential that anti-inflammatory therapies may have some therapeutic role in coronary artery disease. Inhibition of lipo-protein associated phospholipase A2 (Lp-PLA2) represents an alternative approach to modify remodelling of circulating lipoproteins and inhibit inflammatory pathways in the artery wall. In a 12-month study of patients with a recent acute coronary syndrome, administration of the Lp-PLA2 inhibitor darapladib did not slow progression of coronary atherosclerosis. However, the observation that darapladib did have a favorable impact on progression of the necrotic core volume suggests that direct anti-inflammatory therapies may be of potential benefit for patients with coronary artery disease.[107]

Transplant Vasculopathy

The development of coronary artery vasculopathy portends a poor prognosis in heart transplant recipients and represents the leading indication for retransplantation.[108] As a result, considerable interest has focused on the use of arterial imaging to diagnose vas-culopathy and to evaluate medical therapies with regard to their ability to slow its devel-opment. Early studies that employed coronary angiography demonstrated that targeting established atherosclerotic risk factors with statins,[109] calcium channel antagonists,[110] and ACE inhibitors[111] attenuate development and progression of vasculopathy. The ability of intravascular ultrasound to image the entire vessel wall with high resolution has resulted in its incorporation into clinical algorithms for the surveillance of heart transplant recipients. More recently, intravascular ultrasound has demonstrated that the immunomodulatory agent everolimus slows development of transplant vasculopathy, a finding associated with a reduction in rejection, cardiogenic shock, and need for retransplantation.[112]

CONCLUSION

Advances in arterial-wall imaging have provided the opportunity to characterize the factors that influence the natural history of atherosclerosis. The ability to image an arterial bed at different time points permits evaluation of the impact of medical therapies on disease progression. This has provided important insights to define the mechanisms linking therapies with clinical efficacy. The opportunity to incorporate arterial wall imaging in clinical trials also highlights its role in the clinical development of novel antiatherosclerotic agents.

◇◇◇◇◇◇◇◇◇◇◇◇◇

REFERENCES

1. Topol EJ, Nissen SE. Our preoccupation with coronary luminology. The dissociation between clinical and angiographic findings in ischemic heart disease. *Circulation.* 1995;92:2333-2342.
2. Chambless LE, Heiss G, Folsom AR, Rosamond W, Szklo M, Sharrett AR, Clegg LX. Association of coronary heart disease incidence with carotid arterial wall thickness and major risk factors: the Atherosclerosis Risk in Communities (ARIC) Study, 1987-1993. *Am J Epidemiol.* 1997;146:483-494.
3. Lorenz MW, Markus HS, Bots ML, Rosvall M, Sitzer M. Prediction of clinical cardiovascular events with carotid intima-media thickness: a systematic review and meta-analysis. *Circulation.* 2007;115:459-467.
4. Hodis HN, Mack WJ, LaBree L, Selzer RH, Liu CR, Liu CH, Azen SP. The role of carotid arterial intima-media thickness in predicting clinical coronary events. *Ann Intern Med.* 1998;128:262-269.
5. Mintz GS, Painter JA, Pichard AD, Kent KM, Satler LF, Popma JJ, Chuang YC, Bucher TA, Sokolowicz LE, Leon MB. Atherosclerosis in angiographically "normal" coronary artery reference segments: an intravascular ultrasound study with clinical correlations. *J Am Coll Cardiol.* 1995;25:1479-1485.
6. Glagov S, Weisenberg E, Zarins CK, Stankunavicius R, Kolettis GJ. Compensatory enlargement of human atherosclerotic coronary arteries. *N Engl J Med.* 1987;316:1371-1375.
7. Nicholls SJ, Sipahi I, Schoenhagen P, Crowe T, Tuzcu EM, Nissen SE. Application of intravascular ultrasound in anti-atherosclerotic drug development. *Nat Rev Drug Discov.* 2006;5:485-492.
8. Nair A, Kuban BD, Tuzcu EM, Schoenhagen P, Nissen SE, Vince DG. Coronary plaque classification with intravascular ultrasound radiofrequency data analysis. *Circulation.* 2002;106:2200-2206.
9. Greenland P, LaBree L, Azen SP, Doherty TM, Detrano RC. Coronary artery calcium score combined with Framingham score for risk prediction in asymptomatic individuals. *Jama.* 2004;291:210-215.
10. Pletcher MJ, Tice JA, Pignone M, Browner WS. Using the coronary artery calcium score to predict coronary heart disease events: a systematic review and meta-analysis. *Arch Intern Med.* 2004;164:1285-1292.
11. Achenbach S, Daniel WG. Imaging of coronary atherosclerosis using computed tomography: current status and future directions. *Curr Atheroscler Rep.* 2004;6:213-218.
12. Fayad ZA, Fuster V, Fallon JT, Jayasundera T, Worthley SG, Helft G, Aguinaldo JG, Badimon JJ, Sharma SK. Noninvasive in vivo human coronary artery lumen and wall imaging using black-blood magnetic resonance imaging. *Circulation.* 2000;102:506-510.
13. Fayad ZA, Nahar T, Fallon JT, Goldman M, Aguinaldo JG, Badimon JJ, Shinnar M, Chesebro JH, Fuster V. In vivo magnetic resonance evaluation of atherosclerotic plaques in the human thoracic aorta: a comparison with transesophageal echocardiography. *Circulation.* 2000;101:2503-2509.
14. Worthley SG, Helft G, Fuster V, Fayad ZA, Rodriguez OJ, Zaman AG, Fallon JT, Badimon JJ. Noninvasive in vivo magnetic resonance imaging of experimental coronary artery lesions in a porcine model. *Circulation.* 2000;101:2956-2961.
15. Stamper D, Weissman NJ, Brezinski M. Plaque characterization with optical coherence tomography. *J Am Coll Cardiol.* 2006;47:C69-79.
16. Schaar JA, Mastik F, Regar E, den Uil CA, Gijsen FJ, Wentzel JJ, Serruys PW, van der Stehen AF. Current

diagnostic modalities for vulnerable plaque detection. *Curr Pharm Des.* 2007;13:995-1001.

17. Madjid M, Willerson JT, Casscells SW. Intracoronary thermography for detection of high-risk vulnerable plaques. *J Am Coll Cardiol.* 2006;47:C80-85.

18. Rocha R, Silveira L, Jr., Villaverde AB, Pasqualucci CA, Costa MS, Brugnera A, Jr., Pacheco MT. Use of near-infrared Raman spectroscopy for identification of atherosclerotic plaques in the carotid artery. *Photomed Laser Surg.* 2007;25:482-486.

19. Hyafil F, Cornily JC, Feig JE, Gordon R, Vucic E, Amirbekian V, Fisher EA, Fuster V, Feldman LJ, Fayad ZA. Noninvasive detection of macrophages using a nanoparticulate contrast agent for computed tomography. *Nat Med.* 2007;13:636-641.

20. Jaffer FA, Libby P, Weissleder R. Molecular imaging of cardiovascular disease. *Circulation.* 2007;116:1052-1061.

21. Randomised trial of cholesterol lowering in 4444 patients with coronary heart disease: the Scandinavian Simvastatin Survival Study (4S). *Lancet.* 1994;344:1383-1389.

22. Prevention of cardiovascular events and death with pravastatin in patients with coronary heart disease and a broad range of initial cholesterol levels. The Long-Term Intervention with Pravastatin in Ischaemic Disease (LIPID) Study Group. *N Engl J Med.* 1998;339:1349-1357.

23. MRC/BHF Heart Protection Study of cholesterol lowering with simvastatin in 20,536 high-risk individuals: a randomised placebo-controlled trial. *Lancet.* 2002;360:7-22.

24. Downs JR, Clearfield M, Weis S, Whitney E, Shapiro DR, Beere PA, Largendorfer A, Stein EA, Kruyer W, Gotto AM, Jr. Primary prevention of acute coronary events with lovastatin in men and women with average cholesterol levels: results of AFcaps/Texcaps. AirForce/Texas Coronary Atherosclerosis Prevention Study. *JAMA.* 1998;279:1615-1622.

25. Sacks FM, Pfeffer MA, Moye LA, Rouleau JL, Rutherford JD, Cole TG, Brown L, Warnica JW, Arnold JM, Wun CC, Davis BR, Braunwald E. The effect of pravastatin on coronary events after myocardial infarction in patients with average cholesterol levels. Cholesterol and Recurrent Events Trial investigators. *N Engl J Med.* 1996;335:1001-1009.

26. Shepherd J, Cobbe SM, Ford I, Isles CG, Lorimer AR, MacFarlane PW, McKillop JH, Packard CJ. Prevention of coronary heart disease with pravastatin in men with hypercholesterolemia. West of Scotland Coronary Prevention Study Group. *N Engl J Med.* 1995;333:1301-1307.

27. Brensike JF, Levy RI, Kelsey SF, Passamani ER, Richardson JM, Loh IK, Stone NJ, Aldrich RF, Battaglini JW, Moriarty DJ, et al. Effects of therapy with cholestyramine on progression of coronary arteriosclerosis: results of the NHLBI Type II Coronary Intervention Study. *Circulation.* 1984;69:313-324.

28. Watts GF, Lewis B, Brunt JN, Lewis ES, Coltart DJ, Smith LD, Mann JI, Swan AV. Effects on coronary artery disease of lipid-lowering diet, or diet plus cholestyramine, in the St Thomas' Atherosclerosis Regression Study (STARS). *Lancet.* 1992;339:563-569.

29. Buchwald H, Varco RL, Matts JP, Long JM, Fitch LL, Campbell GS, Pearce MB, Yellin AE, Edmiston WA, Smink RD, Jr., et al. Effect of partial ileal bypass surgery on mortality and morbidity from coronary heart disease in patients with hypercholesterolemia. Report of the Program on the Surgical Control of the Hyperlipidemias (POSCH). *N Engl J Med.* 1990;323:946-955.

30. Koga N, Iwata Y. Pathological and angiographic regression of coronary atherosclerosis by LDL-apheresis in a patient with familial hypercholesterolemia. *Atherosclerosis.* 1991;90:9-21.

31. Kitabatake A, Sato H, Hori M, Kamada T, Kubori S, Hoki N, Minamino T, Yamada M, Kato T. Coronary atherosclerosis reduced in patients with familial hypercholesterolemia after intensive cholesterol lowering with low-density lipoprotein-apheresis: 1-year follow-up study. The Osaka LDL-Apheresis Multicenter Trial Group. *Clin Ther.* 1994;16:416-428.

32. Thompson GR, Maher VM, Matthews S, Kitano Y, Neuwirth C, Shortt MB, Davies G, Rees A, Mir A, Prescott RJ, et al. Familial Hypercholesterolaemia Regression Study: a randomised trial of low-density-lipoprotein apheresis. *Lancet.* 1995;345:811-816.

33. Kroon AA, Aengevaeren WR, van der Werf T, Uijen GJ, Reiber JH, Bruschke AV, Stalenhoef AF. LDL-Apheresis Atherosclerosis Regression Study (LAARS). Effect of aggressive versus conventional lipid lowering treatment on coronary atherosclerosis. *Circulation.* 1996;93:1826-1835.

34. Matsuzaki M, Hiramori K, Imaizumi T, Kitabatake A, Hishida H, Nomura M, Fujii T, Sakuma I, Fukami K, Honda T, Ogawa H, Yamagishi M. Intravascular ultrasound evaluation of coronary plaque regression by low density lipoprotein-apheresis in familial hypercholesterolemia: the Low Density Lipoprotein-Apheresis Coronary Morphology and Reserve Trial (LACMART). *J Am Coll Cardiol.* 2002;40:220-227.

35. Furberg CD, Adams HP, Jr., Applegate WB, Byington RP, Espeland MA, Hartwell T, Hunninghake DB, Lefkowitz DS, Probstfield J, Riley WA, et al. Effect

of lovastatin on early carotid atherosclerosis and cardiovascular events. Asymptomatic Carotid Artery Progression Study (ACAPS) Research Group. *Circulation.* 1994;90:1679-1687.

36. Salonen R, Nyyssonen K, Porkkala E, Rummukainen J, Belder R, Park JS, Salonen JT. Kuopio Atherosclerosis Prevention Study (KAPS). A population-based primary preventive trial of the effect of LDL lowering on atherosclerotic progression in carotid and femoral arteries. *Circulation.* 1995;92:1758-1764.

37. Hodis HN, Mack WJ, LaBree L, Selzer RH, Liu C, Alaupovic P, Kwong-Fu H, Azen SP. Reduction in carotid arterial wall thickness using lovastatin and dietary therapy: a randomized controlled clinical trial. *Ann Intern Med.* 1996;124:548-556.

38. de Groot E, Jukema JW, Montauban van Swijndregt AD, Zwinderman AH, Ackerstaff RG, van der Steen AF, Bom N, Lie KI, Bruschke AV. B-mode ultrasound assessment of pravastatin treatment effect on carotid and femoral artery walls and its correlations with coronary arteriographic findings: a report of the Regression Growth Evaluation Statin Study (REGRESS). *J Am Coll Cardiol.* 1998;31:1561-1567.

39. Crouse JR, 3rd, Raichlen JS, Riley WA, Evans GW, Palmer MK, O'Leary DH, Grobbee DE, Bots ML. Effect of rosuvastatin on progression of carotid intima-media thickness in low-risk individuals with subclinical atherosclerosis: the METEOR Trial. *JAMA.* 2007;297:1344-1353.

40. Blankenhorn DH, Azen SP, Kramsch DM, Mack WJ, Cashin-Hemphill L, Hodis HN, DeBoer LW, Mahrer PR, Masteller MJ, Vailas LI, et al. Coronary angiographic changes with lovastatin therapy. The Monitored Atherosclerosis Regression Study (MARS). The MARS Research Group. *Ann Intern Med.* 1993;119:969-976.

41. Pitt B, Mancini GB, Ellis SG, Rosman HS, Park JS, McGovern ME. Pravastatin limitation of atherosclerosis in the coronary arteries (PLAC I): reduction in atherosclerosis progression and clinical events. PLAC I investigation. *J Am Coll Cardiol.* 1995;26:1133-1139.

42. Effect of simvastatin on coronary atheroma: the Multicentre Anti-Atheroma Study (MAAS). *Lancet.* 1994;344:633-638.

43. Kang S, Wu Y, Li X. Effects of statin therapy on the progression of carotid atherosclerosis: a systematic review and meta-analysis. *Atherosclerosis.* 2004;177:433-442.

44. Ballantyne CM, Raichlen JS, Nicholls SJ, Erbel R, Tardif JC, Brener SJ, Cain VA, Nissen SE. Effect of Rosuvastatin Therapy on Coronary Artery Stenoses Assessed by Quantitative Coronary Angiography.

A Study to Evaluate the Effect of Rosuvastatin on Intravascular Ultrasound-Derived Coronary Atheroma Burden. *Circulation.* 2008;117:2458-2466.

45. *http://www.theheart.org/article/837243.do.*

46. Smilde TJ, van Wissen S, Wollersheim H, Trip MD, Kastelein JJ, Stalenhoef AF. Effect of aggressive versus conventional lipid lowering on atherosclerosis progression in familial hypercholesterolaemia (ASAP): a prospective, randomised, double-blind trial. *Lancet.* 2001;357:577-581.

47. Taylor AJ, Kent SM, Flaherty PJ, Coyle LC, Markwood TT, Vernalis MN. ARBITER: Arterial Biology for the Investigation of the Treatment Effects of Reducing Cholesterol: a randomized trial comparing the effects of atorvastatin and pravastatin on carotid intima medial thickness. *Circulation.* 2002;106:2055-2060.

48. Schartl M, Bocksch W, Koschyk DH, Voelker W, Karsch KR, Kreuzer J, Hausmann D, Beckmann S, Gross M. Use of intravascular ultrasound to compare effects of different strategies of lipid-lowering therapy on plaque volume and composition in patients with coronary artery disease. *Circulation.* 2001;104:387-392.

49. Nissen SE, Tuzcu EM, Schoenhagen P, Brown BG, Ganz P, Vogel RA, Crowe T, Howard G, Cooper CJ, Brodie B, Grines CL, DeMaria AN. Effect of intensive compared with moderate lipid-lowering therapy on progression of coronary atherosclerosis: a randomized controlled trial. *JAMA.* 2004;291:1071-1080.

50. Nissen SE, Tuzcu EM, Schoenhagen P, Crowe T, Sasiela WJ, Tsai J, Orazem J, Magorien RD, O'Shaughnessy C, Ganz P. Statin therapy, LDL cholesterol, C-reactive protein, and coronary artery disease. *N Engl J Med.* 2005;352:29-38.

51. Nissen SE, Nicholls SJ, Sipahi I, Libby P, Raichlen JS, Ballantyne CM, Davignon J, Erbel R, Fruchart JC, Tardif JC, Schoenhagen P, Crowe T, Cain V, Wolski K, Goormastic M, Tuzcu EM. Effect of very high-intensity statin therapy on regression of coronary atherosclerosis: the ASTEROID trial. *JAMA.* 2006;295:1556-1565.

52. Okazaki S, Yokoyama T, Miyauchi K, Shimada K, Kurata T, Sato H, Daida H. Early statin treatment in patients with acute coronary syndrome: demonstration of the beneficial effect on atherosclerotic lesions by serial volumetric intravascular ultrasound analysis during half a year after coronary event: the ESTABLISH Study. *Circulation.* 2004;110:1061-1068.

53. Nicholls SJ, Tuzcu EM, Sipahi I, Grasso AW, Schoenhagen P, Hu T, Wolski K, Crowe T, Desai MY, Hazen SL, Kapadia SR, Nissen SE. Statins, high-

density lipoprotein cholesterol, and regression of coronary atherosclerosis. *JAMA.* 2007;297:499-508.

54. Achenbach S, Ropers D, Pohle K, Leber A, Thilo C, Knez A, Menendez T, Maeffert R, Kusus M, Regenfus M, Bickel A, Haberl R, Steinbeck G, Moshage W, Daniel WG. Influence of lipid-lowering therapy on the progression of coronary artery calcification: a prospective evaluation. *Circulation.* 2002;106:1077-1082.

55. Raggi P, Davidson M, Callister TQ, Welty FK, Bachmann GA, Hecht H, Rumberger JA. Aggressive versus moderate lipid-lowering therapy in hypercholesterolemic postmenopausal women: Beyond Endorsed Lipid Lowering with EBT Scanning (BELLES). *Circulation.* 2005;112:563-571.

56. Schmermund A, Achenbach S, Budde T, Buziashvili Y, Forster A, Friedrich G, Henein M, Kerkhoff G, Knollmann F, Kukharchuk V, Lahiri A, Leischik R, Moshage W, Schartl M, Siffert W, Steinhagen-Thiessen E, Sinitsyn V, Vogt A, Wiedeking B, Erbel R. Effect of intensive versus standard lipid-lowering treatment with atorvastatin on the progression of calcified coronary atherosclerosis over 12 months: a multicenter, randomized, double-blind trial. *Circulation.* 2006;113:427-437.

57. Corti R, Fayad ZA, Fuster V, Worthley SG, Helft G, Chesebro J, Mercuri M, Badimon JJ. Effects of lipid-lowering by simvastatin on human atherosclerotic lesions: a longitudinal study by high-resolution, noninvasive magnetic resonance imaging. *Circulation.* 2001;104:249-252.

58. Corti R, Fuster V, Fayad ZA, Worthley SG, Helft G, Smith D, Weinberger J, Wentzel J, Mizsei G, Mercuri M, Badimon JJ. Lipid lowering by simvastatin induces regression of human atherosclerotic lesions: two years' follow-up by high-resolution noninvasive magnetic resonance imaging. *Circulation.* 2002;106:2884-2887.

59. Corti R, Fuster V, Fayad ZA, Worthley SG, Helft G, Chaplin WF, Muntwyler J, Viles-Gonzalez JF, Weinberger J, Smith DA, Mizsei G, Badimon JJ. Effects of aggressive versus conventional lipid-lowering therapy by simvastatin on human atherosclerotic lesions: a prospective, randomized, double-blind trial with high-resolution magnetic resonance imaging. *J Am Coll Cardiol.* 2005;46:106-112.

60. Hatsukami T, Zhao X-Q, Krauss LW. Assessment of rosuvastatin treatment on carotid atherosclerosis in moderately hypercholesterolemic subjects using high-resolution magnetic resonance imaging. *Eur Heart J.* 2005;26:626.

61. Kawasaki M, Sano K, Okubo M, Yokoyama H, Ito Y, Murata I, Tsuchiya K, Minatoguchi S, Zhou X, Fujita H, Fujiwara H. Volumetric quantitative analysis of tissue characteristics of coronary plaques after statin therapy using three-dimensional integrated backscatter intravascular ultrasound. *J Am Coll Cardiol.* 2005;45:1946-1953.

62. Crisby M, Nordin-Fredriksson G, Shah PK, Yano J, Zhu J, Nilsson J. Pravastatin treatment increases collagen content and decreases lipid content, inflammation, metalloproteases, and cell death in human carotid plaques. *Circulation.* 2001;103:926-933.

63. Taylor AJ, Sullenberger LE, Lee HJ, Lee JK, Grace KA. Arterial Biology for the Investigation of the Treatment Effects of Reducing Cholesterol (ARBITER) 2: a double-blind, placebo-controlled study of extended-release niacin on atherosclerosis progression in secondary prevention patients treated with statins. *Circulation.* 2004;110:3512-3517.

64. Brown BG, Zhao X-Q, Chait A, Fisher LD, Cheung MC, Morse JS, Dowdy AA, Marino EK, Bolson EL, Alaupovic P, Frohlich J, Albers JJ. Simvastatin and niacin, antioxidant vitamins, or the combination for the prevention of coronary disease. *N Engl J Med.* 2001;345:1583-1592.

65. Clofibrate and niacin in coronary heart disease. *JAMA.* 1975;231:360-381.

66. Ericsson CG, Hamsten A, Nilsson J, Grip L, Svane B, de Faire U. Angiographic assessment of effects of bezafibrate on progression of coronary artery disease in young male postinfarction patients. *Lancet.* 1996;347:849-853.

67. Effect of fenofibrate on progression of coronary-artery disease in type 2 diabetes: the Diabetes Atherosclerosis Intervention Study, a randomised study. *Lancet.* 2001;357:905-910.

68. Corti R, Osende J, Hutter R, Viles-Gonzalez JF, Zafar U, Valdivieso C, Mizsei G, Fallon JT, Fuster V, Badimon JJ. Fenofibrate induces plaque regression in hypercholesterolemic atherosclerotic rabbits: in vivo demonstration by high-resolution MRI. *Atherosclerosis.* 2007;190:106-113.

69. Bisoendial RJ, Hovingh GK, Levels JHM, Lerch PG, Andresen I, Hayden MR, Kastelein JJP, Stroes ESG. Restoration of Endothelial Function by Increasing High-Density Lipoprotein in Subjects With Isolated Low High-Density Lipoprotein. *Circulation.* 2003;107:2944-2948.

70. Angelin B, Parini P, Eriksson M. Reverse cholesterol transport in man: promotion of fecal steroid excretion by infusion of reconstituted HDL. *Atherosclerosis Supplements.* 2002;3:23-30.

71. Nissen SE, Tsunoda T, Tuzcu EM, Schoenhagen P, Cooper CJ, Yasin M, Eaton GM, Lauer MA, Sheldon

WS, Grines CL, Halpern S, Crowe T, Blankenship JC, Kerensky R. Effect of recombinant ApoA-I Milano on coronary atherosclerosis in patients with acute coronary syndromes: a randomized controlled trial. *JAMA.* 2003;290:2292-2300.

72. Nicholls SJ, Tuzcu EM, Sipahi I, Schoenhagen P, Crowe T, Kapadia S, Nissen SE. Relationship between atheroma regression and change in lumen size after infusion of apolipoprotein A-I Milano. *J Am Coll Cardiol.* 2006;47:992-997.

73. Tardif JC, Gregoire J, L'Allier PL, Ibrahim R, Lesperance J, Heinonen TM, Kouz S, Berry C, Basser R, Lavoie MA, Guertin MC, Rodes-Cabau J. Effects of reconstituted high-density lipoprotein infusions on coronary atherosclerosis: a randomized controlled trial. *JAMA.* 2007;297:1675-1682.

74. *www.theheart.org/article/867025.do.*

75. Kastelein JJ, van Leuven SI, Burgess L, Evans GW, Kuivenhoven JA, Barter PJ, Revkin JH, Grobbee DE, Riley WA, Shear CL, Duggan WT, Bots ML. Effect of torcetrapib on carotid atherosclerosis in familial hypercholesterolemia. *N Engl J Med.* 2007;356:1620-1630.

76. Bots ML, Visseren FL, Evans GW, Riley WA, Revkin JH, Tegeler CH, Shear CL, Duggan WT, Vicari RM, Grobbee DE, Kastelein JJ. Torcetrapib and carotid intima-media thickness in mixed dyslipidaemia (RADIANCE 2 study): a randomised, double-blind trial. *Lancet.* 2007;370:153-160.

77. Nissen SE, Tardif JC, Nicholls SJ, Revkin JH, Shear CL, Duggan WT, Ruzyllo W, Bachinsky WB, Lasala GP, Tuzcu EM. Effect of torcetrapib on the progression of coronary atherosclerosis. *N Engl J Med.* 2007;356:1304-1316.

78. Nicholls SJ, Brennan DM, Wolski K, Kalidindi SR, Moon K-W, Tuzcu EM, Nissen SE. Changes in levels of high-density lipoprotein cholesterol predict the impact of torcetrapib on progression of coronary atherosclerosis: insights from ILLUSTRATE. *Circulation.* 2007;116:II_127.

79. Poredos P. Intima-media thickness: indicator of cardiovascular risk and measure of the extent of atherosclerosis. *Vasc Med.* 2004;9:46-54.

80. Pontremoli R, Viazzi F, Ravera M, Leoncini G, Berruti V, Bezante GP, Del Sette M, Deferrari G. Long term effect of nifedipine GITS and lisinopril on subclinical organ damage in patients with essential hypertension. *J Nephrol.* 2001;14:19-26.

81. Zanchetti A, Rosei EA, Dal Palu C, Leonetti G, Magnani B, Pessina A. The Verapamil in Hypertension and Atherosclerosis Study (VHAS): results of long-term randomized treatment with either verapamil or

chlorthalidone on carotid intima-media thickness. *J Hypertens.* 1998;16:1667-1676.

82. Hosomi N, Mizushige K, Ohyama H, Takahashi T, Kitadai M, Hatanaka Y, Matsuo H, Kohno M, Koziol JA. Angiotensin-converting enzyme inhibition with enalapril slows progressive intima-media thickening of the common carotid artery in patients with non-insulin-dependent diabetes mellitus. *Stroke.* 2001;32:1539-1545.

83. Uchiyama-Tanaka Y, Mori Y, Kishimoto N, Fukui M, Nose A, Kijima Y, Yamahara H, Hasegawa T, Kosaki A, Matsubara H, Iwasaka T. Comparison of the effects of quinapril and losartan on carotid artery intima-media thickness in patients with mild-to-moderate arterial hypertension. *Kidney Blood Press Res.* 2005;28:111-116.

84. Hedblad B, Wikstrand J, Janzon L, Wedel H, Berglund G. Low-dose metoprolol CR/XL and fluvastatin slow progression of carotid intima-media thickness: Main results from the Beta-Blocker Cholesterol-Lowering Asymptomatic Plaque Study (BCAPS). *Circulation.* 2001;103:1721-1726.

85. Wiklund O, Hulthe J, Wikstrand J, Schmidt C, Olofsson SO, Bondjers G. Effect of controlled release/extended release metoprolol on carotid intima-media thickness in patients with hypercholesterolemia: a 3-year randomized study. *Stroke.* 2002;33:572-577.

86. Wikstrand J, Berglund G, Hedblad B, Hulthe J. Antiatherosclerotic effects of beta-blockers. *Am J Cardiol.* 2003;91:25H-29H.

87. Pitt B, O'Neill B, Feldman R, Ferrari R, Schwartz L, Mudra H, Bass T, Pepine C, Texter M, Haber H, Uprichard A, Cashin-Hemphill L, Lees RS. The QUinapril Ischemic Event Trial (QUIET): evaluation of chronic ACE inhibitor therapy in patients with ischemic heart disease and preserved left ventricular function. *Am J Cardiol.* 2001;87:1058-1063.

88. Teo KK, Burton JR, Buller CE, Plante S, Catellier D, Tymchak W, Dzavik V, Taylor D, Yokoyama S, Montague TJ. Long-term effects of cholesterol lowering and angiotensin-converting enzyme inhibition on coronary atherosclerosis: The Simvastatin/Enalapril Coronary Atherosclerosis Trial (SCAT). *Circulation.* 2000;102:1748-1754.

89. Pitt B, Byington RP, Furberg CD, Hunninghake DB, Mancini GB, Miller ME, Riley W. Effect of amlodipine on the progression of atherosclerosis and the occurrence of clinical events. PREVENT Investigators. *Circulation.* 2000;102:1503-1510.

90. Nissen SE, Tuzcu EM, Libby P, Thompson PD, Ghali M, Garza D, Berman L, Shi H, Buebendorf E, Topol EJ. Effect of antihypertensive agents on cardiovascu-

lar events in patients with coronary disease and normal blood pressure: the CAMELOT study: a randomized controlled trial. *JAMA*. 2004;292:2217-2225.

91. Sipahi I, Tuzcu EM, Schoenhagen P, Wolski KE, Nicholls SJ, Balog C, Crowe TD, Nissen SE. Effects of normal, pre-hypertensive, and hypertensive blood pressure levels on progression of coronary atherosclerosis. *J Am Coll Cardiol*. 2006;48:833-838.

92. Rodriguez-Granillo GA, Vos J, Bruining N, Garcia-Garcia HM, de Winter S, Ligthart JM, Deckers JW, Bertrand M, Simoons ML, Ferrari R, Fox KM, Remme W, De Feyter PJ. Long-term effect of perindopril on coronary atherosclerosis progression (from the perindopril's prospective effect on coronary atherosclerosis by angiography and intravascular ultrasound evaluation <PERSPECTIVE] study). *Am J Cardiol*. 2007;100:159-163.

93. Katakami N, Yamasaki Y, Hayaishi-Okano R, Ohtoshi K, Kaneto H, Matsuhisa M, Kosugi K, Hori M. Metformin or gliclazide, rather than glibenclamide, attenuate progression of carotid intima-media thickness in subjects with type 2 diabetes. *Diabetologia*. 2004;47:1906-1913.

94. Arakawa M, Hirose T. <Glinide(s), sulfonylurea(s)]. *Nippon Rinsho*. 2006;64:2107-2112.

95. Oyama T, Saiki A, Endoh K, Ban N, Nagayama D, Ohhira M, Koide N, Miyashita Y, Shirai K. Effect of acarbose, an alpha-glucosidase inhibitor, on serum lipoprotein lipase mass levels and common carotid artery intima-media thickness in type 2 diabetes mellitus treated by sulfonylurea. *J Atheroscler Thromb*. 2008;15:154-159.

96. Hanefeld M, Chiasson JL, Koehler C, Henkel E, Schaper F, Temelkova-Kurktschiev T. Acarbose slows progression of intima-media thickness of the carotid arteries in subjects with impaired glucose tolerance. *Stroke*. 2004;35:1073-1078.

97. Mazzone T, Meyer PM, Feinstein SB, Davidson MH, Kondos GT, D'Agostino RB, Sr., Perez A, Provost JC, Haffner SM. Effect of pioglitazone compared with glimepiride on carotid intima-media thickness in type 2 diabetes: a randomized trial. *JAMA*. 2006;296:2572-2581.

98. Davidson MH, Meyer PM, Haffner SM, Feinstein SB, Kondos GT, D'Agostino RB, Sr., Perez A, Mazzone T. Increases in HDL-C in the CHICAGO study explain the benefits of pioglitazone in reducing CIMT progression in patients with type 2 diabetes. *Circulation*. 2007;116:II_824.

99. Nicholls SJ, Tuzcu EM, Kalidindi S, Wolski K, Moon KW, Sipahi I, Schoenhagen P, Nissen SE. Effect of diabetes on progression of coronary atherosclerosis and arterial remodeling: a pooled analysis of 5 intravascular ultrasound trials. *J Am Coll Cardiol*. 2008;52:255-262.

100. Nissen SE, Nicholls SJ, Wolski K, Nesto R, Kupfer S, Perez A, Jure H, De Larochelliere R, Staniloae CS, Mavromatis K, Saw J, Hu B, Lincoff AM, Tuzcu EM. Comparison of pioglitazone vs glimepiride on progression of coronary atherosclerosis in patients with type 2 diabetes: the PERISCOPE randomized controlled trial. *JAMA*. 2008;299:1561-1573.

101. Rudel LL, Lee RG, Parini P. ACAT2 is a target for treatment of coronary heart disease associated with hypercholesterolemia. *Arterioscler Thromb Vasc Biol*. 2005;25:1112-1118.

102. Delsing DJ, Offerman EH, van Duyvenvoorde W, van Der Boom H, de Wit EC, Gijbels MJ, van Der Laarse A, Jukema JW, Havekes LM, Princen HM. Acyl-CoA:cholesterol acyltransferase inhibitor avasimibe reduces atherosclerosis in addition to its cholesterol-lowering effect in ApoE*3-Leiden mice. *Circulation*. 2001;103:1778-1786.

103. Tardif JC, Gregoire J, L'Allier PL, Anderson TJ, Bertrand O, Reeves F, Title LM, Alfonso F, Schampaert E, Hassan A, McLain R, Pressler ML, Ibrahim R, Lesperance J, Blue J, Heinonen T, Rodes-Cabau J. Effects of the acyl coenzyme A:cholesterol acyltransferase inhibitor avasimibe on human atherosclerotic lesions. *Circulation*. 2004;110:3372-3377.

104. Nissen SE, Tuzcu EM, Brewer HB, Sipahi I, Nicholls SJ, Ganz P, Schoenhagen P, Waters DD, Pepine CJ, Crowe TD, Davidson MH, Deanfield JE, Wisniewski LM, Hanyok JJ, Kassalow LM. Effect of ACAT inhibition on the progression of coronary atherosclerosis. *N Engl J Med*. 2006;354:1253-1263.

105. Feng B, Yao PM, Li Y, Devlin CM, Zhang D, Harding HP, Sweeney M, Rong JX, Kuriakose G, Fisher EA, Marks AR, Ron D, Tabas I. The endoplasmic reticulum is the site of cholesterol-induced cytotoxicity in macrophages. *Nat Cell Biol*. 2003;5:781-792.

106. Tardif JC, Gregoire J, L'Allier PL, Ibrahim R, Anderson TJ, Reeves F, Title LM, Schampaert E, LeMay M, Lesperance J, Scott R, Guertin MC, Brennan ML, Hazen SL, Bertrand OF. Effects of the antioxidant succinobucol (AGI-1067) on human atherosclerosis in a randomized clinical trial. *Atherosclerosis*. 2008;197:480-486.

107. Serruys PW, Garcia-Garcia HM, Buszman P, Erne P, Verheye S, Aschermann M, Duckers H, Bleie O, Dudek D, Botker HE, von Birgelen C, D'Amico D, Hutchinson T, Zambanini A, Mastik F, van Es GA, van der Steen AF, Vince DG, Ganz P, Hamm CW, Wijns W, Zalewski A. Effects of the direct lipoprotein-associated

phospholipase A(2) inhibitor darapladib on human coronary atherosclerotic plaque. *Circulation.* 2008;118: 1172-1182.

108. Kapadia SR, Nissen SE, Tuzcu EM. Impact of intravascular ultrasound in understanding transplant coronary artery disease. *Curr Opin Cardiol.* 1999;14:140-150.

109. Kobashigawa JA, Katznelson S, Laks H, Johnson JA, Yeatman L, Wang XM, Chia D, Terasaki PI, Sabad A, Cogert GA, et al. Effect of pravastatin on outcomes after cardiac transplantation. *N Engl J Med.* 1995;333:621-627.

110. Schroeder JS, Gao SZ, Alderman EL, Hunt SA, Johnstone I, Boothroyd DB, Wiederhold V, Stinson EB. A preliminary study of diltiazem in the prevention of coronary artery disease in heart-transplant recipients. *N Engl J Med.* 1993;328:164-170.

111. Mehra MR, Ventura HO, Smart FW, Stapleton DD. Impact of converting enzyme inhibitors and calcium entry blockers on cardiac allograft vasculopathy: from bench to bedside. *J Heart Lung Transplant.* 1995;14:S246-249.

112. Eisen HJ, Tuzcu EM, Dorent R, Kobashigawa J, Mancini D, Valantine-von Kaeppler HA, Starling RC, Sorensen K, Hummel M, Lind JM, Abeywickrama KH, Bernhardt P. Everolimus for the prevention of allograft rejection and vasculopathy in cardiac-transplant recipients. *N Engl J Med.* 2003;349:847-858.

CHAPTER 12

Use of Imaging in Research on Systolic and Diastolic Function

Thomas H. Marwick, MBBS, PhD

INTRODUCTION

The clinical evaluation of cardiac function is focused on issues related to risk evaluation, distinction of type of heart failure, and etiology. Although the use of imaging tests is central to management, in practical terms these are often reported in a semiquantitative fashion. Research studies often evaluate the responses of systolic or diastolic function to therapy, and are more likely to address aspects that do not yet have a place in standard clinical practice, such as assessment of myocardial texture, myocardial mechanics, energetics, perfusion, and innervations. The requirements of imaging tests in research studies are more stringent than for clinical work. This chapter will consider some generic issues about statistical and imaging considerations before proceeding to discuss the main measurements that are used in research on myocardial function.

STATISTICAL CONSIDERATIONS

The basic characteristics of any test are validity and reliability.[1] Validity (how well the test measures what it should) is measured against an external reference standard. For myocardial function, such standards include implantable crystals and invasive pressure and flow measurements. Discussion of reliability usually focuses on precision (i.e., the control of error, which may originate from random error or bias), but it is important to realize that reliability is the fraction of true variance/(true+error variance). It is easier to show high reliability if the parameter shows some true variation than if it is very stable. Variance is often reported in terms of inter- and intraobserver variability—these parameters are particularly important when image quality constrains accurate measurement, as with echocardiography.

Cardiac function research often involves repeated testing. Repeat imaging is commonplace in many noncardiac settings—for example, repeat imaging of solid tumors is used in the assessment of treatment response.[2] Although the performance of repeat examinations is considered clinically appropriate with echocardiography in some circumstances,[3] it has to be acknowledged that accurate measurement of change can be quite challenging. Test-retest variation is perhaps the more important parameter for understanding whether changes are real or artifactual, but unfortunately this parameter is often neglected. The limitations of reliability of sequential measurements are especially an issue when imaging data are applied on an individual basis (e.g., to inform a treatment decision) and less of a problem when the change is measured across a population (e.g., to measure an average response to treatment).

Finally, the clinical milieu may be as important in interpreting diagnostic test results in experimental settings as it is clinically. This involves an appreciation of the pretest likelihood of disease and the Bayesian incorporation of both clinical and test data.

IMAGING CONSIDERATIONS

A substantial array of imaging tools is now available to the clinical researcher. As in clinical practice, the selection of an imaging technique needs to be grounded on the performance requirements to address the specific question posed, as well as cost, accessibility, and availability. For example, the high spatial and contrast resolution of cardiac magnetic resonance (CMR) makes this a very attractive imaging endpoint, but its selection may be inappropriate for population health studies, studies where large numbers of patients are needed because of clinical variation, or if the results of the study are planned to inform clinical practice in an environment where CMR is unavailable.

The resolution of imaging modalities may be assessed in temporal, spatial, or contrast domains. The highest temporal resolutions are available with M-mode and Doppler echocardiography—often hundreds of frames per second—while the lowest are obtained with three-dimensional echocardiography (3DE), CMR, and some scintigraphic techniques. High temporal resolution is important not only in the evaluation of brief time intervals (e.g., measurement of synchrony or isovolumic phases) but also because undersampling may compromise the ability to measure peak flow and volume measurements. Spatial resolution should be considered in all imaging planes and determines the accuracy of making linear and volume measurements. For example, the spatial resolution of single photon emission computed tomography may be as low as a centimeter, which may particularly pose problems in the measurement of small hearts (e.g., in women). Likewise, M-mode echocardiography has high temporal resolution and high axial resolution, but its inability to image in more than one plane limits the ability to obtain the same cut-plane, and thereby tests reliability for sequential measurements. Finally, contrast resolution relates to the ability of the test to recognize one structure from another, and therefore impacts on spatial resolution. Contrast resolution between myocardium and left ventricular (LV) cavity is a particularly attractive aspect of CMR, and that of echocardiography may be enhanced with LV opacification.[4]

EVALUATION OF LV SYSTOLIC FUNCTION

Simple markers of LV systolic function (such as ejection fraction) are often used for patient selection or stratification in studies. Commonly, more sophisticated measurements are needed to address the evolution of LV function over time, the nature of regional function, or the response of systolic function to stress.

LV Volumes and Ejection Fraction

Although simple and widely understood, these measurements are exquisitely sensitive to loading conditions. As loading is difficult to standardize, this problem is best addressed by simultaneous measurement of ejection and filling pressures to derive elastance. Although classically obtained by invasive monitoring, this may be measured noninvasively.[5] More sophisticated noninvasive approaches involve the use of a transfer function to allow derivation of central pressure from tonometry, as well as echocardiographic techniques for estimating filling pressure.[6]

Irrespective of the imaging technique selected, there are benefits to using a 3D rather than a 2D approach, especially if sequential studies are considered. Difficulty with obtaining the correct imaging axis is particularly an issue for 2DE because of limited imaging windows.[7] Foreshortened images may lead to underestimation of LV volume and variations of imaging planes may produce artifactual changes in LV volume and mass over time—ejection fraction (EF) is usually less susceptible to this problem. The only traditional method that is not at risk from this limitation is radionuclide ventriculography, where EF is derived from scintigraphic counts, but this is susceptible to attenuation. Three-dimensional imaging is now obtainable using 3DE, CMR, SPECT, and cardiac computed tomography (CCT),[8] and it appears that it is the availability of 3D data rather than the nature of the imaging technique (Figure 12.1) that determines the increased reliability of this method.[9] CMR is considered to be the gold standard for LV volume measurement, although caution needs to be paid to tracking the basal segment and a guide-point system appears useful for this purpose.[10] The benefit of lower measurement variability is that smaller sample sizes are required for CMR studies.[11] Nonetheless, CMR is expensive, of limited availability, and unsuitable for some patients—in these circumstances, 3DE is a close second choice for the 60–70% of patients who have adequate images. Comparisons of 3DE with CMR have shown small mean differences in volume measurements, with minor underestimation of CMR volumes related to ambiguity in tracing the trabecular space.[12] Echocardiographic contrast agents improve endocardial detection and increase the accuracy of 2DE,[13, 14] perhaps largely by avoiding foreshortened images. The use of 3DE with contrast requires care to avoid bubble destruction but appears to give the closest approximation to CMR, followed in accuracy by noncontrast 3DE and contrast 2DE.[15]

Contractile Reserve

The substantial reserve of the heart means that the organ's performance under stress may provide information that is not apparent at rest. This is important in both preclinical and established heart disease.

Systolic dysfunction may become apparent under stress when resting function appears to be normal in preclinical disease. An example is in regurgitant valvular disease, where

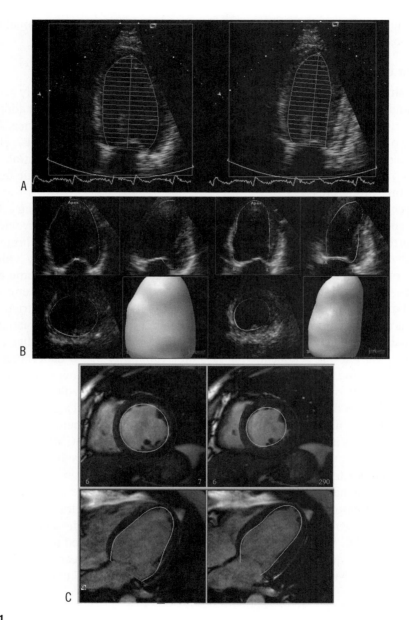

Figure 12.1

Comparison of end-systolic and end-diastolic LV volumes with 2D and 3D echocardiography against the reference standard of cardiac magnetic resonance. Analysis of LV volume using 2DE Simpson's method of discs (A) shows an EDV of 204mls and ESV of 141mls. Analysis of LV volume using 3DE (B) shows an EDV of 262mls and ESV of 165mls. The use of cardiac magnetic resonance (CMR) (C) shows EDV of 272mls and ESV of 174mls. The use of this guide-point CMR approach requires long-axis images for orientation of the apex and base, with measurements performed in the short-axis views. (See Color Plate 33.)

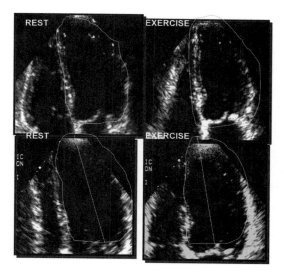

Figure 12.2

Use of 2D echocardiography to measure contractile reserve in response to stress. The upper row shows end-systolic views (with superimposed end-diastolic outlines) at rest and exercise showing reduction of LV volumes and increased ejection fraction poststress. The lower row shows a reduction of ejection fraction poststress.

the volume load may cause LV impairment that may be difficult to recognize in the presence of mitral regurgitation. In this circumstance, exercise 2DE may identify subclinical LV dysfunction, manifest as a failure to increase EF or reduce ESV with stress (Figure 12.2).[16] Exercise is the stressor of choice for this purpose, and although it is possible to exercise patients in the magnet, echo may be more feasible than CMR for this assessment. Nuclear ventriculography is another option.

Noninvasive measurement of contractile reserve in established heart failure (based on ejection fraction or cardiac output) has been shown to be related to outcome.[17] This finding mirrors sympathetic dysfunction,[18] but LV contractile reserve is also dependent on the Frank Starling mechanism and force-frequency effect,[19] so the stress response may not be a surrogate for sympathetic status.

Regional Function

Coronary artery disease is a common cause of LV dysfunction and this disease is typically regional. Because of compensatory hyperkinesis in the uninvolved wall, EF and volumes are not reliable indices of LV involvement and regional parameters are required. In the clinical setting, regional wall motion scoring is performed, but this has significant observer variation—especially with suboptimal image quality[20]—and is not well suited to research work.

The quantitation of regional function is difficult, and requires good spatial and contrast resolution, so the chief protagonists are CMR and 2DE (often with contrast). The venerable centerline approach (measuring the excursion between end-systolic and -diastolic LV contours) is an option but is susceptible to translation.[21] Myocardial thickening in the radial axis can be measured by CMR or echo, and provides the possibility of measuring circumferential fiber shortening,[22] which appears to be a more reliable marker of systolic dysfunction in hypertensive heart disease.

CMR or echocardiography may be used to measure displacement and velocity (which may be influenced by translation and tethering and is therefore not site-specific), strain (an index of deformation), or strain rate as indices of regional function. CMR measurements are based on myocardial tagging. The degree and time-course of lengthening or shortening of tag lines may be measured automatically using a variety of techniques, the most established being harmonic phase (HARP).[23] This technique has been validated in the radial but not the longitudinal plane and may have important technical limitations related to temporal resolution. Strain rate and strain can be derived from color tissue Doppler (Figure 12.3); although limited by angle dependence and signal noise, its measurement of strain rate makes it analogous to regional contractility and high temporal resolution makes it feasible to apply this during stress.[24] Two-dimensional strain is an ultrasound technique based on speckle tracking of the grayscale texture. Although it correlates well with tagged CMR,[25] it is a better technique for measuring strain than strain rate, and its application during stress is constrained by optimal frame-rates of < 80 frames/second (Figure 12.4). The best technique may vary according to the nature of the physiology being measured; TVI-based strain rate is best for measuring timing (e.g., postsystolic thickening) and at high heart rates. Resting imaging of the remodeled heart, where the orientation of the wall and imaging axis may change along the length of the wall, is best done with 2D-strain or MR tagging.

Table 12.1 summarizes the reliability of these myocardial parameters in our laboratory. The smallest variations are associated with systolic and diastolic tissue Doppler measurements. While strain rate and strain are accurate, they are less reproducible in follow-up because they suffer from more signal noise.[26]

LV Morphology

The morphology of the LV describes its mass and shape. Although much of the literature is based upon M-mode echocardiography, LV mass is most accurately measured by CMR[27] and 3DE (Figure 12.5).[28] Cardiac shape is important in LV hypertrophy; distinctions between relative wall thickness and hypertrophy have prognostic significance,[29] which may relate to differences in transmural wall stress. Wall stress (which depends on LV pressure, size, wall thickness, and curvature) is sometimes derived for research purposes, but current techniques assume wall stress is uniform for the entire LV, and 3D measurements of curvature will be needed to obtain regional assessment of wall stress. LV shape—measured as sphericity index (ratio of the maximum longitudinal and short axis dimensions)—is also used as a marker of LV remodeling in heart failure.[30]

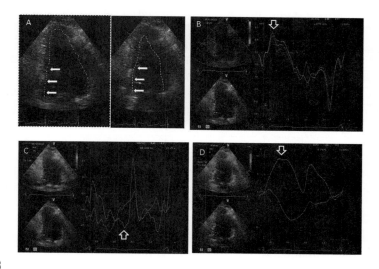

Figure 12.3

Application of quantitative techniques to evaluate regional function after myocardial infarction. Standard 2D echocardiography (A) shows akinesis of the basal and mid inferior walls (arrows). Tissue velocities (B) show a minor gradation of systolic velocity (open arrow) from base to apex, but reduced basal function is not appreciated due to tethering. Strain rate imaging (C) shows reduced and delayed basal inferior systolic strain rate (line marked with open arrow), with minor delay of the midwall segment (turquoise). Tissue velocity-based strain (D) shows lengthening of the basal septal segment (open arrow) and reduction of the midwall segment. (See Color Plate 34.)

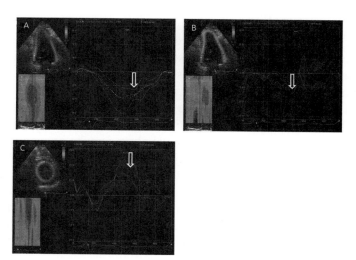

Figure 12.4

Longitudinal (A) and radial (B) assessments of 2D strain from the apical view show delay of the basal inferior systolic strain (line marked with open arrow). The mid-inferior wall dysfunction is more readily appreciated on radial strain in the mid-LV short axis (C). (See Color Plate 35.)

Table 12.1   Reliability of Echocardiographic Measures for Tissue Characterization

	INTRAOBSERVER VARIATION	COEFFICIENT OF VARIATION
Sm	0.4 ± 0.4 cm/s	8%
Em	0.6 ± 0.5 cm/s	5%
Pk systolic SR (TVI)	0.06 ± 0.24	11%
Pk systolic Σ (TVI)	0.5 ± 4.75	15%
Pk systolic SR (2D)	0.00 ± 0.27	11%
Pk systolic Σ (2D)	1.06 ± 0.61	10%
Calibrated IB	2.7 ± 2.0 dB	9%
Cyclic variation of IB	1.5 ± 1.2 dB	15%

Right Ventricular Function

There is increasing interest in the evaluation of right ventricular (RV) function, driven by the availability of new treatment modalities for pulmonary hypertension. Conventional methods have traditionally posed a barrier to RV imaging studies, as this chamber does not conform to a geometric shape. This is not an important consideration for 3D imaging with CMR and 3DE (Figure 12.6), and RV evaluation with CMR has been shown to correlate with outcomes.[31] The evaluation of myocardial deformation may also be independent of RV geometry. The simplest approach to the evaluation of RV function is tissue Doppler,[32] but RV strain assessment is feasible with both tissue velocity and speckle strain.[33]

Other Imaging Information

The imaging of cardiac metabolism and cardiac efficiency may be performed with positron emission tomography (PET) or spectroscopy with CMR. F^{18}-deoxyglucose (FDG) is the best-known PET tracer because of its use in the assessment of myocardial viability. Its ability to trace cellular glucose uptake (it is taken up by the GLUT-transporter and phosphorylated by hexokinase) may provide information about the diabetic heart. Abnormal myocardial metabolism, energy depletion, and reduced mechanical efficiency are hallmarks of the failing heart.[34] Fatty acid metabolism may be imaged with PET (using C^{11} palmitate)[35] or SPECT using beta-methyl-iodophenylpentadecanoic acid (BMIPP). Although these techniques have been used for the assessment of myocardial viability, a more important question would be whether the evidence they could provide of a metabolic switch from fatty acids to glucose utilization influences the outcome of patients with HF. The relationship of global and regional myocardial C^{11} acetate kinetics to cardiac work offers a non-invasive parameter for cardiac efficiency.[36] Analysis of myocardial ATP and phosphocreatine may be performed using MR spectroscopy. While this technique has been available for many years, it remains technically challenging, as spectra may be difficult to quantify. The ready availability of high magnetic field systems may increase the feasibility of this technique.

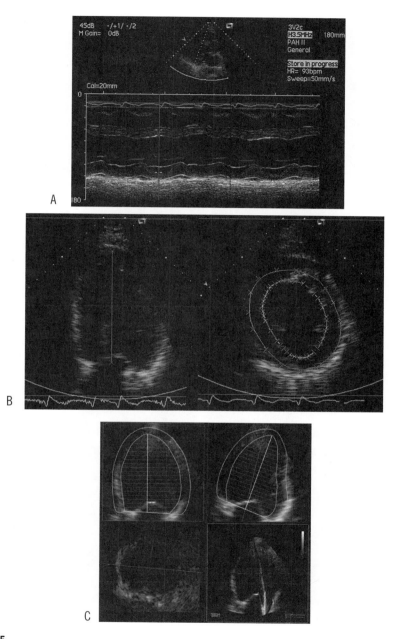

Figure 12.5

Comparison of M-mode, 2DE, and 3DE images of LV mass. Analysis using M-mode (A) showed a mass of 276g. Measurement using 2DE (B) was 277g. LV mass by 3DE (C) was 217g, closest to the CMR measurement of 197g.

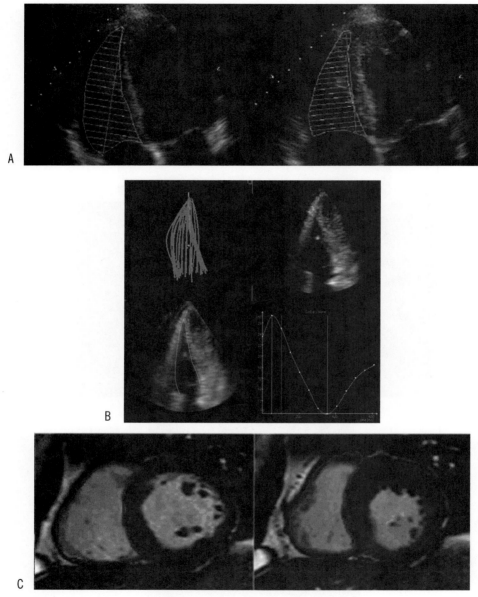

Figure 12.6

Assessment of RV volumes and EF using 2DE, 3DE, and CMR. Analysis of RV volumes using (A) 2DE with Simpson's method. The right panel shows EDV with ESV on the right-hand panel. (B) Real-time 3DE (RT3D); the figure demonstrates selection of one image (upper right), automated contour-tracing (lower left), superimposition of all contours in 3D space (upper left), and the resulting time-volume curve. (C) CMR. The left panel shows EDV, with ESV on the right panel (see Color Plate 36). As the RV is such a non-geometric structure, it appears that 3D approaches will be the optimal bedside measurement strategy.

Cardiac innervation disturbances are associated with heart failure and arrhythmias. Visualization of the parasympathetic system is difficult, but sympathetic imaging may identify high-risk patients. Metaiodobenzylguanidine (MIBG) is a SPECT tracer that undergoes uptake and storage in cardiac nerve terminals, but is not metabolized by monoamine oxidase.[37] Quantification of this agent is relative to the mediastinum or relative to other areas of the heart. Neuronal imaging may also be performed using the PET tracers C-11 hydroxyephedrine (HED) and C-11 epinephrine.

Molecular imaging can be used to visualize angiogenesis, apoptosis, cell migration, and inflammation. While these show promise in the animal laboratory, there will be a number of regulatory hurdles before they are applied in clinical research.

EVALUATION OF LV DIASTOLIC FUNCTION

Heart failure with preserved ejection fraction (HFpEF) is the focus of much LV function research.

Assessment of Diastolic Function

The standard pulse wave Doppler filling profile is the cornerstone of this evaluation.[38] However, the new diagnostic criteria[39] emphasize the echocardiographic estimation of filling pressure,[6] derived from the ratio of passive filling and myocardial velocities (E/E', Figure 12.7), as well as left atrial size.[40]

Many patients with suspected HFpEF have dyspnea only with exertion, and have mild diastolic dysfunction at rest with normal filling pressure. The response of E/E' to stress may be useful in the attribution of exertional dyspnea to diastolic HF.[41] Conversely, the absence of raised filling pressure with exercise makes it difficult to attribute exertional dyspnea to diastolic HF.

LV filling can be measured by all imaging modalities, but not to the same level of sensitivity. Modalities with high temporal resolution are favored (as discussed above, this permits the detection of brief events such as isovolumic time and avoids underestimation of peak flows due to under-sampling). The second important attribute is the ability to distinguish normal from pseudonormal filling. These favor the use of echocardiography rather than other techniques.

The main goals of myocardial tissue characterization are to identify early (Stage B) disease.[42]

Identification of Fibrosis

Two-thirds of myocardial cells are nonmyocytes,[43] and the interstitium is likely an important contributor to LV dysfunction in ischemic cardiomyopathy[44] as well as diastolic dysfunction present in hypertension, diabetes, and the elderly.[45] Pathological hypertrophy is associated with interstitial and perivascular fibrosis, and the fibrous tissue is

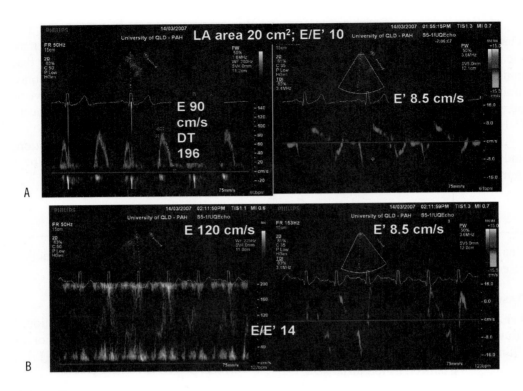

Figure 12.7

Assessment of LV filling pressure using the E/E' ratio at rest (A) and after exercise (B). (See Color Plate 37.)

characterized by an increase in type 1 collagen.[43] Fibrosis is likely a contributor to reduced coronary flow reserve[46], as well as HF and arrhythmias.[43]

CMR Methods

Gadolinium late-enhancement CMR images are useful for the identification of regional fibrosis—for example, after myocardial infarction.[47] However, the recognition of diffuse fibrosis with this technique is not possible, as the technique is based on comparison between the region and a reference normal segment, which is nulled by a prepulse.

Two CMR methods show promise in the recognition of fibrosis. T1 mapping is a means of displaying T1 time, which is shortened by gadolinium, especially in the presence of fibrosis.[48] This finding has been linked with biopsy evidence of fibrosis as well as diastolic function.[49] The second CMR method is the transverse relaxation time of hydrogen protons (T2), which reveal differences in tissue water content.[50]

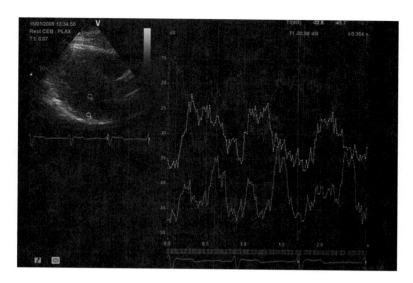

Figure 12.8

Measurement of integrated backscatter (IB) from an image in raw data format. (See Color Plate 38.)

Echocardiographic Methods

Techniques that provide information on myocardial velocity and deformation have been shown to correspond to the presence of fibrosis.[51,52] However, these techniques relate to myocardial motion or thickening, and are therefore influenced by myocyte pathology, rather than being specific for interstitial changes. Ultrasonic integrated backscatter measures the reflection of ultrasound from the myocardium, which is proportionate to its acoustic density, and is increased by fibrosis. As IB varies according to machine settings and patient habitus, this measurement can only be interpreted in the context of a reference density, which is gathered by sample volumes in the pericardium or blood-pool (Figure 12.8). IB is abnormal in a variety of hypertrophic and endocrine conditions.[53-55]

Nuclear Cardiology Techniques

The presence of myocardial fibrosis influences the findings of perfusion scans, and indeed, reduced coronary reserve in nonischemic HF may be due to microvascular dysfunction. However, as many causes of interstitial fibrosis are linked with coronary artery disease, these findings may be attributed to the latter and are nonspecific for fibrosis.

The interstitium can be interrogated with PET. The use of $H_2^{15}O$ and $C^{15}O$, allow measurement of perfusable tissue index (PTI), which is reduced in patients with DCM.[56]

However, the technique is expensive, costly, of limited availability, and technically challenging.

CONCLUSION

A variety of cardiac imaging modalities can be harnessed to provide information for research into systolic and diastolic dysfunction. As it is unlikely that any one modality will provide all necessary information for a study, investigators should be prepared to use multiple modalities, and systems for coregistration of images are important. It should be remembered that not only are the attributes of the technique important, but the selection may be influenced by the circumstances of testing.

◇◇◇◇◇◇◇◇◇◇◇◇

REFERENCES

1. Streiner DL, Norman GR. "Precision" and "accuracy": two terms that are neither. *J Clin Epidemiol* 2006;59:327-30.
2. Eisenhauer EA, Therasse P, Bogaerts J et al. New response evaluation criteria in solid tumours: Revised RECIST guideline (version 1.1). *Eur J Cancer* 2008.
3. Douglas PS, Khandheria B, Stainback RF et al. ACCF/ASE/ACEP/ASNC/ SCAI/SCCT/SCMR 2007 appropriateness criteria for transthoracic and transesophageal echocardiography: a report of the American College of Cardiology Foundation Quality Strategic Directions Committee Appropriateness Criteria Working Group, American Society of Echocardiography, American College of Emergency Physicians, American Society of Nuclear Cardiology, Society for Cardiovascular Angiography and Interventions, Society of Cardiovascular Computed Tomography, and the Society for Cardiovascular Magnetic Resonance endorsed by the American College of Chest Physicians and the Society of Critical Care Medicine. *J Am Coll Cardiol* 2007;50:187-204.
4. Mulvagh SL, Rakowski H, Vannan MA et al. American Society of Echocardiography Consensus Statement on the Clinical Applications of Ultrasonic Contrast Agents in Echocardiography. *J Am Soc Echocardiogr* 2008;21:1179-201.
5. Chen CH, Fetics B, Nevo E et al. Noninvasive single-beat determination of left ventricular end-systolic elastance in humans. *J Am Coll Cardiol* 2001;38:2028-34.
6. Nagueh SF, Mikati I, Kopelen HA, Middleton KJ, Quinones MA, Zoghbi WA. Doppler estimation of left ventricular filling pressure in sinus tachycardia. A new application of tissue doppler imaging. *Circulation* 1998;98:1644-50.
7. King DL, Harrison MR, King DL, Jr., Gopal AS, Martin RP, DeMaria AN. Improved reproducibility of left atrial and left ventricular measurements by guided three-dimensional echocardiography. *J Am Coll Cardiol* 1992;20:1238-45.
8. Lang RM, Mor-Avi V, Sugeng L, Nieman PS, Sahn DJ. Three-dimensional echocardiography: the benefits of the additional dimension. *J Am Coll Cardiol* 2006;48:2053-69.
9. Chuang ML, Hibberd MG, Salton CJ et al. Importance of imaging method over imaging modality in noninvasive determination of left ventricular volumes and ejection fraction: assessment by two- and three-dimensional echocardiography and magnetic resonance imaging. *J Am Coll Cardiol* 2000;35:477-84.
10. Young AA, Cowan BR, Thrupp SF, Hedley WJ, Dell'Italia LJ. Left ventricular mass and volume: fast calculation with guide-point modeling on MR images. *Radiology* 2000;216:597-602.
11. Bellenger NG, Davies LC, Francis JM, Coats AJ, Pennell DJ. Reduction in sample size for studies of remodeling in heart failure by the use of cardiovascular magnetic resonance. *J Cardiovasc Magn Reson* 2000;2:271-8.

12. Mor-Avi V, Jenkins C, Kühl HP et al. Real-time 3D echocardiographic quantification of left ventricular volumes: multicenter study for validation with magnetic resonance imaging and investigation of sources of error. *J Am Coll Cardiol—Cardiovascular Imaging* (in press) 2008;1.

13. Thomson HL, Basmadjian AJ, Rainbird AJ et al. Contrast echocardiography improves the accuracy and reproducibility of left ventricular remodeling measurements: a prospective, randomly assigned, blinded study. *J Am Coll Cardiol* 2001;38:867-75.

14. Hoffmann R, von Bardeleben S, Kasprzak JD et al. Analysis of regional left ventricular function by cineventriculography, cardiac magnetic resonance imaging, and unenhanced and contrast-enhanced echocardiography: a multicenter comparison of methods. *J Am Coll Cardiol* 2006;47:121-8.

15. Jenkins C, Moir S, Chan J, Rakhit D, Haluska B, Marwick TH. Left ventricular volume measurement with echocardiography: a comparison of left ventricular opacification, three-dimensional echocardiography, or both with magnetic resonance imaging. *Eur Heart J* 2008.

16. Leung DY, Griffin BP, Stewart WJ, Cosgrove DM, Thomas JD, Marwick TH. Left ventricular function after valve repair for chronic mitral regurgitation: Predictive value of preoperative assessment of contractile reserve by exercise echocardiography. *J Am Coll Cardiol* 1996;28:1198-205.

17. Naqvi TZ, Goel RK, Forrester JS, Siegel RJ. Myocardial contractile reserve on dobutamine echocardiography predicts late spontaneous improvement in cardiac function in patients with recent onset idiopathic dilated cardiomyopathy. *J Am Coll Cardiol* 1999;34:1537-44.

18. Ohshima S, Isobe S, Izawa H et al. Cardiac sympathetic dysfunction correlates with abnormal myocardial contractile reserve in dilated cardiomyopathy patients. *J Am Coll Cardiol* 2005;46:2061-8.

19. Holubarsch C, Ludemann J, Wiessner S et al. Shortening versus isometric contractions in isolated human failing and non-failing left ventricular myocardium: dependency of external work and force on muscle length, heart rate and inotropic stimulation. *Cardiovasc Res* 1998;37:46-57.

20. Hoffmann R, Marwick TH, Poldermans D et al. Refinements in stress echocardiographic techniques improve inter-institutional agreement in interpretation of dobutamine stress echocardiograms. *Eur Heart J* 2002;23:821-9.

21. Sheehan FH, Bolson EL, Dodge HT, Mathey DG, Schofer J, Woo HW. Advantages and applications of the centerline method for characterizing regional ventricular function. *Circulation* 1986;74:293-305.

22. Grodzicki T, Michalewicz L, Messerli FH. Aging and essential hypertension: effect of left ventricular hypertrophy on cardiac function. *Am J Hypertens* 1998;11:425-9.

23. Garot J, Bluemke DA, Osman NF et al. Fast determination of regional myocardial strain fields from tagged cardiac images using harmonic phase MRI. *Circulation* 2000;101:981-8.

24. Hanekom L, Lundberg V, Leano R, Marwick TH. Optimisation of strain rate imaging for application to stress echocardiography. *Ultrasound Med Biol* 2004;30:1451-60.

25. Cho GY, Chan J, Leano R, Strudwick M, Marwick TH. Comparison of two-dimensional speckle and tissue velocity based strain and validation with harmonic phase magnetic resonance imaging. *Am J Cardiol* 2006;97:1661-6.

26. Marwick TH, Schwaiger M. The future of cardiovascular imaging in the diagnosis and management of heart failure. Part 1 Tasks and tools. *Circ Cardiovasc Imaging* 2008;1:58-69.

27. Grothues F, Smith GC, Moon JC et al. Comparison of interstudy reproducibility of cardiovascular magnetic resonance with two-dimensional echocardiography in normal subjects and in patients with heart failure or left ventricular hypertrophy. *Am J Cardiol* 2002;90:29-34.

28. Jenkins C, Bricknell K, Hanekom L, Marwick TH. Reproducibility and accuracy of echocardiographic measurements of left ventricular parameters using real-time three-dimensional echocardiography. *J Am Coll Cardiol* 2004;44:878-86.

29. Pierdomenico SD, Lapenna D, Bucci A, Manente BM, Cuccurullo F, Mezzetti A. Prognostic value of left ventricular concentric remodeling in uncomplicated mild hypertension. *Am J Hypertens* 2004;17:1035-9.

30. Mannaerts HF, van der Heide JA, Kamp O, Stoel MG, Twisk J, Visser CA. Early identification of left ventricular remodelling after myocardial infarction, assessed by transthoracic 3D echocardiography. *Eur Heart J* 2004;25:680-7.

31. Larose E, Ganz P, Reynolds HG et al. Right ventricular dysfunction assessed by cardiovascular magnetic resonance imaging predicts poor prognosis late after myocardial infarction. *J Am Coll Cardiol* 2007;49:855-62.

32. Meluzin J, Spinarova L, Hude P et al. Prognostic importance of various echocardiographic right ventricular functional parameters in patients with symptomatic heart failure. *J Am Soc Echocardiogr* 2005;18:435-44.

33. Cho EJ, Jiamsripong P, Calleja AM et al. Right ventricular free wall circumferential strain reflects graded elevation in acute right ventricular afterload. *Am J Physiol Heart Circ Physiol* 2008.

34. Neubauer S. The failing heart—an engine out of fuel. *N Engl J Med* 2007;356:1140-51.

35. Schwaiger M, Hicks R. The clinical role of metabolic imaging of the heart by positron emission tomography. *J Nucl Med* 1991;32:565-78.

36. Buxton DB, Nienaber CA, Luxen A, et al. Noninvasive quantitation of regional oxygen consumption in vivo with C-11 acetate and dynamic positron emission tomography. *Circulation* 1989;79:134-42.

37. Carrio I. Cardiac neurotransmission imaging. *J Nucl Med* 2001;42:1062-76.

38. Somaratne JB, Whalley GA, Gamble GD, Doughty RN. Restrictive filling pattern is a powerful predictor of heart failure events postacute myocardial infarction and in established heart failure: a literature-based meta-analysis. *J Card Fail* 2007;13:346-52.

39. Paulus WJ, Tschope C, Sanderson JE et al. How to diagnose diastolic heart failure: a consensus statement on the diagnosis of heart failure with normal left ventricular ejection fraction by the Heart Failure and Echocardiography Associations of the European Society of Cardiology. *Eur Heart J* 2007;28:2539-50.

40. Tsang TS, Barnes ME, Gersh BJ, Bailey KR, Seward JB. Left atrial volume as a morphophysiologic expression of left ventricular diastolic dysfunction and relation to cardiovascular risk burden. *Am J Cardiol* 2002;90:1284-9.

41. Burgess MI, Jenkins C, Sharman JE, Marwick TH. Diastolic stress echocardiography: hemodynamic validation and clinical significance of estimation of ventricular filling pressure with exercise. *J Am Coll Cardiol* 2006;47:1891-900.

42. Hunt SA, Abraham WT, Chin MH et al. ACC/AHA 2005 Guideline Update for the Diagnosis and Management of Chronic Heart Failure in the Adult: a report of the American College of Cardiology/American Heart Association Task Force on Practice Guidelines (Writing Committee to Update the 2001 Guidelines for the Evaluation and Management of Heart Failure): developed in collaboration with the American College of Chest Physicians and the International Society for Heart and Lung Transplantation: endorsed by the Heart Rhythm Society. *Circulation* 2005;112:e154-e235.

43. Weber KT. Targeting pathological remodeling: concepts of cardioprotection and reparation. *Circulation* 2000;102:1342-5.

44. Beltrami CA, Finato N, Rocco M et al. Structural basis of end-stage failure in ischemic cardiomyopathy in humans. *Circulation* 1994;89:151-63.

45. Grodzicki T, Messerli FH. The heart in the hypertensive elderly. *J Hum Hypertens* 1998;12:593-7.

46. Brilla CG, Matsubara L, Weber KT. Advanced hypertensive heart disease in spontaneously hypertensive rats. Lisinopril-mediated regression of myocardial fibrosis. *Hypertension* 1996;28:269-75.

47. Kim RJ, Fieno DS, Parrish TB et al. Relationship of MRI delayed contrast enhancement to irreversible injury, infarct age, and contractile function. *Circulation* 1999;100:1992-2002.

48. Messroghli DR, Plein S, Higgins DM et al. Human myocardium: single-breath-hold MR T1 mapping with high spatial resolution—reproducibility study. *Radiology* 2006;238:1004-12.

49. Iles L, Pfluger H, Phrommintikul A et al. Evaluation of diffuse myocardial fibrosis in heart failure with cardiac magnetic resonance contrast-enhanced T1 mapping. *J Am Coll Cardiol* 2008;52:1574-80.

50. Miller S, Helber U, Kramer U et al. Subacute myocardial infarction: assessment by STIR T2-weighted MR imaging in comparison to regional function. *MAGMA* 2001;13:8-14.

51. Picano E, Pelosi G, Marzilli M et al. In vivo quantitative ultrasonic evaluation of myocardial fibrosis in humans. *Circulation* 1990;81:58-64.

52. Park TH, Nagueh SF, Khoury DS et al. Impact of myocardial structure and function postinfarction on diastolic strain measurements: implications for assessment of myocardial viability. *Am J Physiol Heart Circ Physiol* 2006;290:H724-H731.

53. Di B, V, Giorgi D, Viacava P et al. Severe aortic stenosis and myocardial function: diagnostic and prognostic usefulness of ultrasonic integrated backscatter analysis. *Circulation* 2004;110:849-55.

54. Di B, V, Giorgi D, Talini E et al. Incremental value of ultrasonic tissue characterization (backscatter) in the evaluation of left ventricular myocardial structure and mechanics in essential arterial hypertension. *Circulation* 2003;107:74-80.

55. Bogazzi F, Di B, V, Palagi C et al. Improvement of intrinsic myocardial contractility and cardiac fibrosis degree in acromegalic patients treated with somatostatin analogues: a prospective study. *Clin Endocrinol* (Oxf) 2005;62:590-6.

56. Knaapen P, Boellaard R, Gotte MJ et al. Perfusable tissue index as a potential marker of fibrosis in patients with idiopathic dilated cardiomyopathy. *J Nucl Med* 2004;45:1299-304.

CHAPTER 13

Atrial Pathobiology and Electroanatomic Mapping for Research

Hany Dimitri, MBBS, FRACP
Prashanthan Sanders, MBBS, PhD, FRACP
Jonathan M. Kalman, MBBS, PhD, FRACP

INTRODUCTION

Atrial fibrillation (AF) has been associated with several key causative factors including age, hypertension, myocardial infarction congestive heart failure, and valvular heart disease.[1-4] In more recent years, other important pathologic associations have become evident, such as that with obstructive sleep apnea and obesity.[5-8] Furthermore, a group of patients without obvious structural heart disease on imaging, nor a precipitating associated condition may also develop atrial fibrillation. They are known as lone fibrillators, indicating this lack of associated disease or cardiac pathology.[9]

The changes to the atria that predispose to atrial fibrillation and the changes inflicted by atrial fibrillation itself may be considered in two broad categories—electrophysiologic and electroanatomic. The mechanisms for these phenomena are atrial cellular, ionic, and ultrastructural changes.

This chapter will focus on the electroanatomic changes caused by various cardiac pathologies as investigated and researched in the cardiac electrophysiology laboratory primarily using 3D electroanatomical mapping systems.

REMODELING DUE TO ATRIAL ARRHYTHMIA AND STRUCTURAL DISEASE

Morillo et al. induced atrial fibrillation in mongrel dogs by continuously pacing the right atrial appendage at 400 beats per minute for 6 weeks. They demonstrated marked biatrial enlargement in these chronically rapidly paced animals, and this increased atrial area was strongly correlated with AF inducibility. Light microscopy demonstrated focal and early hypertrophy, associated with increase in the number and size of the mitochondria and disruption of the sarcoplasmic reticulum on electron microscopy. There was

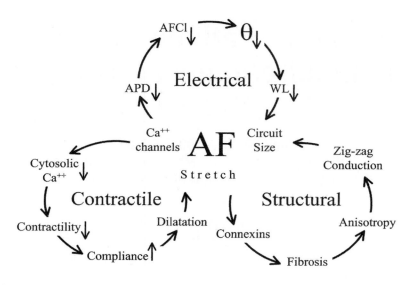

Figure 13.1

Three proposed positive feedback loops of atrial remodeling in AF. Down-regulation of the L-type Ca²⁺ channels is considered to be the primary cause for electrical and contractile remodeling. Stretch of the atrial myocardium, which is the result of loss of contractility and increase in compliance of the fibrillating atria, is hypothesized to act as a stimulus for structural remodeling of the atria.

Printed with permission from Allessie et al.[14]

no identified increase in connective tissue content.[10] Elvan et al. showed an increase in the expression and distribution of gap protein Cx43 in rapidly paced dogs[11] and similar findings were made by Van der Velden in goats.[12] Ausma et al. extensively investigated the ultrastructural changes in the atrial myocardium of a chronically-paced goat model. Marked changes were identified in the cellular structure of the atrial myocyte including loss of myofibrils, glycogen accumulation, and mitochondrial morphologic changes as well as sarcoplasmic reticulum fragmentation and nuclear chromatic dispersion.[13] Allesie et al. proposed three positive feedback loops of atrial remodeling: electrical, contractile, and structural with down-regulation of the L-type Ca²⁺ channels and atrial stretch being key components in this model (Figure 13.1).[14]

The central mechanism of chronic arrhythmogenic structural remodeling is fibrosis. This was demonstrated in a study on mongrel dogs with experimentally induced congestive heart failure. Apart from the histologic findings of sarcomere disruption and loss of myofibrils, quantitative analysis demonstrated significantly more fibrosis in all atrial regions of CHF dogs compared to control. There was localized slowing of conduction and increased conduction heterogeneity contributing to the substrate for atrial fibrillation.[15] In humans, Kamada et al. showed a significantly higher percent area of left atrial fibrosis in the specimens from patients with dilated cardiomyopathy compared to patients with an old myocardial infarction. The generation of fibrotic atrial tissue is the end point of a multifactorial process involving at least four interrelated pathways: the renin-angiotension system, transforming growth factor β, inflammation, and oxidative stress pathways. The latter two are the important physiologic stresses contributing to atrial extracellular matrix turnover and atrial fibrotic progression.[16] Xu et al. studied atrial myocardial samples from explanted hearts, in patients undergoing heart transplantation. They studied maintenance and recurrence of AF with the increased level of collagen I associated with selective down-regulation of tissue inhibitors of metalloproteinases with upregulation of metalloproteinases-2 expression.[17] Correlating with the interstitial fibrosis causing impairment of myocyte coupling is the reduction in expression and function of connexon 43.[18] Alongside the fibrotic changes occurring in the atrial tissue, there is myocyte loss through apoptosis.[19] The end result of these fibrotic and apoptotic processes is disruption of myocardial electrical continuity and alteration of conduction.

The progressive and heterogenous loss of atrial tissue and presence of fibrosis results in the recording of signals with low voltage amplitude when an electrophysiologic recording catheter is brought into contact with the endocardial surface. Another characteristic feature of the underlying modified atrial substrate is the observation that the recorded electrograms maybe fractionated (complex fractionated atrial electrograms [CFAE]). These CFAE are found in areas described in detail by Konings et al. that harbor slow conduction and/or pivot points where the wavelets turn around at the end of arcs of functional block.[20, 21] CFAE may also represent points of localized reentry important to the sustenance of atrial fibrillation, and hence have become a target for radiofrequency ablation in the cure of atrial fibrillation.[22, 23] The definition of the electrogram morphology that constitutes fractionated has varied. In Nademanee's laboratory, CFAE are defined as fractionated electrograms comprised of ≥ 2 deflections, perturbation of the baseline with continuous deflection of a prolonged activation complex, or atrial electrograms with a cycle length $\leq 120ms$.[23] Studies have demonstrated that simple visual observation of these CFAE and their ablation can result in success rates in the cure of atrial fibrillation as high as 91% at 12 months follow-up postablation,[23] however, these results have been difficult to reproduce. Other investigators have defined CFAE as fractionated potentials with ≥ 3 deflections from the isoelectric line or continuous activity[24] or electrograms with a cycle length $\leq 120ms$ or shorter than the coronary sinus, or those that were fractionated or displayed continuous electrical activity.[22] Takahashi et al. attempted to define the characteristics of electrograms that identified successful ablation sites. They found that ablation of sites with a temporal activation gradient of $> 70ms$ or continuous activity had a significant effect on atrial fibrillatory cycle length indicating favorable sites for effective ablation.[25]

SITE-SPECIFIC CONDUCTION

Apart from the changes that may predispose to atrial fibrillation, and the changes that atrial fibrillation may cause to the atria, there are regions where predictable alterations in conduction occur, contributing to the heterogeneity that is central to the theories on atrial fibrillation propagation. In the right atria, important structures include the crista terminalis, which has unique conduction properties because of anisotropy[26] resulting from the displacement of gap junctions to the poles of the myocardial cells resulting in a higher degree of end-to-end connections. Another area of the right atrium that demonstrates nonuniform anisotropy implicated as a critical substrate for induction of atrial fibrillation is the posterior triangle of Koch, where there are multiple inputs to the atrioventricular node.[27, 28] Bachmann's bundle, one of the structures responsible for interatrial conduction and has been shown to have a faster velocity of conduction and higher effective refractory period in animals.[29] In humans, interatrial bundles are not limited to the anteriorly located Bachmann's bundle, but are present in all parts of the interatrial septum. In Platanov et al.'s examination of 84 postmortem human hearts, the subset of specimens from patients with a known history of AF did not show any distinct difference in myoarchitecture when compared to subjects without AF.[30] Within the left atrium, the septopulmonary bundle has been identified as a crista-equivalent. Markides et al. demonstrated a vertical line of block in the posterior left atrium. In these postmortem hearts, this corresponded to a region of abrupt change in myocardial fiber orientation.[31] In patients with structural heart disease and a dilated left atrium, Roberts-Thompson et al. have described a consistent posterior left atrial vertical line of functional conduction delay (Figure 13.2). Suggesting a potential role in arrhythmogenesis, this line facilitates circuitous wave-front propagation.[32]

ELECTROANATOMIC MAPPING IN RESEARCH

Anatomic Mapping Systems

Anatomic mapping systems are now extensively used not only in the mapping and ablation of atrial fibrillation, but other arrhythmias such as atrial flutter and ventricular tachycardia. The ability to visualize a catheter in three dimensions relative to important cardiac structures allows nonfluoroscopic guidance of catheter movement, and, in particular, tagging of sites of radiofrequency ablation.

The CARTO™ (Biosense Webster, Diamond Bar, CA) system is based on a metal coil generating an electrical circuit when placed in a magnetic field. The strength of this circuit, i.e. the current, depends on the strength of the magnetic field and the orientation for the coil within.[33] The low-intensity magnetic field is emitted from three coils under the operating table on which the patient is supine. The catheter (NaviStar™) has a location sensor in its tip that allows its real-time navigation within the three dimensional space.

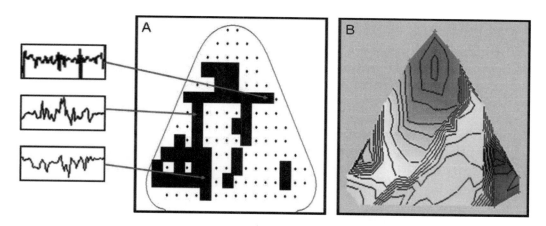

Figure 13.2

Relationship between complex fractionated atrial electrograms and slow conduction during pacing. In panel **A**, fractinated electrograms during atrial fibrillation are illustrated in black. In panel **B**, isochronal crowding denotes lines of conduction block during pacing. The distribution of fractionated electrograms during atrial fibrillation corresponds to the lines of conduction block during pacing.

Roberts-Thomson KC, Stevenson I, Kistler PM, Haqqani HM, Spence SJ, Goldblatt JC, Sanders P, Kalman JM. The role of chronic atrial stretch and atrial fibrillation on posterior left atrial wall conduction. *Heart Rhythm* 2009;6(8):1109-1117 with permission from Elsevier.

Validation in both in-vitro and in-vivo studies has demonstrated catheter accuracy to < 1mm.[34] As the catheter tip makes contact with the endocardium, using stable coronary sinus recordings as a reference, a color-coded activation map may be created. Local electrogram voltage at the point of contact is also stored and this allows a voltage map to be superimposed on the constructed anatomy (Figure 13.3).

Ensite (St. Jude Medical, Minneapolis, MN), allows noncontact via a multi-electrode array comprised of 64 intracavitary polyamide-insulated 0.003-inch diameter wires. Each wire has a 0.025-inch break in insulation producing a noncontact unipolar electrode.[35] This allows for the construction of more than 3000 virtual electrograms (based on an inverse salutation to Laplace's equation by use of a boundary element method)[35] of activation points from the raw cavity potentials, which can be displayed on a preconstructed geometry. The accuracy of electrogram reconstruction decreases in increasing distance between the electrode array and the endocardium becoming significant at distances greater than 34mm. The Ensite system also allows contact mapping (NavX™). This system requires three pairs of cutaneously applied patches, which create a three-dimensional coordinate system. The mapping catheter location is determined by measuring field strength from the matches, which emit low-amplitude 5.7kHz signals.[36] NavX Fusion™ aims to fuse the virtual anatomy created by the mapping catheter to the patient's computed tomographic

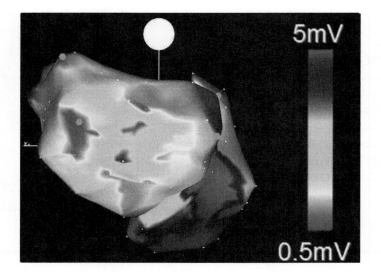

Figure 13.3

Voltage map created with the CARTO mapping system. Using a Navistar mapping/ablation catheter, which has a location sensor in its tip, contact with the myocardial wall allows the recording of a local bipolar electrogram. The maximum amplitude of the voltage may be represented on the constructed anatomy as a continuum of color from low voltage (0.5mV) to high voltage (5mV). (See Color Plate 39.)

(CT) image. Validation studies have shown this to be highly accurate and associated with a reduction in fluoroscopic time relative to procedural duration.[37] Further advances in this technology allows automated CFE mapping and representation of this information in a color-coded fashion on a constructed anatomic map fused to the CT scan (Figure 13.4). This algorithm measures the time between multiple discrete deflections (-dV/dT) in a local AF electrogram recording over a specified length of time (5 seconds) and then averages these interdeflection time intervals to calculate a mean cycle length of the local electrogram during atrial fibrillation.[38]

The Use of Electroanatomical Mapping for Research

Congestive Heart Failure

In heart failure, the prevalence of atrial fibrillation is 10–30%, increasing with worsening disease state.[39, 40] Atrial fibrillation confers an additional morbidity and mortality to that already inherent in congestive heart failure (CHF).[41, 42] Animal studies have demonstrated interstitial fibrosis, cellular hypertrophy and degeneration, larger left atria with increased susceptibility to atrial fibrillation, and heterogeneity of conduction.[15, 43, 44] Sanders et al.[45] studied 21 patients with symptomatic congestive heart failure and left ventricular ejection fraction ≤ 35%, in order to determine the electroanatomic and electrophysiologic

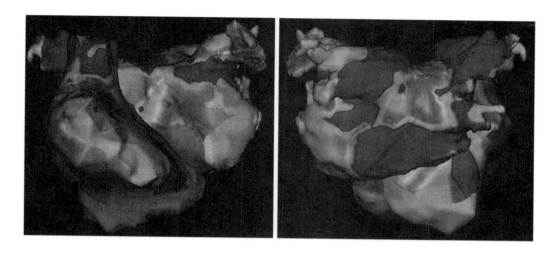

Figure 13.4

Automated complex fractionated electrogram mapping with NavX Fusion. (See Color Plate 40.)

properties characteristic of their atria. Using the CARTO system, high-density endocardial contact points (231.5 ± 57.5) were mapped in order to analyze regional atrial voltages and conduction velocity. Areas of scar (electrically silent) were defined as absence of recordable activity or a bipolar voltage amplitude ≤ 0.05mV with low-voltage areas being defined as those contiguous areas with a bipolar voltage of ≤ 0.5mV. In order to analyze regional difference, the right atrium was examined in six areas: high and low septum, high and low lateral wall, high and low posterior wall. An index of heterogeneity of bipolar voltage was obtained by calculating the coefficient of variation of voltage of all points. To determine regional velocity, isochronal maps (5ms intervals) were created. An average of the conduction velocity between five pairs of points through areas of least isochronal crowding was performed in each of the six segments. The mean RA bipolar voltage amplitude was significantly reduced in patients with CHF compared with controls (1.4 ± 0.4mV vs 1.9 ± 0.2mV, p = 0.01). Six out of eight CHF patients, but no control patients, demonstrated areas of electrical silence suggestive of atrial myocardial scar. There were regional differences with areas of scar observed predominantly in the low-posterior RA and lateral RA forming 5.1 ± 8.5% of points in the CHF group. Furthermore, there were more fractionated potentials (defined as complex activity of long duration [≥ 50ms]) identified in patients with CHF (Figure 13.5).

Distal CS pacing demonstrated earliest activation of the RA in control patients was uniform over a wide area of the septum consistent with described areas in interatrial connection superiorly at Bachmann's bundle, inferiorly at the CS ostium and in some, the region of the fossa ovalis. However, in patients with CHF, there was altered interatrial

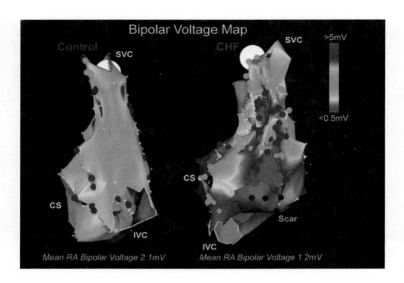

Figure 13.5

Bipolar voltage mapping in congestive cardiac failure. Bipolar right atrial voltage mapping using the CARTO mapping system in congestive cardiac failure. Voltage is color coded. In congestive cardiac failure, the mapping defined areas of low atrial voltage, electrical silence, and widespread fractionated signals. (See Color Plate 41.)

Printed with permission from Sanders at al.[45]

conduction with relatively late activation in the superior region near Bachmann's bundle (Figure 13.6). Total RA activation time was prolonged in CHF patients compared to control (125.3 ± 14.9 vs 103.3 ± 12.1ms; $p = 0.006$).

In summary, with regard to the atrial structural remodeling, Sanders et al. defined extensive abnormalities characterized by low atrial voltage, areas of electrical silence suggesting scarred myocardium, and widespread regions of fractionated signals. These findings suggest inhomogeneous and slowed conduction delay or block, as previously described, the arrhythmic substrate necessary for reentry.

Age

Atrial fibrillation is the most commonly sustained atrial arrhythmia and increases in prevalence with advancing age.[46] The incidence of atrial fibrillation in the Cardiovascular Health Study in the 65–74 years age group was 18 per 1000 (men) and 10 per 1000 (women), however, in the 75–84 years age group, the incidence more than doubled to 43 per 1000 (men) and 22 per 1000 (women).[4] Hayashi et al., in a rat model, demonstrated that heterogeneous atrial interstitial fibrosis and cell hypertrophy contributed to the increase in atrial conduction slowing, conduction block, and inducibility of atrial fibrillation ion in the old rat model.[47] Kistler et al. detailed the electrophysiologic and electroanatomic characteris-

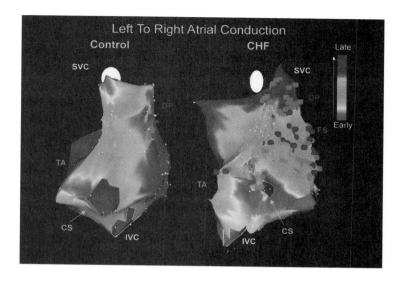

Figure 13.6

Left to right atrial conduction in patients with congestive cardiac failure. Distal coronary sinus pacing in control patients showed RA activation occurred over a wide area of the septum consistent with described interatrial connection superiorly at Bachmann's bundle, inferiorly at the CS ostium, and in some, the region of the fossa ovalis. In patients with congestive cardiac failure, this was altered with relatively late conduction in the superior region near Bachmann's bundle. (See Color Plate 42.)

Printed with permission from Sanders at al.[45]

tics of atrial remodeling seen with human age.[48] Three groups of patients were identified prospectively: > 60 years (n = 13, 9 males), 31–59 years (n = 13, 5 males), and ≤ 30 years old (n = 15, 6 males). Among the three groups, there were no differences in the left atrial of ventricular dimensions or left ventricular ejection fraction. Apart from electrophysiologic analysis, electroanatomic mapping of the right atrium was done during constant pacing from a stable bipole on a coronary sinus placed recording catheter. Atrial points were acquired from six RA sites: high and low septal, high and low lateral, high and low posterior. Voltage and regional conduction velocity was performed offline. Electroanatomic mapping revealed more extensive double potentials and fractionated electrograms in the two older age groups, with a strong correlation with advancing age. Figure 13.7 shows clustering of these fractionated signals along the posterior right atrium. The mapped bipolar voltage was significantly lower at all right atrial sites in the older age groups.

In summary, this work demonstrated structural and anatomic abnormalities associated with increasing age characterized by global and regional reductions in atrial voltage and an increase in the heterogeneity of voltage. This is likely to represent the increasing presence of fibrosis associated with age. Associated with increased conduction delay with age was anatomically determined functional conduction delay noted at the crista terminalis

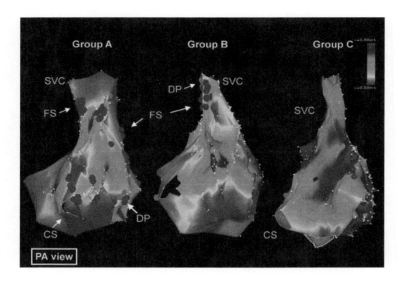

Figure 13.7

Electroanatomical bipolar voltage mapping in three age groups. (Group A ≥ 60, Group B 31–59, Group C ≤ 30.) Voltage is color coded (see Color Plate 43). The mapped bipolar voltage was significantly lower at all right atrial sites in the older age groups. Notice the clustering of fractionated signals and double potentials on the right atrial posterior wall. CS = coronary sinus; DP = double potentials; FS = fractionated signals; SVC = superior vena cava.

Printed with permission from Kistler et al.[48]

Mitral Stenosis

Rheumatic mitral stenosis is associated with atrial fibrillation in 40% of sufferers,[49] which significantly increases the complication of thromboembolism.[50] Associated electrophysiologic abnormalities previously identified have included short effective refractory times and sinus node dysfunction.[51] More recently, John et al. delineated the electrophysiologic and electroanatomic changes in the atria among a group of patients undergoing mitral valvuloplasty for mitral stenosis, a surrogate model of chronic atrial stretch. Twenty-four patients presenting for percutaneous intervention for severe mitral stenosis were compared to a group of patients with left-sided accessory pathways and no evidence of mitral valve disease. In a similar fashion to what has been outlined in previous sections, the left and right atria were evaluated in regional fashion. Electrically silent areas were identified with an atrial voltage of ≤ 0.05mV, while areas of low voltage were ≤ 0.5mV. Isochronal activation maps (5ms intervals) were created and regional conduction velocity determined in the direction of the wave front. The CARTO system determines the conduction velocity as a function of the difference in the local activation time between two specified points. Delayed conduction was defined by fractionated electrograms (≥ 50ms duration) and double potentials separated by an isoelectric interval of ≥ 50ms. Electroanatomic mapping identified patients with severe mitral stenosis to have markedly enlarged left atria with significant right atrial compression (Figure 13.8). Furthermore, the mean bipolar voltage was reduced in both the left and right atria of patients with mitral stenosis compared to controls (Figure 13.9). Areas of electrical silence were identified in the posterior wall adjacent to the pulmonary veins, anterior left atrium, septal left atrium, and lateral right atrial wall.

In summary, the identified changes in these patients suggested a loss of atrial myocardium culminating in lower voltages and areas of scar. This was associated with conduction abnormalities and regions with double potentials, fractionated electrograms and conduction delay.

Sinus Node Disease

Sanders et al. have demonstrated diffuse atrial remodeling in 16 patients with sinus node disease,[52] a condition characterized by disordered impulse generation within or impaired conduction of impulses from the sinus node to the surrounding atrial tissue. This disease's association with atrial fibrillation is well established.

Electrophysiologic and electroanatomic characteristic of these patients were compared to that of controls without sinus node disease or structural atrial abnormality. Bipolar voltage mapping revealed areas of low voltage and spontaneous scarring

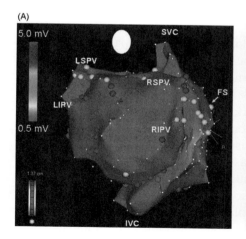
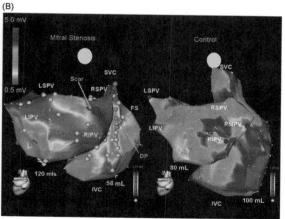

Figure 13.8

Electroanatomical map of a patient with mitral stenosis (A) Voltage is color-coded on the left-hand scale (see Color Plate 44). (B) Note the markedly enlarged LA (100ml) resulted in significant deformation and compression of the RA (58ml). In this extreme example observed, both atria demonstrate extensive regions of low voltage associated with regions of scar and fractionated signals.

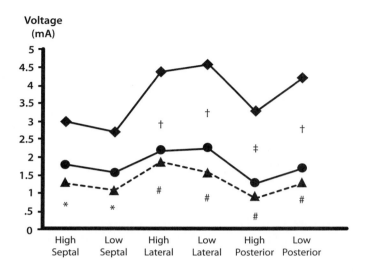

Figure 13.9

Electroanatomical voltage mapping according to right atrial regions demonstrating a significant reduction in regional atrial voltage at six of six sites in group A compared with group C and four of six sites in group B vs C. (▲ = group A; ● = group B; ◆ = group C) *p < 0.05 for group A vs C; #p < 0.01 for group A vs C; ‡p < 0.05 for group B vs C; †p < 0.01 for group B vs C.

Printed with permission from Kistler et al.[48]

associated with fractionated electrograms and double potentials in patients with sinus node disease compared to relatively healthy atria in the control patients (Figure 13.10). Activation and propagation mapping was performed in seven patients with sinus node disease and compared to controls. Patients with sinus node disease demonstrated 1.6 ± 1 sinus activation sites with unicentric activation in five, however, all seven control patients revealed multicentric sinus node activation (3.6 ± 1.7 sites) with greater intersite separation than those in sites identified in the diseased patients. Furthermore, in sinus node disease, the sinus pacemaker complex was located significantly more caudally than in controls. Propagation maps during a sinus impulse in patients with sinus node disease demonstrated areas of marked conduction delay and conduction block, especially along the crista terminalis. The wavefront propagated around these areas resulting in circuitous depolarization. Interestingly, in controls, the sinus node impulse exited simultaneously on either side of the crista terminalis with rapid activation septally and anteriorly, however, in contrast, the anteroinferior margin of the crista terminalis was a site of sinus impulse exit in five of seven patients with sinus node disease and activation was delayed in the septal direction with activation fronts breaking cranially, caudally, and through gaps in this anatomic structure (Figure 13.11).

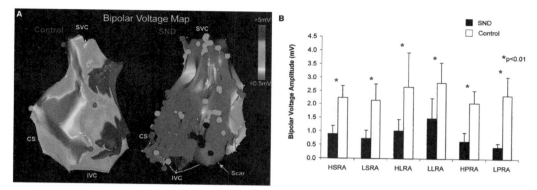

Figure 13.10

Bipolar voltage mapping in a patient with sinus node disease compared to controls. (A) Bipolar voltage mapping in a patient with sinus node disease (right) and an age-matched control (left). The patient with sinus node disease demonstrates significantly greater number of double potentials and fractionated signals. (B), Regional bipolar voltage showing a reduction in average voltage in each atrial site analyzed. (See Color Plate 45.)

Printed with permission from Sanders et al.[52]

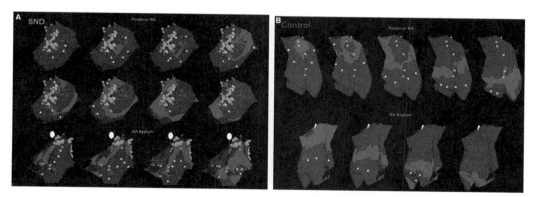

Figure 13.11

Propagation map across the right atrium in sinus node disease (SND) compared to controls. In sinus node disease (A), there are numerous sites of slowed conduction (fractionated signals) and conduction block (double potentials) with marked heterogeneity in depolarisation septally and anteriorly. In controls (B), there is simultaneous activation of the crista terminalis with rapid depolarization septally and anteriorly. (See Color Plate 46.)

Printed with permission from Sanders et al.[52]

In summary, patients with sinus node disease were found to have widespread atrial structural abnormalities with loss of functioning myocardium identified by low voltages and myocardial scarring, particularly seen in the crista terminalis causing collision of activation wavefronts and deviation in their propagation. This forms a structural basis for the development of atrial fibrillation in this group of patients.

Paroxysmal Atrial Fibrillation

Stiles et al.[53] have identified an abnormal atrial substrate associated with disease progression in 13 patients with paroxysmal atrial fibrillation presenting for radiofrequency ablation. Both right and left atrial volumes were higher in patients with paroxysmal atrial fibrillation compared to the control group without. Furthermore, the mean bipolar voltage was reduced in affected patients (Figure 13.12). A mixed linear model identified regional differences in bipolar voltage with significant areas being the high-lateral right atrium, posterior left atrium, and the left atrial roof. There were no areas of myocardial scar identified by electrical silence seen in this group of patients. Fractionated electrograms and double potentials were seen in greater numbers in all atrial regions with clustering at the high-posterior and high-septal right atrial regions and the left-atrial septum and roof.

High-Density Mapping of Atrial Fibrillation

Given the association of diseased myocardium with areas with slowed conduction and conduction block, Stiles et al. investigated the association of these with specific reference to atrial fibrillation. The study compromised 20 patients with drug-refractory atrial fibrillation presenting for radiofrequency ablation. A five-spline 20-pole catheter (1mm electrodes separated by 4-4-4mm interelectrode spacing; PentaRay; Biosense-Webster, Diamond Bar, CA USA) was used to map both atria during either spontaneous or induced atrial fibrillation, which was sustained for more than 10 minutes. At each point, 8 seconds of electrograms were recorded and their location locked into a three-dimensional map annotated using the diagnostic landmark mapping feature of the NavX system (St. Jude Medical Systems, MN). Complex fractionated atrial electrograms were identified as those potentials exhibiting multiple deflections from the isoelectric line and were quantified using the CFE-mean contact mapping tool on the NavX system. This provided a measure of electrogram fractionation as the average time duration between consecutive deflections during the 8 second recorded electrogram. Dominant frequency was analyzed from frequency spectra collected by computing a fast Fourier transform with a spectral resolution of 0.07Hz via an offline automated system. The left atrium was found to be more fractionated than the right atrium and patients with persistent disease had greater fraction than those with paroxysmal. These findings were similar to those of Dimitri et al.[54] Activation frequency was high in the left atrium than the right and high in persistent than paroxysmal atrial fibrillation. There was significant regional variation in frequency especially in paroxysmal disease. Electrogram fractionation was observed in close proximity to sites of high-frequency activation, an example of this is seen in Figure 13.13.

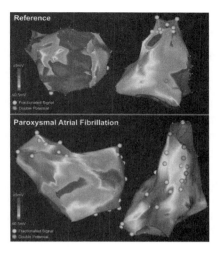

Figure 13.12

Electroanatomical mapping in paroxysmal atrial fibrillation. Representative CARTO maps of a patient with atrial fibrillation (bottom) and a reference patient (top). In addition to having greater regions of low voltage, the patient with atrial fibrillation has more evidence of conduction abnormalities in the form of fractionated signals and double potentials. There were mainly found clustered at the high-posterior and high-septal right atrial regions and the left atrial septum and roof. (See Color Plate 47.)

Printed from Stiles M et al. Paroxysmal lone atrial fibrillation is associated with an abnormal atrial substrate: characterizing the "second factor." *J Am Coll Cardiol* 2009;53:14 with permission from Elsiever.

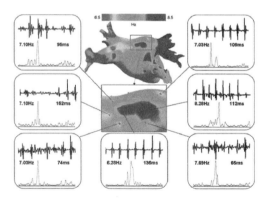

Figure 13.13

Relationship between dominant frequency and complex fractionated electrograms in drug-refractory atrial fibrillation. Anterosuperior view of the left atrium with the roof en face displaying dominant frequency (DF) data on a color spectrum (see Color Plate 48). High DF areas are seen in the pulmonary veins, basal left atrial appendage, and the left atrial roof. A zoomed view of the area of high DF at the roof is shown with the corresponding points (inset). One second electrograms, frequency spectra (3–15Hz), and corresponding DF and complex fractionated electrogram-mean (CFE-mean) values for each of the local seven points contributing to the color map are shown in linked boxes. The central point of highest DF is fast and regular, with surrounding points showing either increased CFE-mean suggesting increased fractionation of electrograms in that area, lower DF, or both.

Printed with permission from Stiles et al.

CONCLUSION

The utilization of electroanatomic mapping of the atria to characterize the atrial myocardial substrate in age, heart failure, mitral stenosis, sinus node disease, and paroxysmal atrial fibrillation have provided important insights into the underlying mechanism of disease particularly leading to atrial arrhythmias. The important findings of areas of low voltage suggesting atrial fibrosis and evidence of its pathophysiologic effect including slowed conduction and conduction block form the foundation of the second factor concept that interplays with the electrophysiologic changes in refractoriness originally implicated in the pathogenesis of atrial fibrillation. The use of electroanatomic mapping in the electrophysiology laboratory has been instrumental in evaluating and characterizing disease atria allowing for acquisition of critical data, tagging of interesting points for future scrutiny and offline analysis. High-density mapping of atrial fibrillation to determine the relationship between activation frequency, complex fractionated electrograms and the anatomical substrate has furthered our understanding of the complexities predisposing to atrial arrhythmias.

◇◇◇◇◇◇◇◇◇◇◇◇

REFERENCES

1. Kannel WB, Abbott RD, Savage DD, McNamara PM. Epidemiologic features of chronic atrial fibrillation: the Framingham study. *The New England journal of medicine.* 1982;306(17):1018-1022.

2. Onundarson PT, Thorgeirsson G, Jonmundsson E, Sigfusson N, Hardarson T. Chronic atrial fibrillation—epidemiologic features and 14 year follow-up: a case control study. *European Heart Journal.* 1987;8(5):521-527.

3. Benjamin EJ, Levy D, Vaziri SM, D'Agostino RB, Belanger AJ, Wolf PA. Independent risk factors for atrial fibrillation in a population-based cohort. The Framingham Heart Study. *Jama.* 1994;271(11):840-844.

4. Psaty BM, Manolio TA, Kuller LH, Kronmal RA, Cushman M, Fried LP, White R, Furberg CD, Rautaharju PM. Incidence of and risk factors for atrial fibrillation in older adults. *Circulation.* 1997;96(7):2455-2461.

5. Stevenson IH, Teichtahl H, Cunnington D, Ciavarella S, Gordon I, Kalman JM. Prevalence of sleep disordered breathing in paroxysmal and persistent atrial fibrillation patients with normal left ventricular function. *European Heart Journal.* 2008;29(13):1662-1669.

6. Gami AS, Somers VK. Implications of obstructive sleep apnea for atrial fibrillation and sudden cardiac death. *Journal of Cardiovascular Electrophysiology.* 2008.

7. Gami AS, Hodge DO, Herges RM, Olson EJ, Nykodym J, Kara T, Somers VK. Obstructive sleep apnea, obesity, and the risk of incident atrial fibrillation. *Journal of the American College of Cardiology.* 2007;49(5):565-571.

8. Gami AS, Pressman G, Caples SM, Kanagala R, Gard JJ, Davison DE, Malouf JF, Ammash NM, Friedman PA, Somers VK. Association of atrial fibrillation and obstructive sleep apnea. *Circulation.* 2004;110(4):364-367.

9. Gersh BJ, Solomon A. Lone atrial fibrillation: epidemiology and natural history. *American Heart Journal.* 1999;137(4 Pt 1):592-595.

10. Morillo CA, Klein GJ, Jones DL, Guiraudon CM. Chronic rapid atrial pacing. Structural, functional, and electrophysiological characteristics of a new model of sustained atrial fibrillation. *Circulation.* 1995;91(5):1588-1595.

11. Elvan A, Huang XD, Pressler ML, Zipes DP. Radiofrequency catheter ablation of the atria eliminates pacing-induced sustained atrial fibrillation and reduces connexin 43 in dogs. *Circulation.* 1997;96(5):1675-1685.

12. van der Velden HM, van Kempen MJ, Wijffels MC, van Zijverden M, Groenewegen WA, Allessie MA, Jongsma HJ. Altered pattern of connexin40 distribution in persistent atrial fibrillation in the goat. *Journal of Cardiovascular Electrophysiology.* 1998;9(6):596-607.

13. Ausma J, Wijffels M, Thone F, Wouters L, Allessie M, Borgers M. Structural changes of atrial myocardium due to sustained atrial fibrillation in the goat. *Circulation.* 1997;96(9):3157-3163.

14. Allessie M, Ausma J, Schotten U. Electrical, contractile and structural remodeling during atrial fibrillation. *Cardiovascular Research.* 2002;54(2):230-246.

15. Li D, Fareh S, Leung TK, Nattel S. Promotion of atrial fibrillation by heart failure in dogs: atrial remodeling of a different sort. *Circulation.* 1999;100(1):87-95.

16. Lin CS, Pan CH. Regulatory mechanisms of atrial fibrotic remodeling in atrial fibrillation. *Cell Mol Life Sci.* 2008;65(10):1489-1508.

17. Xu J, Cui G, Esmailian F, Plunkett M, Marelli D, Ardehali A, Odim J, Laks H, Sen L. Atrial extracellular matrix remodeling and the maintenance of atrial fibrillation. *Circulation.* 2004;109(3):363-368.

18. Akar FG, Spragg DD, Tunin RS, Kass DA, Tomaselli GF. Mechanisms underlying conduction slowing and arrhythmogenesis in nonischemic dilated cardiomyopathy. *Circulation Research.* 2004;95(7):717-725.

19. Cardin S, Li D, Thorin-Trescases N, Leung TK, Thorin E, Nattel S. Evolution of the atrial fibrillation substrate in experimental congestive heart failure: angiotensin-dependent and -independent pathways. *Cardiovascular Research.* 2003;60(2):315-325.

20. Konings KT, Smeets JL, Penn OC, Wellens HJ, Allessie MA. Configuration of unipolar atrial electrograms during electrically induced atrial fibrillation in humans. *Circulation.* 1997;95(5):1231-1241.

21. Konings KT, Kirchhof CJ, Smeets JR, Wellens HJ, Penn OC, Allessie MA. High-density mapping of electrically induced atrial fibrillation in humans. *Circulation.* 1994;89(4):1665-1680.

22. Oral H, Chugh A, Good E, Wimmer A, Dey S, Gadeela N, Sankaran S, Crawford T, Sarrazin JF, Kuhne M, Chalfoun N, Wells D, Frederick M, Fortino J, Benloucif-Moore S, Jongnarangsin K, Pelosi F, Jr., Bogun F, Morady F. Radiofrequency catheter ablation of chronic atrial fibrillation guided by complex electrograms. *Circulation.* 2007;115(20):2606-2612.

23. Nademanee K, McKenzie J, Kosar E, Schwab M, Sunsaneewitayakul B, Vasavakul T, Khunnawat C, Ngarmukos T. A new approach for catheter ablation of atrial fibrillation: mapping of the electrophysiologic substrate.[see comment]. *Journal of the American College of Cardiology.* 2004;43(11):2044-2053.

24. Rostock T, Rotter M, Sanders P, Takahashi Y, Jais P, Hocini M, Hsu LF, Sacher F, Clementy J, Haissaguerre M. High-density activation mapping of fractionated electrograms in the atria of patients with paroxysmal atrial fibrillation.[see comment]. *Heart Rhythm.* 2006;3(1):27-34.

25. Takahashi Y, O'Neill MD, Hocini M, Dubois R, Matsuo S, Knecht S, Mahapatra S, Lim KT, Jais P, Jonsson A, Sacher F, Sanders P, Rostock T, Bordachar P, Clementy J, Klein GJ, Haissaguerre M. Characterization of electrograms associated with termination of chronic atrial fibrillation by catheter ablation. *Journal of the American College of Cardiology.* 2008;51(10):1003-1010.

26. Saffitz JE, Kanter HL, Green KG, Tolley TK, Beyer EC. Tissue-specific determinants of anisotropic conduction velocity in canine atrial and ventricular myocardium. *Circulation Research.* 1994;74(6):1065-1070.

27. Papageorgiou P, Monahan K, Boyle NG, Seifert MJ, Beswick P, Zebede J, Epstein LM, Josephson ME. Site-dependent intra-atrial conduction delay. Relationship to initiation of atrial fibrillation. *Circulation.* 1996;94(3):384-389.

28. McGuire MA, Bourke JP, Robotin MC, Johnson DC, Meldrum-Hanna W, Nunn GR, Uther JB, Ross DL. High resolution mapping of Koch's triangle using sixty electrodes in humans with atrioventricular junctional (AV nodal) reentrant tachycardia. *Circulation.* 1993;88(5 Pt 1):2315-2328.

29. Platonov PG. Interatrial conduction in the mechanisms of atrial fibrillation: from anatomy to cardiac signals and new treatment modalities. *Europace.* 2007;9 Suppl 6:vi10-16.

30. Platonov PG, Mitrofanova L, Ivanov V, Ho SY. Substrates for intra-atrial and interatrial conduction in the atrial septum: anatomical study on 84 human hearts. *Heart Rhythm.* 2008;5(8):1189-1195.

31. Markides V, Schilling RJ, Ho SY, Chow AW, Davies DW, Peters NS. Characterization of left atrial activation in the intact human heart. *Circulation.* 2003;107(5):733-739.

32. Roberts-Thomson KC, Stevenson IH, Kistler PM, Haqqani HM, Goldblatt JC, Sanders P, Kalman JM. Anatomically determined functional conduction delay in the posterior left atrium relationship to structural heart disease. *Journal of the American College of Cardiology.* 2008;51(8):856-862.

33. Ben-Haim SA, Osadchy D, Schuster I, Gepstein L, Hayam G, Josephson ME. Nonfluoroscopic, in vivo navigation and mapping technology. *Nature medicine.* 1996;2(12):1393-1395.

34. Gepstein L, Hayam G, Ben-Haim SA. A novel method for nonfluoroscopic catheter-based electroanatomical mapping of the heart. In vitro and in vivo accuracy results. *Circulation.* 1997;95(6):1611-1622.

35. Schilling RJ, Peters NS, Davies DW. Simultaneous endocardial mapping in the human left ventricle using a noncontact catheter: comparison of contact and reconstructed electrograms during sinus rhythm. *Circulation.* 1998;98(9):887-898.

36. Sra J, Hauck J, Krum D, Schweitzer J. Three-dimensional right atrial geometry construction and catheter tracking using cutaneous patches. *Journal of cardiovascular electrophysiology.* 2003;14(8):897.

37. Brooks AG, Wilson L, Kuklik P, Stiles MK, John B, Shashidhar, Dimitri H, Lau DH, Roberts-Thomson RL, Wong CX, Young GD, Sanders P. Image integration using NavX Fusion: initial experience and validation. *Heart Rhythm.* 2008;5(4):526-535.

38. Verma A, Novak P, Macle L, Whaley B, Beardsall M, Wulffhart Z, Khaykin Y. A prospective, multicenter evaluation of ablating complex fractionated electrograms (CFEs) during atrial fibrillation (AF) identified by an automated mapping algorithm: acute effects on AF and efficacy as an adjuvant strategy. *Heart Rhythm.* 2008;5(2):198-205.

39. Dries DL, Exner DV, Gersh BJ, Domanski MJ, Waclawiw MA, Stevenson LW. Atrial fibrillation is associated with an increased risk for mortality and heart failure progression in patients with asymptomatic and symptomatic left ventricular systolic dysfunction: a retrospective analysis of the SOLVD trials. Studies of Left Ventricular Dysfunction. *Journal of the American College of Cardiology.* 1998;32(3):695-703.

40. Stevenson WG, Stevenson LW, Middlekauff HR, Fonarow GC, Hamilton MA, Woo MA, Saxon LA, Natterson PD, Steimle A, Walden JA, Tillisch JH. Improving survival for patients with atrial fibrillation and advanced heart failure. *Journal of the American College of Cardiology.* 1996;28(6):1458-1463.

41. Middlekauff HR, Stevenson WG, Stevenson LW. Prognostic significance of atrial fibrillation in advanced heart failure. A study of 390 patients. *Circulation.* 1991;84(1):40-48.

42. Wang TJ, Larson MG, Levy D, Vasan RS, Leip EP, Wolf PA, D'Agostino RB, Murabito JM, Kannel WB, Benjamin EJ. Temporal relations of atrial fibrillation and congestive heart failure and their joint influence on mortality: the Framingham Heart Study. *Circulation.* 2003;107(23):2920-2925.

43. Boyden PA, Tilley LP, Albala A, Liu SK, Fenoglio JJ, Jr., Wit AL. Mechanisms for atrial arrhythmias associated with cardiomyopathy: a study of feline

hearts with primary myocardial disease. *Circulation.* 1984;69(5):1036-1047.

44. Power JM, Beacom GA, Alferness CA, Raman J, Wijffels M, Farish SJ, Burrell LM, Tonkin AM. Susceptibility to atrial fibrillation: a study in an ovine model of pacing-induced early heart failure. *Journal of Cardiovascular Electrophysiology.* 1998;9(4):423-435.

45. Sanders P, Morton JB, Davidson NC, Spence SJ, Vohra JK, Sparks PB, Kalman JM. Electrical remodeling of the atria in congestive heart failure: electrophysiological and electroanatomic mapping in humans. *Circulation.* 2003;108(12):1461-1468.

46. Brand FN, Abbott RD, Kannel WB, Wolf PA. Characteristics and prognosis of lone atrial fibrillation. 30-year follow-up in the Framingham Study. *Jama.* 1985;254(24):3449-3453.

47. Hayashi H, Wang C, Miyauchi Y, Omichi C, Pak HN, Zhou S, Ohara T, Mandel WJ, Lin SF, Fishbein MC, Chen PS, Karagueuzian HS. Aging-related increase to inducible atrial fibrillation in the rat model. *Journal of Cardiovascular Electrophysiology.* 2002;13(8):801-808.

48. Kistler PM, Sanders P, Fynn SP, Stevenson IH, Spence SJ, Vohra JK, Sparks PB, Kalman JM. Electrophysiologic and electroanatomic changes in the human atrium associated with age. *Journal of the American College of Cardiology.* 2004;44(1):109-116.

49. Selzer A, Cohn KE. Natural history of mitral stenosis: a review. *Circulation.* 1972;45(4):878-890.

50. Wolf PA, Dawber TR, Thomas HE, Jr., Kannel WB. Epidemiologic assessment of chronic atrial fibrillation and risk of stroke: the Framingham study. *Neurology.* 1978;28(10):973-977.

51. Fan K, Lee KL, Chow WH, Chau E, Lau CP. Internal cardioversion of chronic atrial fibrillation during percutaneous mitral commissurotomy: insight into reversal of chronic stretch-induced atrial remodeling. *Circulation.* 2002;105(23):2746-2752.

52. Sanders P, Kistler PM, Morton JB, Spence SJ, Kalman JM. Remodeling of sinus node function in patients with congestive heart failure: reduction in sinus node reserve. *Circulation.* 2004;110(8):897-903.

53. Stiles MJ, B; Wong, C; Kuklik, P; Young, G; Sanders, P. Paroxysmal Lone Atrial Fibrillation is Associated with an Abnormal Substrate: The "Second Factor" *Heart, Lung and Circulation* 2008;17:S120.

54. Dimitri HS, M; John, B; Lau, D; Shashidhar; Mackenize, L; Brooks, A; Wilson, L; Roberts-Thompson, K; Wong, C; Willoughby, S; Young, G; Sanders, P. Atrial Remodelling in Paroxysmal Versus Permanent Atrial Fibrillation: Comparison of Electrogram Fragmentation and Voltage Reduction *Heart, Lung and Circulation* 2007;16:S201.

Part IV

Imaging in Clinical Management

CHAPTER 14

Clinical Use of Imaging for Cardiovascular Risk Assessment

Vijay Nambi, MD

Stephen G. Worthley, MBBS, PhD, FRACP

INTRODUCTION

Despite significant advances in the management of atherosclerotic cardiovascular disease, it still remains the leading cause of death in Western society. Although traditional risk factors are extremely useful in the prediction of cardiovascular disease, about 20% of individuals who have acute coronary syndromes have been reported to have no preceding risk factors.[1] Hence, in order to improve risk prediction, a lot of effort has focused on evaluating whether novel biomarkers and imaging markers can improve risk prediction. Biomarkers such as C-reactive protein (CRP) and lipoprotein associated phospholipase A2 (LpPLA2) have been shown to be capable of improving coronary heart disease and/or stroke risk prediction.[2,3] Similarly, the use of imaging has also been shown to improve risk prediction beyond traditional Framingham risk scores. Below we review the imaging modalities with specific reference to carotid initma media thickness (CIMT) and coronary calcium score (CAC) in risk stratification for coronary artery disease (CAD).

THE NEED FOR ADDITIONAL RISK STRATIFICATION

Several risk scores such as the Framingham risk score[4,5] are routinely used in the prediction of cardiovascular risk. These risk scores use traditional risk factors such as hypertension, tobacco use, total cholesterol (TC), high-density lipoprotein cholesterol (HDL-C), age, and sex to predict 10-year risk for coronary heart disease. Although these risk scores are overall very effective for CHD risk prediction, there still remains significant room for the improvement of CHD risk.

Limitations of Traditional Risk Scores

It has been reported that about 25% of the individuals who experience sudden cardiac death or a nonfatal myocardial infarction have no preceding symptoms.[6] Traditional risk factors (TRF) although excellent in predicting incident CHD events have limitations. TRF predict only about 70% of the incident CHD events.[7] Further, the majority of the events (> 60%) occur in individuals who are low or intermediate in risk[8] who in turn represent the majority of the population.[8] Additionally, in one study, only about 25% of the men and 18% of the women (young individuals [age < 55 years]) who presented with an acute myocardial infarction would have met criteria for pharmacotherapy based on their 10-year risk estimate prior to their acute myocardial infarction.[9] Finally, the FRS calculates a 10-year risk for CHD and does not take into account the lifetime risk for CHD[10] or the family history of CHD and race of the individual in risk estimation. Alternate risk scores such as the Reynolds risk score,[2] which uses family history and C-reactive protein to improve risk prediction have been proposed and been demonstrated to improve risk prediction over and above FRS.

THE SHAPE GUIDELINE RECOMMENDATIONS

The Screening for Heart Attack Prevention and Education (SHAPE) Task Force therefore presented a guideline [11, 12] calling for noninvasive screening of all asymptomatic men between the ages of 45 and 75 years and asymptomatic women between the ages of 55 and 75 years who are not considered very low risk to further stratify risk, then treatment for them based on the imaging and clinical characteristics of an individual. They proposed that those with a CAC score of 0 or a CIMT < 50th percentile and no plaque be considered lower risk if they had no conventional risk factors and moderate risk if they had conventional risk factors. Similarly, they identified a CAC score of > 0 to < 100 or a CIMT in the 50th to 75th percentile and without carotid artery plaque to represent a moderately high risk category, while a CAC score of 100–399, CIMT > 75th percentile or the presence of carotid plaque to represent a high-risk category, and finally, a CAC score ≥ 400 or a carotid plaque causing > 50% stenosis to represent a very-high-risk category. However, this recommendation was not based on any supporting literature for such a strategy. We review the available evidence for the use of imaging in risk stratification and provide a useful construct to incorporate imaging into clinical risk stratification.

CRITERIA TO EVALUATE IMPROVED RISK STRATIFICATION

The ultimate goal of any risk stratification tool is to prevent hard cardiovascular end points, such as myocardial infarction (MI) and cardiovascular death. There are no data as yet to suggest that *therapy* based on the results of an imaging test is superior to current preventive strategies. However, both CAC and CIMT have been shown to be associated with CHD and further improve risk prediction, over and above Framingham risk scores. In evaluating any new marker's ability to improve risk prediction two important statistical characteristics will need to be evaluated, namely predictivity (discrimination) and calibration. The predictivity of a model can be evaluated using the area under a receiver operator characteristic curve (AUC of a ROC curve), which is a test of the diagnostic accuracy of a test. The test plots sensitivity or true positives on the y-axis against 1-specificity, or false positives, on the x-axis. A perfect test (which does not exist) would have a value of 1 (all true positives and no false positives) while a test with a value of 0.5 is practically of no use (equal number of true and false positives). In addition, one would need to examine the number of individuals who would be reclassified by the addition of the new test and, finally, examine if the expected number of adverse events using the new model correlates well with the observed number of events.

CORONARY ARTERY CALCIUM SCORE

CAC scores have been shown to be associated with incident CHD events in multiple observational studies and have also been shown to be additive to Framingham risk scores.[13-16] Higher calcium scores have consistently shown a relationship with increased incidence of CHD events[14, 15, 17] with the annual MI or CHD death rates reported in one study[14] being 0.4%, 1.3%, and 2.4% for CAC scores < 100, 100–399, and ≥ 400 respectively, suggesting that a CAC score ≥ 400 identifies the high-risk individual. Recently, Budoff et al. [18] reported that in an observational cohort of about 25,000 individuals followed for a mean of 6.8 years, presence of coronary artery calcium was significantly associated with mortality with a relative risk of 62.58 (95% CI 43.04 to 91.00), (p < 0.0001) for a CAC score > 1000 when compared with a CAC score = 0. Approximately 99.4% compared to 87.8% of individuals with CAC = 0 and CAC > 1000 were respectively alive at 10 years.[18]

Studies have also evaluated the presence of calcium across risk groups. Nasir et al. showed that among 1611 asymptomatic individuals referred for CAC estimation, 25% of the individuals with CAC scores between 100 and 399 and ≥ 400 were classified as low risk based on NCEP/ATP-III guidelines.[19] Further, they reported that about 60% of the individuals with CAC scores ≥ 400 would not have been eligible for pharmacotherapy based on NCEP/ATP-III estimated risk alone.

Arad et al. reported that CAC score predicted CHD events better than the FRS with the AUC of the ROC curve being 0.79 ± 0.03 for the CAC score versus 0.68 ± 0.03 for the Framingham index (p < 0.0006).[17] However, the CHD events, of which there were 119, included nonfatal MI or coronary death (n = 40), coronary revascularization (bypass surgery or percutaneous angioplasty) (n = 59), nonhemorrhagic stroke (n = 7), and peripheral vascular surgery (n = 13) raising the question as to whether the identification of coronary calcium lead to further testing and eventually revascularization. The overall event rate was reported to be 0.54% in individuals with a CAC score = 0 and 14% in those with a CAC score ≥ 400.

On the other hand, Detrano et al. compared CAC scores with TRF assessment in the prediction of incident CHD in asymptomatic high-risk individuals (≥ 2 risk factors and 10-year FRS > 10%).[20] In these individuals two-thirds had detectable coronary calcium with a median score of 44. They reported that CAC scores were equivalent to TRF in the prediction of coronary death or infarction. Additionally, they reported that the addition of CAC scores to TRF assessment did not seem to improve risk prediction. However, this study was limited by the fact that the majority of the individuals were males older than 45 years of age and a follow-up of about only 41 months. Similarly, in another study, Schenker et al. included individuals referred for the evaluation of ischemia, (i.e., high-risk symptomatic individuals) and performed a rest-stress Rubidium-82 positron emission tomography (PET) perfusion imaging and CAC scoring.[21] They reported that of 606 individuals included for their analysis, 165 individuals had ischemia detected on their PET scan. Of those individuals, 34 (about 20%) had a CAC score = 0. In all, 213 individuals had a CAC score = 0 and, of these 213 individuals, 16% had ischemia detected on the PET scan. Incident CHD events did occur in both ischemic and nonischemic individuals with CAC score = 0 and these rates were significantly higher than that reported in the literature for asymptomatic individuals.

The majority of the studies,[14, 22-24] however, indicate that CAC scores may improve risk prediction beyond FRS especially in the intermediate risk group. Greenland et al. evaluated data from the South Bay Heart Watch Study,[14] a prospective observational study of 1461 asymptomatic, nondiabetic individuals with at least one CHD risk factor followed for 8.5 years. Over this time period, there were 84 hard CHD end points (MI or CHD death). Among those with a FRS of 0–9% (n = 98) there were no events among those with a CAC score of ≤ 300 while there was only one event among those with a CAC score > 300. They further reported that CAC risk score modified risk prediction only in individuals with a FRS > 10% (i.e., in the intermediate-risk group and not in those with a FRS < 10%). The ACCF/AHA consensus document[25] reported that in a secondary analysis of four studies[14, 22-24] a CAC score ≥ 400 would elevate an intermediate risk individual to a high risk or CHD equivalent. Finally, most recently, the Heinz Nixdorf Recall study was presented at the annual meeting of the American College of Cardiology (March 2009). This analysis, which included ~4100 individuals followed prospectively, showed that log transformed CAC measures significantly improved the AUC (from 0.667 to 0.754) when added to the ATP III risk stratification scheme. However, again, there were only 93 events in the follow-up period of time.

Hence, overall, it seems that CAC scoring in intermediate-risk individuals can help in improving risk stratification of that individual.

However, there are several important caveats that one must keep in mind:

a. There are no data as of now to suggest that a strategy using CAC scores to treat individuals will decrease incident CHD.

b. Merely by indicating the presence of atherosclerosis in the coronary arteries, CAC scores may trigger unnecessary testing, such as stress tests or coronary angiograms and revascularization in asymptomatic individual.

c. Although small, CAC score estimation with computed tomography (CT) scans is associated with a small amount of exposure to radiation (about four chest x-rays).

d. CAC scores are highly associated with age and gender. Younger individuals, especially women, invariably have no calcium. Hence, there may be limited value in younger individuals.

Given the available information, in an editorial, Greenland and Bonow[26] highlight the importance of factoring in the pretest probability to effectively use CAC scores in risk stratification. Various cut-points have been suggested as to which value one would "reclassify" an individual to a higher risk group. Gaziano and Greenland[27] initially suggested using a CAC score of < 80 to stratify to a lower risk group and a score of > 80 to stratify to a higher risk group. The American College of Cardiology/American Heart Association in their 2007 statement suggested that a score > 400 be considered as high risk (i.e., same status as somebody with diabetes or peripheral arterial disease).[25] The use of CAC scoring may in fact be an important motivator to help individuals effect lifestyle changes. In one study,[28] the impact of CAC screening on statin and aspirin usage was tested in 1640 men aged 40–50 years. Those with CAC, over a period of 6 years, were three times more likely to be on a statin (48.5% vs 15.5%, p < 0.001) and also significantly more likely to be on aspirin (53.0% vs 32.3%, p < 0.001) therapy. However, in smaller analysis, the presence of CAC was not enough to motivate patients to improve their modifiable risk over 1 year.[29] In summary, the use of CAC scores in an appropriate population (intermediate risk for CHD) can help better stratify CHD risk but data are currently lacking if treatment based on this risk stratification (i.e., using CAC scoring in addition to traditional risk scoring) will prevent further CHD events.

Carotid Intima Media Thickness

The carotid intima media thickness, or CIMT, is a well-validated imaging surrogate that has been associated with both prevalent and incident CHD and stroke.[30-32] Further, CIMT has been used in multiple studies to track the progression/regression of atherosclerosis.[33-36]

The National Cholesterol Education Panel/Adult Treatment Panel III (NCEP/ATP-III) identified the measurement of CIMT as an option to identify individuals at higher risk than that identified by major risk factors alone.[37]

Several studies of various populations have examined the value of using CIMT in risk prediction. Baldassarre et al.[38] reported that in 1969 individuals who attended their lipid clinic, 242 had a FRS < 20%, and in this cohort there were 24 individuals who had a cardiovascular event within a follow-up period of 5.1 ± 2.3 years. Both CIMT and Framingham risk score were independent predictors of cardiovascular events. Among individuals in the 10–20% 10-year FRS category (i.e., intermediate rsik group by ATP-III), an increased maximum CIMT (> 60th percentile for men, > 80th percentile for women) was associated with a risk similar to those in the 20–30% 10-year FRS category by traditional risk statification. However, the measurement of CIMT did not increase the hazard ratio in those with a FRS < 10%. Other than the low number of events (n = 24), the study was additionally limited by the use of the maximum CIMT of any segment rather than the mean of the maximum CIMT, no adjustment for age and sex, and the fact that all individuals were dyslipidemic. Similarly, Bernard et al.[39] reported that CIMT was an independent predictor of incident cardiovascular events (n = 34; 28 coronary events and 6 strokes) among 229 patients with diabetes mellitus. Further, the predictive ability of CIMT was similar to that of the FRS (AUC of the ROC curve 0.720 vs 0.715 respectively). However, given the individuals studied, neither of these studies can be applied to the general population. Bard et al.[40] examined 95 individuals who were inter-mediate in risk for CHD (10-year FRS 6–19%) and reported that the addition of CIMT and carotid plaque area resulted in the reclassification of about 63% of the individuals. However, the study did not address if the addition of CIMT improved risk prediction in this intermediate-risk population.

More recently, in the Northern Manhattan Study (NOMAS), an ongoing population-based study of stroke incidence,[41] examined the contribution of carotid plaque (defined as an area of focal wall thickening 50% greater than surrounding wall thickness) to ischemic cardiovascular events. In their cohort of 2189 individuals, during a mean follow-up of 6.9 years, there were 319 ischemic strokes, MI, or vascular death. Overall, the age-adjusted incidence rate of combined vascular outcome in our study was 12/1,000 person-years for subjects without carotid plaque, 16/1,000 person-years for subjects with plaque but a maximum plaque thickness of < 1.9mm, and 35/1,000 person-years for those with a maximum plaque thickness 1.9mm. The 10-year risk of adverse cardiovascular outcome in the low FRS group ranged from 5.8% in those without a plaque to 18.3% in those with plaque and a maximum plaque thickness of < 1.9mm and 24.7% in those with plaque and a maximum plaque thickness of > 1.9mm. In the intermediate risk group, the 10-year event rates for the same categories were 11.5%, 18.6%, and 25.1% respectively, sug-gesting that the presence of plaque is significantly associated with future risk of adverse cardiovascular events.

We more recently examined the utility of CIMT ± plaque in risk prediction in a healthy, middle-aged population enrolled in the Atherosclerosis Risk In Communities (ARIC) study.[42] ARIC is a study of cardiovascular disease incidence that enrolled 15,792 individuals aged 45–64 years from 1987–1989. In all, for our analysis, there were 13,145 individuals without baseline CHD or stroke followed for a mean of 13.8 years. The addi-tion of CIMT, categorized (sex-specific) as < 25th percentile, 25th to 75th percentile, and > 75th percentile and plaque, to traditional risk factors (TRFs) (age, systolic blood pressure, use of antihypertensive medication, total cholesterol, HDL-C, gender, diabetes and smoking status) significantly improved the AUC from 0.742 (TRFs only) to 0.750 (95% confidence interval [CI] for increase in AUC 0.005, 0.012) (TRFs + CIMT) and 0.755 (95% C.I. 0.008, 0.017) (TRF's + CIMT + plaque). The addition of CIMT + plaque reclassified 8.6%, 37.5%, 38.3%, and 21.5% of individuals in the < 5%, 5–10%, 10–20%, and > 20% risk categories, respectively. No individual was reclassified from the > 20% risk category to the < 5% category and vice versa. Of the individuals reclassified in the intermediate-risk group (5–20%), about 61% were reclassified to a lower-risk group. Overall, the addition of CIMT and plaque resulted in a better model when observed and expected risk was compared. Finally, the addition of CIMT and plaque resulted in an improved net reclassification index (NRI), a statistical test that examines the net effect of "good" and "bad" reclassification. Adding CIMT and plaque resulted in a NRI of 9.1% and a clinical NRI (NRI in the intermediate, 5–20% risk group) of 21.7%. Hence, the addition of CIMT and plaque information did improve the ability to predict incident CHD in a middle-aged population. However, again, it must be noted that such a strategy of targeting therapy based on the predicted CHD risk after the addition of CIMT has not been tested in clinical trials to determine if treatment based on such a strategy will decrease incident CHD events.

Vascular Age

Another way CIMT has been used in risk stratification is through the estimation of the vascular age.[43] To estimate the vascular age, an individual's mean CIMT is estimated; then using race and sex specific normograms available from studies such as the ARIC, a determination is made of the age to which the individuals CIMT would be at the 50th percentile. The vascular age is used with other TRF to calculate the FRS. For example, if a 50-year-old male has a mean CIMT value, that would be the 50th percentile in a 65-year age group, then his vascular age is 65 years while his chronological age is 50 years. Using this model, Gepner et al.[44] showed in an observational study that almost 57% of the individuals in the 5–20% 10-year risk category would be reclassified using the vascular age. Other studies[45] have similarly shown that using the vascular age can result in reclassification of FRS in several individuals. However, all these studies have been disadvantaged due to the small number of incident CHD events and by lack of prospective data suggesting that the use of vascular age instead of chronological age will improve patient outcomes.

The American Society of Echocardiography[46] stated in their consensus documented that "measuring CIMT and identifying carotid plaque by ultrasound are most useful for refining CVD risk assessment in patients at intermediate CVD risk." They further suggested that "patients with the following clinical circumstances also might be considered for CIMT measurement and carotid plaque detection: (1) family history of premature CVD in a first degree relative (men < 55 years old, women < 65 years old); (2) individuals younger than 60 years old with severe abnormalities in a single risk factor (e.g., genetic dyslipidemia) who otherwise would not be candidates for pharmacotherapy; or (3) women younger than 60 years old with at least two CVD risk factors." Hence, like coronary calcium scores, CIMT can also be used in improving risk stratification of individuals who are intermediate or indeterminate in risk with FRS alone. However, it must be noted that in a recent systematic review, the U.S. Preventive Task Force concluded that current evidence did not support the use of coronary calcium score or CIMT or 7 other novel markers including CRP in risk stratification of intermediate risk individuals[47] as the data available did not meet all the criteria required for a marker to be considered clinically useful. With more data emerging, including some presented here, these may be reconsidered in the future.

Comparison of Coronary Calcium Score and Carotid Intima Media Thickness

Coronary calcium score and CIMT are only moderately correlated within the same individual.[48-52] There have been a few studies in which individuals have had both modalities CAC and CIMT. One study[53] of patients with coronary angiography documented CAD > 50%, presence of coronary artery calcium and thickened (mean of the maximum) CIMT both predicted the presence of CAD although CAC was better. This is not surprising given that, anatomically, CAC images the coronary artery while CIMT the carotid arteries. However, in another study of 42 patients,[54] carotid plaque area > 0, measured on a carotid ultrasound, was more sensitive (72% vs 58%) and had a better negative predictive value (74% vs 65%) when compared with CAC for detecting the presence of significant coronary artery stenosis (> 50%). A 2008 study[55] compared the ability of CAC and CIMT to predict incident cardiovascular (CVD) events in 6698 individuals without CHD enrolled in the Multi-Ethnic Study of Atherosclerosis (MESA). Over a follow up of 3.9 years (median), there were 222 CVD events. Of the 222 incident CVD events, 159 were CHD events (61 MI, 81 angina, 3 resuscitated cardiac arrests, 13 CHD deaths), 59 were stroke events (3 of which included a CHD event), and 7 were other atherosclerotic CVD deaths. Overall, CAC had a stronger association (hazard ratio [HR] increased 2.1 fold [95% confidence interval [CI], 1.8–2.5] for every 1 SD increase of log transformed CAC) with incident CVD when compared to CIMT (hazard ratio [HR] increased 1.3 fold [95% confidence interval [CI], 1.1–1.4] for every one SD increase of maximum CIMT). CAC also better predicted incident CHD events while CIMT seemed to be a modestly better predictor of stroke than CAC. However, it must be noted that angina (although stringent measures were used as criteria for angina) was one of the CVD end points and the overall period of follow-up was rather short. Further, the presence of an abnormal CAC is more likely to result in stress testing that is an abnormal CIMT. The investigators reported all high CAC (17%) and CIMT (1%) to the participants and referred them to their primary care physicians. Finally, the presence of absence of plaque was not considered. Hence, although it is likely that CAC is better than CIMT in the prediction of incident CVD events (specifically CHD) this would have to weighed against the potential for increased unnecessary testing (stress tests) and/or revascularization that may accompany the same.

Coronary Calcium Score and C-Reactive Protein

The addition of CAC scores to CRP has also been evaluated. In an analysis from the South Bay Heart Watch study,[56] 967 asymptomatic nondiabetic participants without CHD and a

CRP < 10mg/L had undergone CAC scoring. Over a follow-up period 6.4 ± 1.3 years, 104 participants experienced any cardiovascular event (MI, coronary death, revascularization, or stroke). After categorizing CAC scores by tertiles and CRP by < or > 75th percentile (4.05mg/L), the adjusted relative risk for MI/coronary event was noted to be increased across increasing CAC scores at low or higher CRP levels. Having the highest CRP and CAC score was associated with the highest relative risk of 6.1 (p < 0.05). This analysis suggested the potential for the complementary value of adding CRP to CAC scoring in asymptomatic nondiabetic individuals.

FUTURE IMAGING TECHNOLOGIES

The future of risk prediction will likely be further refined by the identification of novel genetic variants such as the variant on chromosome 9p21[57, 58] that was described in 2007. In addition, multibiomarker strategies,[59] and strategies combining imaging, biomarkers, and genetics will likely be used to further refine risk and personalize medicine.

Advances in imaging technologies are already allowing for accurate identification of plaque characteristics and the evaluation of endothelial function. Whether these technologies will allow for improved risk prediction remains to be seen.

CONCLUSION

Prediction of cardiovascular risk using traditional risk factors is very helpful but has its limitations. Improvement in cardiovascular risk prediction will likely be with the use of additional biomarkers, genetic markers, and imaging. Currently there is evidence that the addition of CAC scores and CIMT improve risk prediction. However, it is important to remember that although the addition of imaging will improve cardiovascular risk prediction, it is likely to impact therapy only in the intermediate-risk group. In other words, the knowledge of the prior probability of CHD risk is very important in deciding from whom to obtain additional testing. Further, we will have to consider how lifetime risk estimates will influence the imaging tests in low-risk individuals. A recent study suggested that among low-risk individuals, ~50% have a high and ~50% have a low lifetime risk for CHD. Furthermore, those with the high lifetime risk estimates had a higher risk of having sub-clinical atherosclerosis and greater progression of disease.[60]

In summary, as of today, we recommend using traditional risk factors to first assess risk and in those who are intermediate in risk and with LDL-C > 100mg/dL consider additional testing to help further stratify risk. We must also recognize that there is no data suggesting that such a strategy of reclassifying risk and therapy based on the reclassified risk has not been studied in clinical trials to evaluate if it would decrease incident cardiovascular events.

◇◇◇◇◇◇◇◇◇◇◇◇◇

REFERENCES

1. Khot UN, Khot MB, Bajzer CT, Sapp SK, Ohman EM, Brener SJ, Ellis SG, Lincoff AM, Topol EJ. Prevalence of conventional risk factors in patients with coronary heart disease. *JAMA* 2003; 290(7):898–904.

2. Ridker PM, Buring JE, Rifai N, Cook NR. Development and validation of improved algorithms for the assessment of global cardiovascular risk in women: the Reynolds Risk Score. *JAMA* 2007; 297(6):611–619.

3. Nambi V, Hoogeveen RC, Chambless L, Hu Y, Bang H, Coresh J, Ni H, Boerwinkle E, Mosley T, Sharrett R, Folsom AR, Ballantyne CM. Lipoprotein-associated phospholipase A2 and high-sensitivity C-reactive protein improve the stratification of ischemic stroke risk in the Atherosclerosis Risk in Communities (ARIC) study. *Stroke* 2009; 40(2):376–381.

4. Wilson PW, D'Agostino RB, Levy D, Belanger AM, Silbershatz H, Kannel WB. Prediction of coronary heart disease using risk factor categories. *Circulation* 1998; 97(18):1837–1847.

5. D'Agostino RB, Russell MW, Huse DM, Ellison RC, Silbershatz H, Wilson PW, Hartz SC. Primary and subsequent coronary risk appraisal: new results from the Framingham study. *Am Heart J* 2000; 139(2 Pt 1):272–281.

6. Myerburg RJ, Kessler KM, Castellanos A. Sudden cardiac death: epidemiology, transient risk, and intervention assessment. *Ann Intern Med* 1993; 119(12):1187–1197.

7. Greenland P, Smith SC, Jr., Grundy SM. Improving coronary heart disease risk assessment in asymptomatic people: role of traditional risk factors and noninvasive cardiovascular tests. *Circulation* 2001; 104(15):1863–1867.

8. Ford ES, Giles WH, Mokdad AH. The distribution of 10-Year risk for coronary heart disease among US adults: findings from the National Health and Nutrition Examination Survey III. *J Am Coll Cardiol* 2004; 43(10):1791–1796.

9. Akosah KO, Schaper A, Cogbill C, Schoenfeld P. Preventing myocardial infarction in the young adult in the first place: how do the National Cholesterol Education Panel III guidelines perform? *J Am Coll Cardiol* 2003; 41(9):1475–1479.

10. Lloyd-Jones DM, Wilson PW, Larson MG, Beiser A, Leip EP, D'Agostino RB, Levy D. Framingham risk score and prediction of lifetime risk for coronary heart disease. *Am J Cardiol* 2004; 94(1):20–24.

11. Rybicki FJ, Gerson DS, Bettmann M, Yucel EK. Screening programs for individuals at risk of cardiovascular disease. *Am J Cardiol* 2007; 99(10):1481–1482.

12. Naghavi M, Falk E, Hecht HS, Jamieson MJ, Kaul S, Berman D, Fayad Z, Budoff MJ, Rumberger J, Naqvi TZ, Shaw LJ, Faergeman O, Cohn J, Bahr R, Koenig W, Demirovic J, Arking D, Herrera VL, Badimon J, Goldstein JA, Rudy Y, Airaksinen J, Schwartz RS, Riley WA, Mendes RA, Douglas P, Shah PK. From vulnerable plaque to vulnerable patient--Part III: Executive summary of the Screening for Heart Attack Prevention and Education (SHAPE) Task Force report. *Am J Cardiol* 2006; 98(2A):2H–15H.

13. Pletcher MJ, Tice JA, Pignone M, Browner WS. Using the coronary artery calcium score to predict coronary heart disease events: a systematic review and meta-analysis. *Arch Intern Med* 2004; 164(12):1285–1292.

14. Greenland P, LaBree L, Azen SP, Doherty TM, Detrano RC. Coronary artery calcium score combined with Framingham score for risk prediction in asymptomatic individuals. *JAMA* 2004; 291(2):210–215.

15. Shaw LJ, Raggi P, Schisterman E, Berman DS, Callister TQ. Prognostic value of cardiac risk factors and coronary artery calcium screening for all-cause mortality. *Radiology* 2003; 228(3):826–833.

16. Wong ND, Budoff MJ, Pio J, Detrano RC. Coronary calcium and cardiovascular event risk: evaluation by age- and sex-specific quartiles. *Am Heart J* 2002; 143(3):456–459.

17. Arad Y, Goodman KJ, Roth M, Newstein D, Guerci AD. Coronary calcification, coronary disease risk factors, C-reactive protein, and atherosclerotic cardiovascular disease events: the St. Francis Heart Study. *J Am Coll Cardiol* 2005; 46(1):158–165.

18. Budoff MJ, Shaw LJ, Liu ST, Weinstein SR, Mosler TP, Tseng PH, Flores FR, Callister TQ, Raggi P, Berman DS. Long-term prognosis associated with coronary calcification: observations from a registry of 25,253 patients. *J Am Coll Cardiol* 2007; 49(18):1860–1870.

19. Nasir K, Michos ED, Blumenthal RS, Raggi P. Detection of high-risk young adults and women by coronary calcium and National Cholesterol Education Program Panel III guidelines. *J Am Coll Cardiol* 2005; 46(10):1931–1936.

20. Detrano RC, Wong ND, Doherty TM, Shavelle RM, Tang W, Ginzton LE, Budoff MJ, Narahara KA. Coronary calcium does not accurately predict near-term

future coronary events in high-risk adults. *Circulation* 1999; 99(20):2633–2638.

21. Schenker MP, Dorbala S, Hong EC, Rybicki FJ, Hachamovitch R, Kwong RY, Di Carli MF. Interrelation of coronary calcification, myocardial ischemia, and outcomes in patients with intermediate likelihood of coronary artery disease: a combined positron emission tomography/computed tomography study. *Circulation* 2008; 117(13):1693–1700.

22. Vliegenthart R, Oudkerk M, Hofman A, Oei HH, van Dijck W, van Rooij FJ, Witteman JC. Coronary calcification improves cardiovascular risk prediction in the elderly. *Circulation* 2005; 112(4):572–577.

23. LaMonte MJ, FitzGerald SJ, Church TS, Barlow CE, Radford NB, Levine BD, Pippin JJ, Gibbons LW, Blair SN, Nichaman MZ. Coronary artery calcium score and coronary heart disease events in a large cohort of asymptomatic men and women. *Am J Epidemiol* 2005; 162(5):421–429.

24. Kondos GT, Hoff JA, Sevrukov A, Daviglus ML, Garside DB, Devries SS, Chomka EV, Liu K. Electron-beam tomography coronary artery calcium and cardiac events: a 37-month follow-up of 5635 initially asymptomatic low- to intermediate-risk adults. *Circulation* 2003; 107(20):2571–2576.

25. Greenland P, Bonow RO, Brundage BH, Budoff MJ, Eisenberg MJ, Grundy SM, Lauer MS, Post WS, Raggi P, Redberg RF, Rodgers GP, Shaw LJ, Taylor AJ, Weintraub WS, Harrington RA, Abrams J, Anderson JL, Bates ER, Grines CL, Hlatky MA, Lichtenberg RC, Lindner JR, Pohost GM, Schofield RS, Shubrooks SJ, Jr., Stein JH, Tracy CM, Vogel RA, Wesley DJ. ACCF/AHA 2007 clinical expert consensus document on coronary artery calcium scoring by computed tomography in global cardiovascular risk assessment and in evaluation of patients with chest pain: a report of the American College of Cardiology Foundation Clinical Expert Consensus Task Force (ACCF/AHA Writing Committee to Update the 2000 Expert Consensus Document on Electron Beam Computed Tomography). *Circulation* 2007; 115(3):402–426.

26. Greenland P, Bonow RO. How low-risk is a coronary calcium score of zero? The importance of conditional probability. *Circulation* 2008; 117(13):1627–1629.

27. Gaziano JM, Buring JE, Breslow JL, Goldhaber SZ, Rosner B, VanDenburgh M, Willett W, Hennekens CH. Moderate alcohol intake, increased levels of high-density lipoprotein and its subfractions, and decreased risk of myocardial infarction. *N Engl J Med* 1993; 329(25):1829–1834.

28. Taylor AJ, Bindeman J, Feuerstein I, Le T, Bauer K, Byrd C, Wu H, O'Malley PG. Community-based provision of statin and aspirin after the detection of coronary artery calcium within a community-based screening cohort. *J Am Coll Cardiol* 2008; 51(14):1337–1341.

29. O'Malley PG, Feuerstein IM, Taylor AJ. Impact of electron beam tomography, with or without case management, on motivation, behavioral change, and cardiovascular risk profile: a randomized controlled trial. *JAMA* 2003; 289(17):2215–2223.

30. Chambless LE, Heiss G, Folsom AR, Rosamond W, Szklo M, Sharrett AR, Clegg LX. Association of coronary heart disease incidence with carotid arterial wall thickness and major risk factors: the Atherosclerosis Risk in Communities (ARIC) Study, 1987–1993. *Am J Epidemiol* 1997; 146(6):483-494.

31. Hodis HN, Mack WJ, LaBree L, Selzer RH, Liu CR, Liu CH, Azen SP. The role of carotid arterial intima-media thickness in predicting clinical coronary events. *Ann Intern Med* 1998; 128(4):262–269.

32. O'Leary DH, Polak JF, Kronmal RA, Manolio TA, Burke GL, Wolfson SK, Jr., Cardiovascular Health Study Collaborative Research Group. Carotid-artery intima and media thickness as a risk factor for myocardial infarction and stroke in older adults. *N Engl J Med* 1999; 340(1):14–22.

33. Taylor AJ, Kent SM, Flaherty PJ, Coyle LC, Markwood TT, Vernalis MN. ARBITER: Arterial Biology for the Investigation of the Treatment Effects of Reducing Cholesterol: a randomized trial comparing the effects of atorvastatin and pravastatin on carotid intima medial thickness. *Circulation* 2002; 106(16):2055–2060.

34. Crouse JR, III, Raichlen JS, Riley WA, Evans GW, Palmer MK, O'Leary DH, Grobbee DE, Bots ML. Effect of rosuvastatin on progression of carotid intima-media thickness in low-risk individuals with subclinical atherosclerosis: the METEOR Trial. *JAMA* 2007; 297(12):1344–1353.

35. Smilde TJ, van Wissen S, Wollersheim H, Trip MD, Kastelein JJ, Stalenhoef AF. Effect of aggressive versus conventional lipid lowering on atherosclerosis progression in familial hypercholesterolaemia (ASAP): a prospective, randomised, double-blind trial. *Lancet* 2001; 357(9256):577–581.

36. de Groot E, van Leuven SI, Duivenvoorden R, Meuwese MC, Akdim F, Bots ML, Kastelein JJ. Measurement of carotid intima-media thickness to assess progression and regression of atherosclerosis. *Nat Clin Pract Cardiovasc Med* 2008; 5(5):280–288.

37. Expert Panel on Detection, Evaluation, and Treatment of High Blood Cholesterol in Adults. Executive summary of the third report of the National Cholesterol

Education Program (NCEP) Expert Panel on Detection, Evaluation, and Treatment of High Blood Cholesterol in Adults (Adult Treatment Panel III). *JAMA* 2001; 285:2486–2497.

38. Baldassarre D, Amato M, Pustina L, Castelnuovo S, Sanvito S, Gerosa L, Veglia F, Keidar S, Tremoli E, Sirtori CR. Measurement of carotid artery intima-media thickness in dyslipidemic patients increases the power of traditional risk factors to predict cardiovascular events. *Atherosclerosis* 2007; 191(2):403–408.

39. Bernard S, Serusclat A, Targe F, Charriere S, Roth O, Beaune J, Berthezene F, Moulin P. Incremental predictive value of carotid ultrasonography in the assessment of coronary risk in a cohort of asymptomatic type 2 diabetic subjects. *Diabetes Care* 2005; 28(5):1158–1162.

40. Bard RL, Kalsi H, Rubenfire M, Wakefield T, Fex B, Rajagopalan S, Brook RD. Effect of carotid atherosclerosis screening on risk stratification during primary cardiovascular disease prevention. *Am J Cardiol* 2004; 93(8):1030–1032.

41. Rundek T, Arif H, Boden-Albala B, Elkind MS, Paik MC, Sacco RL. Carotid plaque, a subclinical precursor of vascular events: the Northern Manhattan Study. *Neurology* 2008; 70(14):1200–1207.

42. Nambi V, Chambless L, Folsom AR, He M, Hu Y, Mosley T, Volcik K, Boerwinkle E, Ballantyne CM. Carotid intima-media thickness and presence or absence of plaque improves prediction of coronary heart disease risk in the Atherosclerosis Risk in Communities (ARIC) study. *J Am Coll Cardiol* In press.

43. Stein JH, Fraizer MC, Aeschlimann SE, Nelson-Worel J, McBride PE, Douglas PS. Vascular age: integrating carotid intima-media thickness measurements with global coronary risk assessment. *Clin Cardiol* 2004; 27(7):388–392.

44. Gepner AD, Keevil JG, Wyman RA, Korcarz CE, Aeschlimann SE, Busse KL, Stein JH. Use of carotid intima-media thickness and vascular age to modify cardiovascular risk prediction. *J Am Soc Echocardiogr* 2006; 19(9):1170–1174.

45. Junyent M, Zambon D, Gilabert R, Nunez I, Cofan M, Ros E. Carotid atherosclerosis and vascular age in the assessment of coronary heart disease risk beyond the Framingham Risk Score. *Atherosclerosis* 2008; 196(2):803–809.

46. Stein JH, Korcarz CE, Hurst RT, Lonn E, Kendall CB, Mohler ER, Najjar SS, Rembold CM, Post WS. Use of carotid ultrasound to identify subclinical vascular disease and evaluate cardiovascular disease risk: a consensus statement from the American Society of Echocardiography Carotid Intima-Media Thickness Task Force. Endorsed by the Society for Vascular Medicine. *J Am Soc Echocardiogr* 2008; 21(2):93–111; quiz 189–190.

47. U.S. Preventive Services Task Force. Using nontraditional risk factors in coronary heart disease risk assessment: U.S. Preventive Services Task Force recommendation statement. *Ann Intern Med* 2009; 151(7):474–482.

48. Newman AB, Naydeck BL, Sutton-Tyrrell K, Edmundowicz D, O'Leary D, Kronmal R, Burke GL, Kuller LH. Relationship between coronary artery calcification and other measures of subclinical cardiovascular disease in older adults. *Arterioscler Thromb Vasc Biol* 2002; 22(10):1674–1679.

49. Oei HH, Vliegenthart R, Hak AE, Iglesias del Sol A, Hofman A, Oudkerk M, Witteman JC. The association between coronary calcification assessed by electron beam computed tomography and measures of extracoronary atherosclerosis: the Rotterdam Coronary Calcification Study. *J Am Coll Cardiol* 2002; 39(11):1745–1751.

50. Wagenknecht LE, Langefeld CD, Carr JJ, Riley W, Freedman BI, Moossavi S, Bowden DW. Race-specific relationships between coronary and carotid artery calcification and carotid intimal medial thickness. *Stroke* 2004; 35(5):e97–99.

51. Barrett-Connor E, Laughlin GA, Connor C. Coronary artery calcium versus intima-media thickness as a measure of cardiovascular disease among asymptomatic adults (from the Rancho Bernardo Study). *Am J Cardiol* 2007; 99(2):227–231.

52. Arad Y, Spadaro LA, Roth M, Scordo J, Goodman K, Sherman S, Lledo A, Lerner G, Guerci AD. Correlations between vascular calcification and atherosclerosis: a comparative electron beam CT study of the coronary and carotid arteries. *J Comput Assist Tomogr* 1998; 22(2):207–211.

53. Terry JG, Carr JJ, Tang R, Evans GW, Kouba EO, Shi R, Cook DR, Vieira JL, Espeland MA, Mercuri MF, Crouse JR, 3rd. Coronary artery calcium outperforms carotid artery intima-media thickness as a noninvasive index of prevalent coronary artery stenosis. *Arterioscler Thromb Vasc Biol* 2005; 25(8):1723–1728.

54. Brook RD, Bard RL, Patel S, Rubenfire M, Clarke NS, Kazerooni EA, Wakefield TW, Henke PK, Eagle KA. A negative carotid plaque area test is superior to other noninvasive atherosclerosis studies for reducing the likelihood of having underlying significant coronary artery disease. *Arterioscler Thromb Vasc Biol* 2006; 26(3):656–662.

55. Folsom AR, Kronmal RA, Detrano RC, O'Leary DH, Bild DE, Bluemke DA, Budoff MJ, Liu K,

Shea S, Szklo M, Tracy RP, Watson KE, Burke GL. Coronary artery calcification compared with carotid intima-media thickness in the prediction of cardiovascular disease incidence: the Multi-Ethnic Study of Atherosclerosis (MESA). *Arch Intern Med* 2008; 168(12):1333–1339.

56. Park R, Detrano R, Xiang M, Fu P, Ibrahim Y, LaBree L, Azen S. Combined use of computed tomography coronary calcium scores and C-reactive protein levels in predicting cardiovascular events in nondiabetic individuals. *Circulation* 2002; 106(16):2073–2077.

57. Helgadottir A, Thorleifsson G, Manolescu A, Gretarsdottir S, Blondal T, Jonasdottir A, Sigurdsson A, Baker A, Palsson A, Masson G, Gudbjartsson DF, Magnusson KP, Andersen K, Levey AI, Backman VM, Matthiasdottir S, Jonsdottir T, Palsson S, Einarsdottir H, Gunnarsdottir S, Gylfason A, Vaccarino V, Hooper WC, Reilly MP, Granger CB, Austin H, Rader DJ, Shah SH, Quyyumi AA, Gulcher JR, Thorgeirsson G, Thorsteinsdottir U, Kong A, Stefansson K. A common variant on chromosome 9p21 affects the risk of myocardial infarction. *Science* 2007; 316(5830):1491–1493.

58. McPherson R, Pertsemlidis A, Kavaslar N, Stewart A, Roberts R, Cox DR, Hinds DA, Pennacchio LA, Tybjaerg-Hansen A, Folsom AR, Boerwinkle E, Hobbs HH, Cohen JC. A common allele on chromosome 9 associated with coronary heart disease. *Science* 2007; 316(5830):1488–1491.

59. Wang TJ, Gona P, Larson MG, Tofler GH, Levy D, Newton-Cheh C, Jacques PF, Rifai N, Selhub J, Robins SJ, Benjamin EJ, D'Agostino RB, Vasan RS. Multiple biomarkers for the prediction of first major cardiovascular events and death. *N Engl J Med* 2006; 355(25):2631–2639.

60. Berry JD, Liu K, Folsom AR, Lewis CE, Carr JJ, Polak JF, Shea S, Sidney S, O'Leary DH, Chan C, Lloyd-Jones DM. Prevalence and progression of subclinical atherosclerosis in younger adults with low short-term but high lifetime estimated risk for cardiovascular disease: the coronary artery risk development in young adults study and multi-ethnic study of atherosclerosis. *Circulation* 2009; 119(3):382–389.

CHAPTER 15

Chest Pain Evaluation

Theodore D. Karamitsos, MD, PhD
Tammy J. Pegg, MRCP
Joseph B. Selvanayagam, MBBS (Hons), FRACP, DPhil

INTRODUCTION

One of the most difficult challenges in cardiology is determining whether chest pain has a cardiovascular origin. Only 10–30% of patients with chest pain are clearly defined at presentation as having acute coronary syndromes based on history, electrocardiographic changes, and serial enzyme elevations.[1,2] The majority of patients have a less clear clinical picture and the initial evaluation does not often yield a definitive diagnosis. Because of the limitation of clinical, electrocardiographic, and biochemic data, many of these patients are finally admitted to the hospital, with major logistic and financial implications for healthcare providers. Despite this low threshold for admission, up to 8% of patients with acute myocardial infarction are erroneously sent home.[3] The triage of such patients with inconclusive initial evaluation from conventional investigations such as electrocardiograms (ECG) and cardiac biomarkers can be aided significantly by the appropriate use of noninvasive imaging. Imaging techniques such as echocardiography, single photon emission computed tomography (SPECT), multidector computed tomography (MDCT), and cardiac magnetic resonance (CMR) have all been demonstrated to have favorable diagnostic and, in some cases, prognostic value in the setting of chest pain. In the case of suspected coronary artery disease (CAD), each of these techniques interrogate different stages of the ischemic cascade (see Figure 15.1). The application of these techniques in chest pain patients could potentially improve the efficiency of evaluation, reduce unnecessary admissions and yield a more rapid and accurate diagnosis. In this chapter we will discuss the advantages and disadvantages of these imaging modalities and their ability to improve the triage of patients with acute chest pain.

ECHOCARDIOGRAPHY

The use of two-dimensional echocardiography in the acute chest pain setting is based on its ability to detect direct (perfusion abnormalities) and indirect (wall motion abnormalities) measures of myocardial ischemia both at rest and during stress.

Early studies evaluating the usefulness of echocardiography in patients presenting with chest pain and a nondiagnostic ECG found that analyses of wall motion at rest had

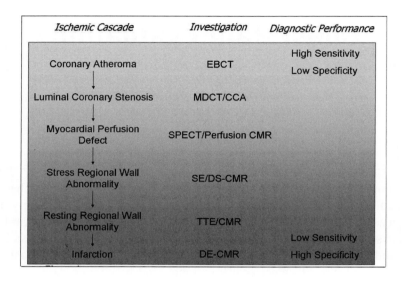

Figure 15.1

A flow diagram illustrating the utility of currently available noninvasive imaging modalities to interrogate various stages of the ischemic cascade in patients with chest pain and suspected coronary artery disease. EBCT: electron beam computed tomography; MDCT: multi-detector computed tomography; CMR: cardiovascular magnetic resonance; SE: stress echocardiography; TTE: transthoracic echocardiography; SPECT: single photon emission computed tomography; DE-CMR: delayed enhancement cardiovascular magnetic resonance.

high sensitivity for detecting acute myocardial infarction (92–93%) and cardiac ischemia (88%).[4, 5] However, the specificity was limited to 53–57% for acute myocardial infarction and 78% for cardiac ischemia. One of the limitations of assessing wall motion only at rest is that for optimal sensitivity, the patient must have active chest pain although some patients may still have late abnormalities, despite spontaneous reperfusion, and restoration of normal antegrade flow, as a result of myocardial stunning.

Trippi et al. were the first to assess the practicality and accuracy of dobutamine stress echocardiography (DSE) in the emergency department on 25 low-risk patients with chest pain.[6] The sensitivity and specificity of DSE versus clinical and cardiac catheterization findings were 90% and 89%, respectively, with a negative predictive value for DSE of 99%. Patients experienced frequent mild side effects (55%), but few (6%) caused the test to be discontinued prematurely. Two other studies have assessed the feasibility and the prognostic value of DSE in patients with acute chest pain and nondiagnostic ECG and both concluded that stress echocardiography is a feasible, safe, and effective tool for early stratification of patients admitted to the ER with acute chest pain and nonischemic ECG.[7, 8] Nevertheless, both these studies have some limitations in the real emergency department world. Obtaining a stress echocardiogram requires a highly experienced operator and sometimes wall motion abnormalities may be subtle and difficult to identify, particularly in patients with poor echocardiographic windows. The former issue has been addressed (at least in part) with the use of ultrasound contrast agents. Recent studies evaluated the clinical utility, diagnostic accuracy, and prognostic value of myocardial contrast echocardiography (MCE) in patients with acute chest pain.[9, 10] Tsutsui et al. studied 158 chest pain patients with MCE during dobutamine stress.[9] They found that dobutamine stress MCE was highly accurate in detecting patients with significant CAD (88% diagnostic accuracy), and was an independent predictor of recurrent cardiac events in follow-up. The use of contrast allows the simultaneous assessment of myocardial perfusion as well as contrast-enhanced wall motion.[11] This approach significantly increases the sensitivity of echocardiography in identifying patients with significant CAD. Moreover, the portability of MCE to the bedside makes it a very powerful tool in the assessment of patients with acute chest pain, as it is possible to rapidly stratify patients to high and low risk in the emergency setting.

Echocardiographic assessment of global cardiac function in patients evaluated for suspected cardiac ischemia also provides prognostic information. The presence of systolic dysfunction has been shown to be an independent prognostic variable in predicting both short- and long-term cardiac events.[12, 13] In a prospective study by Rinkevich et al., patients with suspected cardiac chest pain and no ST-segment elevation were evaluated in the emergency department for regional left ventricular function using MCE.[13] The authors found that assessment of regional function had incremental prognostic value over demographic, clinical, and ECG data.

Echocardiography is also well suited for the evaluation of patients with suspected aortic dissection. Transthoracic echocardiography has been found to have high sensitivity for dissections involving the ascending aorta, ranging from 78% to 100%,[14, 15] whereas for dissections of the descending aorta its sensitivity was as low as 55% in one series[15] and only 31% in the study by Nienaber et al.[14] Transesophageal echocardiography, by virtue of its design, overcomes many of the difficulties and technical limitations associated with transthoracic echocardiography. Therefore, it is the method of choice for evaluating patients with suspected or known aortic dissection, and with the use of a biplane transducer most of the ascending aorta can be studied.[16] A number of studies have demonstrated a sensitivity of 97% to 100% for identifying an intimal flap[17, 18] and 77% to 87% for identifying the site of entry.[18, 19]

In conclusion, in the emergency department an early, bedside echocardiographic examination is a safe technique to further evaluate patients with chest pain and elusive clinical findings, and nondiagnostic electrocardiograms. Dobutamine stress can further enhance the diagnostic accuracy of echocardiography, but acute myocardial infarction should first be excluded. MCE, combining a simultaneous visualization of left ventricular wall motion and perfusion, offers a comprehensive assessment of patients with chest pain.

CARDIOVASCULAR MAGNETIC RESONANCE

Cardiovascular magnetic resonance is a powerful and versatile imaging modality and is considered the gold standard for the assessment of cardiovascular anatomy, right and left ventricular function (cine CMR), and myocardial viability (delayed enhancement CMR).[20] The major advantages of CMR compared to all other noninvasive imaging modalities are its multiparametric nature (allowing for concurrent evaluation of cardiac anatomy, function, viability, perfusion, and coronary arteries), absence of ionizing radiation, high spatial resolution enabling easy delineation of the endocardium, and ability to image the heart in any plane.

Notwithstanding these advantages, CMR historically has not been widely used for the assessment of acute chest pain patients and very few studies have assessed perfusion CMR in the acute chest pain setting. Safety concerns related to longer imaging times during which patients are removed from the emergency department or coronary care setting have been limiting factors. As a general principle, patients with ongoing chest pain, hemodynamic instability, arrhythmias, acute heart failure, or ischemic ECG changes should not be removed from a monitored setting to undergo CMR. After a period of initial observation (> 12 hours), particularly if the ECG and biomarkers remain normal or are nondiagnostic, myocardial perfusion CMR can be performed safely.

In myocardial perfusion CMR, a bolus of gadolinium-based contrast agent is injected into a peripheral vein and a sequence of images is then obtained to follow the dynamic passage of the dye through the heart. Vasodilatation with adenosine or dipyridamole induces an increase of blood flow (hyperemia) in myocardial areas subtended by normal coronary arteries, whereas no or only minimal changes are found in areas supplied by stenotic coronary arteries. This relative hypoenhancement in underperfused areas is usually evident visually and constitutes a perfusion defect. Several single-center studies[21-23] and a published multicenter trial[24] have compared perfusion CMR favorably to existing nuclear methods (SPECT) or invasive cardiac catheterization for the detection of myocardial ischemia in the setting of chronic chest pain.

Two studies to date have evaluated the feasibility and diagnostic performance of CMR in patients presenting with acute chest pain to the emergency department.[25, 26] Patients with ST-elevation myocardial infarction were excluded. A comprehensive CMR study assessing ventricular function, myocardial perfusion at rest (but not stress perfusion), and delayed enhancement CMR for myocardial infarction detection (see Figure 15.2) was performed. Twenty-five patients (16%) had a final diagnosis of acute coronary syndrome, with CMR correctly identifying 21 of them (sensitivity 84%), whereas specificity was 85%. Multivariate logistic regression analysis showed that abnormal CMR was the strongest predictor of acute coronary syndromes and added significant diagnostic information to the other tests (risk factors, ECG, troponin). In a study from the same center, Ingkanisorn et al. evaluated the diagnostic value of adenosine stress CMR on

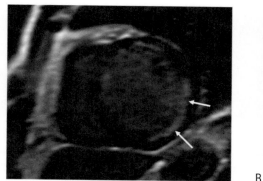
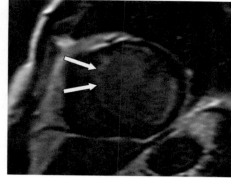

A   B

Figure 15.2

A patient example of delayed hyperenhancement CMR (DE-CMR) in coronary artery disease (CAD). This patient presented with 3-month history of exertional angina with no clinical or biochemical evidence of acute myocardial infarction. Panel A demonstrates infero-lateral DHE (white arrows) in a subendocardial pattern suggestive of old myocardial infarction. Panel B demonstrates transmural anteroseptal DHE (block arrows) suggestive of CAD also in left anterior descending artery territory.

135 troponin-negative patients with chest pain.[26] The imaging protocol included regional and global function, adenosine stress perfusion, and infarct imaging within 72 hours of presentation to the emergency department with chest pain. Patients were followed for 1 year for composite adverse outcomes defined as interval diagnosis of > 50% stenoses on coronary angiography, abnormal correlative stress test, new MI, or death. During the follow-up, 20 patients (15%) experienced an end-point event. Adenosine CMR perfusion abnormalities had 100% sensitivity and 93% specificity for the detection of CAD—no patient with a normal adenosine CMR study had a subsequent diagnosis of CAD or an adverse outcome. These encouraging preliminary findings need to be confirmed by larger, multicenter studies.

Greenwood and colleagues have reported on the safety and diagnostic accuracy of stress CMR imaging early after ST-segment elevation myocardial infarction.[27] Thirty-five patients admitted with first acute ST-segment elevation myocardial infarction underwent a comprehensive CMR imaging protocol at a median of 4 days (rest and adenosine-stress perfusion, viability, and cardiac functional assessment) and exercise tolerance testing before standard x-ray coronary angiography. All patients completed the CMR protocol and no complications occurred. CMR was more sensitive (86% vs 48%, p = 0.007) and more specific than ETT (100% vs 50%, p < 0.0001) to detect significant coronary stenoses and more sensitive to predict revascularization (94% vs 56%, p = 0.04).

Acute myocarditis may present with acute chest pain masquerading as an acute coronary syndrome (Figure 15.3). CMR imaging has been shown to have a definitive role in establishing the diagnosis of acute myocarditis. Mahrholdt et al. studied 32 patients

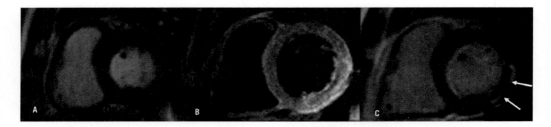

Figure 15.3

An CMR example of acute myocarditis. This 44-year-old male smoker presented to the emergency department with severe retro-sternal chest pain. ECG showed ST elevation in all precordial chest and limb leads. Urgent diagnostic coronary angiography was normal. CMR scan shows failure of infero-lateral wall contraction and thickening at peak systole (panel A). T1 weighted triple inversion recovery sequence (panel B) demonstrates high signal in the infero-lateral wall indicative of high water content/tissue edema. Panel C delayed hyperenhancement image following bolus injection of 0.1mmol/kg gadodiamide based contrast agent, show corresponding area of hyperenhancement also suggestive of tissue necrosis/odema (arrow).

Image courtesy of the Oxford Centre for Clinical Magnetic Resonance Research (OCMR).

with suspected myocarditis and found that 88% of them showed patchy, epicardial, and lateral wall contrast enhancement.[28] Importantly, CMR provides information on the exact localization of myocardial damage caused by myocarditis, which can be used to guide biopsy, enhancing sensitivity and specificity.

Aortic diseases and particularly aortic dissection should be ruled out in a patient presenting in the emergency department with abrupt onset chest pain. CMR has the highest accuracy, sensitivity, and specificity, for the detection of all forms of aortic dissection except subtle/discrete forms.[29] However, the distribution and availability of CMR is limited particularly in emergency situations and a CMR study is more time consuming compared to a MDCT scan. Therefore, CMR is usually used in hemodynamically stable patients, and in chronic aortic dissections for follow-up imaging.[30]

In conclusion, CMR and particularly adenosine stress studies, provide valuable diagnostic and prognostic information on selected patients with chest pain, in whom myocardial infarction has been excluded. Although in such patients CMR scanning appears to be safe, patients with ongoing chest pain, hemodynamic instability, arrhythmias, or dynamic ECG changes should not be removed from a monitoring setting to undergo CMR.

NUCLEAR MEDICINE TECHNIQUES

Single photon emission computed tomography remains the mainstay of myocardial perfusion imaging (MPI) in most units. The technique is accessible, and unlike newer imag-

Table 15.1   Effective Radiation Dose for Cardiac Diagnostic Imaging Methods

INVESTIGATION	ESTIMATED EFFECTIVE RADIATION DOSE (mSv)
Chest radiograph	0.1mSv
Background radiation	3mSv/year
Conventional coronary angiography	5mSv
[99m]Tc-tetrofosmin rest/stress	11mSv
[99m]Tc-sestamibi rest/stress	12mSv
64 slice MDCT coronary CTA	2–20mSV*
[201]TI rest/stress	25mSV

*Variable effective radiation dose due to varying protocols (ECG pulsing) and significant intersex difference (see section on MDCT).

ing methods, has a comprehensive evidence base supporting its use in the detection of significant CAD.

Although the first common tracer agent was [201]TI (Thallium-201), modern [99m]Tc (Technetium) labeled tracers have now superseded [201]TI in most centers, with reductions in effective radiation dose from less radiation scatter (Table 15.1). Furthermore ^{99m}Tc tracers are better suited to use with a gamma radiation camera as they produce less attenuation artifact improving the specificity. Two forms of ^{99m}Tc have gained widespread use; ^{99m}Tc-sestamibi and ^{99m}Tc-tetrofosmin.

Most units have adopted a 1-day rest/stress protocol. After the administration of a small amount of tracer agent for the rest study, there is then a prolonged delay while the tracer is redistributed. Ideally, exercise (commonly with a bicycle) provides the tachycardic stress, which precedes a repeat injection of a higher dose tracer for the stress study. Visual assessment of myocardial scintigrams using this protocol has a reported sensitivity of 82% and specificity of 88% for the identification of significant coronary artery disease.[31] If a patient is unable to exercise adequately (i.e., achieve 80% of target heart rate) then pharmacologic stress using a direct vasodilator agent, such as adenosine and dipyridamole; or an inotropic agent such as dobutamine will provide similar diagnostic performance.[32] Although nuclear methods have a good overall diagnostic accuracy for the detection of CAD, there are a certain factors/subgroups of patients where this is reduced (Table 15.2).

Improving Image Quality

Image quality is optimally achieved by ECG gated SPECT images using a ^{99m}Tc contrast agent. Advantages of using ECG gating for image acquisition include the simultaneous assessment of global left ventricular function and regional systolic thickening. Artifact problems associated with LBBB may be resolved by the utilization of adenosine pharamacologic stress, which may also improve the specificity of this technique in women.[33]

Table 15.2 Factors that Reduce the Sensitivity and Specificity of Nuclear Based MPI Assessment

COMMON REASONS FOR FALSE NEGATIVES	COMMON REASONS FOR FALSE POSITIVES
• Single vessel disease	• Breast tissue (anterior wall attenuation)
• Left circumflex disease	• Obesity
• Mild coronary artery stenosis (luminal stenosis 50–70%)	• High diaphragm (inferior wall attenuation)
• Distal vessel or branch disease	• Left bundle-branch block (septal attenuation)
• Inadequate heart rate response to physiological/pharmacological stress	
• Prior use of nitrates/Ca channel blockers	

Table 15.3 Features on SPECT Study that Indicate Prognostically Important CAD

COMMON REASONS FOR FALSE NEGATIVES	COMMON REASONS FOR FALSE POSITIVES
• Large defect (≥ 20% area of LV)	
• Defects in > 1 coronary artery territory (multivessel disease)	
• Defect reversibility (inducible ischemia)	
• Transient or persistent LV dilation following stress	
• LVEF ≤ 40%	
• Increased uptake of ^{201}Tl by lung parenchyma	

Prognosis Data

A normal SPECT study has an excellent negative predictive value for the detection of CAD and a negative result is associated with a good prognosis (annual mortality and nonfatal MI rate < 1% compared to 7% in patients with an abnormal test).[34, 35]

Conclusions

SPECT is a well-established technique with a good evidence-based background, not only in terms of diagnosis, but prognosis as well. ECG gated SPECT provides information on perfusion, and additionally on global and regional LV function. It provides an intermediate dose of radiation which may not be suitable for younger patients or as a screening tool.

COMPUTED TOMOGRAPHY

Electron Beam Computed Tomography

Electron beam computed tomography (EBCT) was the forerunner of multidetector computed tomography and was pioneered by Agaston et al.[36] Its utility is restricted to risk stratification for coronary artery disease through the quantification of coronary artery calcium (CAC). CAC is an indicator of atherosclerotic plaque burden, and very high levels confer an increased risk of future cardiac events.[37] A score greater than 130 Hounsefield units is generally considered to be abnormal[38, 39] but scores should be indexed to gender and age. However, absolute event rates are relatively low (1% to 2% per year) even in the highest-risk group, thus the routine clinical use of CAC scoring has yet to be defined clearly. There is no correlation between CAC and physiologic or anatomic significance of a stenosis. Furthermore, there is significant intrinsic variability in repeated measurements, and therefore coronary artery calcification scores are not suitable for treatment monitoring or assessing disease progression.[40, 41]

Multidetector Computed Tomography

MDCT has rapidly advanced from the introduction of the first four-slice MDCT in 1999 to the recent release of 320-slice MDCT in 2008. No other area of cardiovascular imaging has experienced such accelerated growth. Scanners with 64 detectors (Figure 15.4) and now dual-source 64-detector scanners are becoming more widely available; thus, temporal and spatial resolutions are steadily improving with a concomitant reduction in unreadable segments and false-positive studies (Table 15.4).

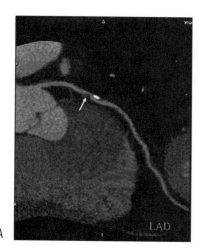
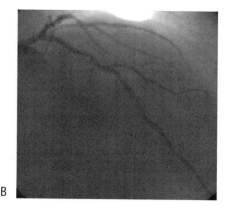

Figure 15.4

An example of CT coronary angiogram. This 54-year-old man presented with acute chest pain and had normal cardiac biomarkers and ECG. He had an equivocal exercise test. He underwent CT coronary angiography as part of a research study protocol. This shows significant LAD disease (A, arrow), which was later confirmed by x-ray angiography (B).

Table 15.4   Common Reasons for a False Positive or Negative

COMMON REASONS FOR A FALSE POSITIVE	COMMON REASONS FOR FALSE NEGATIVE
• Extensive coronary calcification without luminal stenosis	• Low contrast to noise ratio
• Reconstruction artifact	• Motion artifact
	• Suboptimal contrast (especially in distal vessels)
	• Disease in distal vessels
	• Overlapping greater cardiac vein (especially important for circumflex lesions)

Studies are under way to determine which patient populations are best served by CT angiography (CTA). To date, it has shown to be useful in the following groups (in single center studies): low- to intermediate-risk patients seen in the emergency department with acute chest pain,[42] patients with left bundle-branch block; and patients before cardiac valve surgery. MDCT has no role in the assessment of patients at high risk of myocardial ischemia as they should proceed directly to invasive coronary angiography.

Data on the clinical efficacy of MDCT for assessment of patients with intermediate risk of CAD is encouraging but still preliminary. A recent meta-analysis of MDCT to identify significant CAD reported a sensitivity of 76% (95% CI 63–89%) and specificity of 95% (95% CI 94–97%) for 16-slice MDCT, however 64-slice MDCT showed a much better sensitivity of 87% (95% CI 80–94%) and specificity 96% (95–97%).[43] The excellent specificity reported in these studies reflects the very high prevalence of CAD within the sampled population. In addition, all but one study excluded segments that were uninterpretable because of heavy calcification. In a real-world situation, these areas would be reported and would tend to overdiagnose significant luminal stenosis, hence the additional false positives would reduce the specificity. *The value of MDCT centers on its excellent negative predictive value for significant coronary stenosis, however prognostic follow-up studies are needed.*

MDCT in the Emergency Room Setting

Currently, only a few studies have examined the use of 16–64-slice MDCT for diagnostic purposes of *acute* chest pain in the setting of the emergency department. A small randomized study[44] showed that early triage with MDCT was a safe and effective alternative to standard practice (clinical assessment, observation and serial assessment of cardiac enzymes and ECG changes) providing a rapid and cost-effective treatment strategy. However 25% of patients randomized to MDCT required further risk stratification with nuclear scintigraphy due to the inability of MDCT to evaluate intermediate lesions. Similarly, other studies of MDCT in an emergency room setting show only moderate specificity (74%), however the sensitivity and negative predictive value remain excellent (both 100%).[42] Studies so far have enrolled small numbers, with a low prevalence of ACS (reflecting the emergency room population). From these few patients, it is difficult to derive understanding about the full capability of coronary MDCT in the detection of ACS, especially in younger patients where unstable plaques are seen as nonocclusive and noncalcified lesions. This difference has already been highlighted by studies of electron beam computed tomography and coronary calcium scores. Coronary calcium scores are able to exclude significant CAD with a high degree of precision, but in the sensitivity of the technique is diminished in younger patients presenting with acute chest pain, reflecting the difference in plaque calcium content.[45] In conclusion, although early pilot studies suggest early triage with MDCT was effective and reduced the need for hospitalization, the personal cost in terms of unnecessary investigations and repeated radiation exposure has not been addressed. Furthermore more robust assessment of the sensitivity is required for all patients presenting with chest pain, with particular attention to atypical or younger patients.

Limitations of MDCT

The high effective radiation dose administered remains the major limitation of this technique. This is especially so in women where the effective radiation dose is double that of men. The intersex difference arises because of the direct interposition of radiosensitive breast tissue into the imaging field, and indirect exposure of the female gonads from internal radiation scatter. Ongoing developments are focused upon limiting radiation exposure. One of the more important advances is prospective ECG gating: systems incorporate ECG data and prospectively pulse radiation emissions during the image acquisition phase of each cardiac cycle (diastole). This protocol requires ECG gating and a stable cardiac rhythm, but can reduce the effective radiation dose to 2–10mSv (in keeping with conventional coronary angiography), at the expense of some image quality.

CONCLUSION

Cardiac imaging in patients with chest pain is rapidly becoming an essential component of the diagnostic triage. New imaging techniques like CMR and MDCT have been added to our imaging armamentarium and, together with echocardiography and radionuclide perfusion imaging, offers additional diagnostic and prognostic information on patients with chest pain. Nevertheless, the diagnosis of acute chest pain in the emergency department remains primarily clinical and guided by history, risk factors, ECG findings, and cardiac biomarkers. Imaging-based diagnostic strategies with either of the aforementioned modalities appear to increase the diagnostic accuracy in such patients, but larger multicenter studies are required in the emergency department setting. A major limitation is that most institutions cannot offer a 24-hour service for performing and interpreting cardiac imaging. Emergency imaging may also increase not only the initial cost of patient evaluation but also result in a large number of repeat investigations for both cardiac and extracardiac incidentalomas, the cost of which, in terms of cumulative radiation exposure and financial implications, has yet to be fully evaluated. Hence, clinical outcome data are urgently needed in evaluating the efficacy of these imaging techniques for chest pain evaluation.

◇◇◇◇◇◇◇◇◇◇◇◇

REFERENCES

1. Gibler WB, Lewis LM, Erb RE, Makens PK, Kaplan BC, Vaughn RH, Biagini AV, Blanton JD, Campbell WB. Early detection of acute myocardial infarction in patients presenting with chest pain and nondiagnostic ECGs: serial CK-MB sampling in the emergency department. *Ann Emerg Med.* 1990;19(12):1359-1366.

2. Gibler WB, Young GP, Hedges JR, Lewis LM, Smith MS, Carleton SC, Aghababian RV, Jorden RO, Allison EJ, Jr., Otten EJ, et al. Acute myocardial infarction in chest pain patients with nondiagnostic ECGs: serial CK-MB sampling in the emergency department. The Emergency Medicine Cardiac Research Group. *Ann Emerg Med.* 1992;21(5):504-512.

3. Lee TH, Rouan GW, Weisberg MC, Brand DA, Acampora D, Stasiulewicz C, Walshon J, Terranova G, Gottlieb L, Goldstein-Wayne B, et al. Clinical characteristics and natural history of patients with acute myocardial infarction sent home from the emergency room. *The American journal of cardiology.* 1987;60(4):219-224.

4. Peels CH, Visser CA, Kupper AJ, Visser FC, Roos JP. Usefulness of two-dimensional echocardiography for immediate detection of myocardial ischemia in the emergency room. *Am J Cardiol.* 1990;65(11):687-691.

5. Sasaki H, Charuzi Y, Beeder C, Sugiki Y, Lew AS. Utility of echocardiography for the early assessment of patients with nondiagnostic chest pain. *Am Heart J.* 1986;112(3):494-497.

6. Trippi JA, Lee KS, Kopp G, Nelson DR, Yee KG, Cordell WH. Dobutamine stress tele-echocardiography for evaluation of emergency department patients with chest pain. *J Am Coll Cardiol.* 1997;30(3):627-632.

7. Geleijnse ML, Elhendy A, Kasprzak JD, Rambaldi R, van Domburg RT, Cornel JH, Klootwijk AP, Fioretti PM, Roelandt JR, Simoons ML. Safety and prognostic value of early dobutamine-atropine stress echo-

cardiography in patients with spontaneous chest pain and a non-diagnostic electrocardiogram. *Eur Heart J.* 2000;21(5):397-406.

8. Bedetti G, Pasanisi EM, Tintori G, Fonseca L, Tresoldi S, Minneci C, Jambrik Z, Ghelarducci B, Orlandini A, Picano E. Stress echo in chest pain unit: the SPEED trial. *Int J Cardiol.* 2005;102(3):461-467.

9. Tsutsui JM, Xie F, O'Leary EL, Elhendy A, Anderson JR, McGrain AC, Porter TR. Diagnostic accuracy and prognostic value of dobutamine stress myocardial contrast echocardiography in patients with suspected acute coronary syndromes. *Echocardiography.* 2005;22(6):487-495.

10. Jeetley P, Burden L, Greaves K, Senior R. Prognostic value of myocardial contrast echocardiography in patients presenting to hospital with acute chest pain and negative troponin. *Am J Cardiol.* 2007;99(10):1369-1373.

11. Dijkmans PA, Senior R, Becher H, Porter TR, Wei K, Visser CA, Kamp O. Myocardial contrast echocardiography evolving as a clinically feasible technique for accurate, rapid, and safe assessment of myocardial perfusion: the evidence so far. *J Am Coll Cardiol.* 2006;48(11):2168-2177.

12. Sabia P, Abbott RD, Afrookteh A, Keller MW, Touchstone DA, Kaul S. Importance of two-dimensional echocardiographic assessment of left ventricular systolic function in patients presenting to the emergency room with cardiac-related symptoms. *Circulation.* 1991;84(4):1615-1624.

13. Rinkevich D, Kaul S, Wang XQ, Tong KL, Belcik T, Kalvaitis S, Lepper W, Dent JM, Wei K. Regional left ventricular perfusion and function in patients presenting to the emergency department with chest pain and no ST-segment elevation. *Eur Heart J.* 2005;26(16):1606-1611.

14. Nienaber CA, von Kodolitsch Y, Nicolas V, Siglow V, Piepho A, Brockhoff C, Koschyk DH, Spielmann RP. The diagnosis of thoracic aortic dissection by noninvasive imaging procedures. *N Engl J Med.* 1993;328(1):1-9.

15. White RD, Ullyot DJ, Higgins CB. MR imaging of the aorta after surgery for aortic dissection. *Ajr.* 1988;150(1):87-92.

16. Armstrong WF, Bach DS, Carey LM, Froehlich J, Lowell M, Kazerooni EA. Clinical and echocardiographic findings in patients with suspected acute aortic dissection. *American Heart Journal.* 1998;136(6):1051-1060.

17. Ballal RS, Nanda NC, Gatewood R, D'Arcy B, Samdarshi TE, Holman WL, Kirklin JK, Pacifico AD. Usefulness of transesophageal echocardiography in assessment of aortic dissection. *Circulation.* 1991;84(5):1903-1914.

18. Adachi H, Omoto R, Kyo S, Matsumura M, Kimura S, Takamoto S, Yokote Y. Emergency surgical intervention of acute aortic dissection with the rapid diagnosis by transesophageal echocardiography. *Circulation.* 1991;84(5 Suppl):III14-19.

19. Adachi H, Kyo S, Takamoto S, Kimura S, Yokote Y, Omoto R. Early diagnosis and surgical intervention of acute aortic dissection by transesophageal color flow mapping. *Circulation.* 1990;82(5 Suppl):IV19-23.

20. Constantine G, Shan K, Flamm SD, Sivananthan MU. Role of MRI in clinical cardiology. *Lancet.* 2004;363(9427):2162-2171.

21. Nagel E, Klein C, Paetsch I, Hettwer S, Schnackenburg B, Wegscheider K, Fleck E. Magnetic resonance perfusion measurements for the noninvasive detection of coronary artery disease. *Circulation.* 2003;108(4):432-437.

22. Paetsch I, Jahnke C, Wahl A, Gebker R, Neuss M, Fleck E, Nagel E. Comparison of dobutamine stress magnetic resonance, adenosine stress magnetic resonance, and adenosine stress magnetic resonance perfusion. *Circulation.* 2004;110(7):835-842.

23. Cheng AS, Pegg TJ, Karamitsos TD, Searle N, Jerosch-Herold M, Choudhury RP, Banning AP, Neubauer S, Robson MD, Selvanayagam JB. Cardiovascular magnetic resonance perfusion imaging at 3-tesla for the detection of coronary artery disease: a comparison with 1.5-tesla. *Journal of the American College of Cardiology.* 2007;49(25):2440-2449.

24. Schwitter J, Wacker CM, van Rossum AC, Lombardi M, Al-Saadi N, Ahlstrom H, Dill T, Larsson HB, Flamm SD, Marquardt M, Johansson L. MR-IMPACT: comparison of perfusion-cardiac magnetic resonance with single-photon emission computed tomography for the detection of coronary artery disease in a multicentre, multivendor, randomized trial. *Eur Heart J.* 2008;29(4):480-489.

25. Kwong RY, Schussheim AE, Rekhraj S, Aletras AH, Geller N, Davis J, Christian TF, Balaban RS, Arai AE. Detecting acute coronary syndrome in the emergency department with cardiac magnetic resonance imaging. *Circulation.* 2003;107(4):531-537.

26. Ingkanisorn WP, Kwong RY, Bohme NS, Geller NL, Rhoads KL, Dyke CK, Paterson DI, Syed MA, Aletras AH, Arai AE. Prognosis of negative adenosine stress magnetic resonance in patients presenting to an emergency department with chest pain. *J Am Coll Cardiol.* 2006;47(7):1427-1432.

27. Greenwood JP, Younger JF, Ridgway JP, Sivananthan MU, Ball SG, Plein S. Safety and diagnostic accuracy of stress cardiac magnetic resonance imaging vs exercise tolerance testing early after acute ST elevation myocardial infarction. *Heart.* 2007;93(11):1363-1368.

28. Mahrholdt H, Goedecke C, Wagner A, Meinhardt G, Athanasiadis A, Vogelsberg H, Fritz P, Klingel K, Kandolf R, Sechtem U. Cardiovascular magnetic resonance assessment of human myocarditis: a comparison to histology and molecular pathology. *Circulation.* 2004;109(10):1250-1258.

29. Kersting-Sommerhoff BA, Higgins CB, White RD, Sommerhoff CP, Lipton MJ. Aortic dissection: sensitivity and specificity of MR imaging. *Radiology.* 1988;166(3):651-655.

30. Erbel R, Alfonso F, Boileau C, Dirsch O, Eber B, Haverich A, Rakowski H, Struyven J, Radegran K, Sechtem U, Taylor J, Zollikofer C, Klein WW, Mulder B, Providencia LA. Diagnosis and management of aortic dissection. *European Heart Journal.* 2001;22(18):1642-1681.

31. Mahmarian J. *State of the art for coronary artery disease detection: thallium-201.* 2nd ed. St Louis: Mosby; 1999.

32. O'Keefe JH, Jr., Barnhart CS, Bateman TM. Comparison of stress echocardiography and stress myocardial perfusion scintigraphy for diagnosing coronary artery disease and assessing its severity. *Am J Cardiol.* 1995;75(11):25D-34D.

33. Cerqueira MD, Verani MS, Schwaiger M, Heo J, Iskandrian AS. Safety profile of adenosine stress perfusion imaging: results from the Adenoscan Multicenter Trial Registry. *J Am Coll Cardiol.* 1994;23(2):384-389.

34. Gibbons RS. American Society of Nuclear Cardiology project on myocardial perfusion imaging: measuring outcomes in response to emerging guidelines. *J Nucl Cardiol.* 1996;3(5):436-442.

35. Iskander S, Iskandrian AE. Risk assessment using single-photon emission computed tomographic technetium-99m sestamibi imaging. *J Am Coll Cardiol.* 1998;32(1):57-62.

36. Agatston AS, Janowitz WR, Hildner FJ, Zusmer NR, Viamonte M, Jr., Detrano R. Quantification of coronary artery calcium using ultrafast computed tomography. *J Am Coll Cardiol.* 1990;15(4):827-832.

37. Greenland P, LaBree L, Azen SP, Doherty TM, Detrano RC. Coronary artery calcium score combined with Framingham score for risk prediction in asymptomatic individuals. *Jama.* 2004;291(2):210-215.

38. Hausleiter J, Meyer T, Hadamitzky M, Kastrati A, Martinoff S, Schomig A. Prevalence of noncalcified coronary plaques by 64-slice computed tomography in patients with an intermediate risk for significant coronary artery disease. *J Am Coll Cardiol.* 2006;48(2):312-318.

39. Haberl R, Becker A, Leber A, Knez A, Becker C, Lang C, Bruning R, Reiser M, Steinbeck G. Correlation of coronary calcification and angiographically documented stenoses in patients with suspected coronary artery disease: results of 1,764 patients. *J Am Coll Cardiol.* 2001;37(2):451-457.

40. Lu B, Zhuang N, Mao SS, Child J, Carson S, Bakhsheshi H, Budoff MJ. EKG-triggered CT data acquisition to reduce variability in coronary arterial calcium score. *Radiology.* 2002;224(3):838-844.

41. Achenbach S, Ropers D, Mohlenkamp S, Schmermund A, Muschiol G, Groth J, Kusus M, Regenfus M, Daniel WG, Erbel R, Moshage W. Variability of repeated coronary artery calcium measurements by electron beam tomography. *Am J Cardiol.* 2001;87(2):210-213, A218.

42. Hoffmann U, Nagurney JT, Moselewski F, Pena A, Ferencik M, Chae CU, Cury RC, Butler J, Abbara S, Brown DF, Manini A, Nichols JH, Achenbach S, Brady TJ. Coronary multidetector computed tomography in the assessment of patients with acute chest pain. *Circulation.* 2006;114(21):2251-2260.

43. Hamon M, Biondi-Zoccai GG, Malagutti P, Agostoni P, Morello R, Valgimigli M, Hamon M. Diagnostic performance of multislice spiral computed tomography of coronary arteries as compared with conventional invasive coronary angiography: a meta-analysis. *J Am Coll Cardiol.* 2006;48(9):1896-1910.

44. Goldstein JA, Gallagher MJ, O'Neill WW, Ross MA, O'Neil BJ, Raff GL. A randomized controlled trial of multi-slice coronary computed tomography for evaluation of acute chest pain. *J Am Coll Cardiol.* 2007;49(8):863-871.

45. Georgiou D, Budoff MJ, Kaufer E, Kennedy JM, Lu B, Brundage BH. Screening patients with chest pain in the emergency department using electron beam tomography: a follow-up study. *J Am Coll Cardiol.* 2001;38(1):105-110.

CHAPTER 16

Evaluation of Dyspnea

Ben K. Dundon, MBBS
Matthew I. Worthley, MBBS, PhD, FRACP

INTRODUCTION

Dyspnea is one of the most pervasive symptoms encountered in clinical medicine, and is defined most simply as the awareness of breathlessness. Although common in healthy individuals during physical activity, dyspnea may be caused by myriad cardiac, respiratory, and systemic pathologies. Initially intended solely for the assessment of dyspnea in congestive cardiac failure, the New York Heart Association (NYHA) functional grading system is the most widely utilized classification of dyspnea, regardless of underlying etiology. This system provides a universally recognized, semiquantitative benchmark for clinicians and trialists in the assessment and management of breathless patients (Table 16.1).

The differential diagnosis for dyspnea is long, and often the etiology is multifactorial, particularly in elderly, comorbid patients. As such, imaging plays a crucial role in distinguishing between cardiac, pulmonary, and systemic contributors. This chapter will focus on the investigation of cardiovascular contributors to dyspnea, as an exhaustive discussion of pulmonary parenchymal and the myriad potential endocrine and metabolic contributors to dyspnea are beyond the scope of this text. While cardiac causes of dyspnea can be broadly classified into impairment of systolic and/or diastolic function, a pathoanatomic approach has been adopted in listing the common causes in Table 16.2.

INVESTIGATING DYSPNEA

The investigation of dyspnea, as with most symptoms, requires careful consideration of the clinical context—the nature and timing of symptoms, the relationship to exacerbating and relieving factors and relevant medical history and clinical examination. Simple and easily accessible investigations such as 12-lead electrocardiography (ECG) and chest x-ray (CXR) should be considered a standard component of the extended clinical examination of all dyspneic patients, in addition to targeted hematology and biochemic assays (such as brain natriuretic peptide [BNP]), particularly in the acute setting. Such an approach provides a preliminary or definitive diagnosis in a substantial proportion of dyspneic patients, and usually allows appropriately targeted preliminary treatment to commence. Furthermore, noncardiac contributors to the patient's symptoms may often be identified, or excluded, by such an approach. Echocardiography should be considered a routine,

Table 16.1   Updated NYHA Functional Classification of Dyspnea

Class 1	No limitation in physical activity.
Class 2	Slight limitation of physical activity due to dyspnea, comfortable at rest.
Class 3	Marked limitation of physical activity. Dyspnea with minimal exertion.
Class 4	Inability to carry out any physical activity without discomfort. Dyspnea at rest.

Table 16.2   Cardiovascular Contributors to Dyspnea

Myocardial
Myocardial Ischemia/Infarction
Nonischemic Dilated Cardiomypoathy
Restrictive Cardiompoathy
Hypertrophic Cardiomyopathy
Hypertensive Heart Disease
Valvular
Stenosis
Regurgitation
Pericardial
Constriction/Infiltration
Effusion
Cardiac Dysrhythmia
Atrial Fibrillation/Flutter
Atrial/AV Node Reentrant Tachycardia
Bradyarrhythmia—intrinsic or iatrogenic
Ventricular ectopy/Nonsustained Ventricular Tachycardia
Vascular
Systemic Vascular
Pulmonary Vascular
Congenital
Masses

second-line investigation to evaluate cardiac structure and function in the dyspneic patient. Moreover, where clinically indicated, stress echocardiography and nuclear techniques have become valuable components of the diagnostic pathway for the exclusion of myocardial ischemia as a contributor to patient symptoms. Newer imaging modalities such as real-time three-dimensional echo, cardiovascular magnetic resonance imaging and computed tomography continue to emerge as valuable diagnostic tools in the extended evaluation of the dyspneic patient. These noninvasive imaging modalities may play an important additional role in the exploration of etiology and disease severity, potentially providing invaluable guidance to clinicians planning targeted therapeutic strategies.

Electrocardiography

A normal ECG is uncommon in the presence of significant cardiac structural pathology. As such, this "electrical imaging" of the heart is safe, simple, and readily available and provides an essential starting point in the assessment of cardiovascular dyspnea. Certain abnormalities carry significant prognostic implications (e.g., left bundle-branch block is associated with increased mortality in a variety of patient cohorts), or may guide further investigation and therapeutic decision-making (e.g., myocardial ischemia/infarction). Indeed, myocardial ischemia/infarction is one of the most common causes of systolic and/or diastolic cardiac dysfunction.

Although not necessary in all patients, exercise ECG testing may provide further assistance to the clinician, both in the assessment of disease severity (and sometimes validity), but also in unmasking contributors to dyspnea not apparent at rest (e.g., coronary ischemia, frequent ventricular ectopy, or an inability to appropriately increase heart rate with exercise—so called chronotropic incompetence). Moreover, 24-hour ambulatory ECG monitoring is occasionally useful to exclude paroxysmal arrhythmia in sporadic breathlessness where no obvious symptom pattern can be determined.

Limitations of ECG

The resting ECG, although useful, is unable to provide a definitive diagnosis in the majority of cases of dyspnea. Its greatest utility is in the exclusion of cardiac ischemia or significant arrhythmia and serves as an essential screening test. The classical ECG finding of pulmonary embolus (PE) (S1Q3T3) is quite rare, and isolated sinus tachycardia is a far more common finding in PE patients.

Chest X-Ray

CXR is an essential component of the evaluation of acute breathlessness, and commonly identifies noncardiac contributors to dyspnea, including pulmonary parenchymal, vascular, musculoskeletal, and even subdiaphragmatic pathology. The role of CXR in the evaluation of chronic dyspnea may be considered in a more targeted fashion than ECG. Similarly, CXR may reveal important diagnostic and prognostic information not apparent on clinical examination, such as pulmonary nodules, consolidation, or increased pulmonary venous markings that may direct further investigation and management. Often-overlooked findings include thoracic restriction caused by vertebral fractures, and features of pulmonary hypertension: proximal pulmonary artery prominence with peripheral oligemia (pruning), right ventricular enlargement (seen on the lateral film as an obliteration of the normal retrosternal airspace), and right atrial enlargement (right heart border projection into

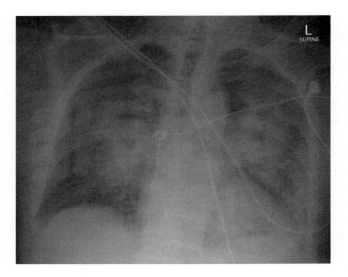

Figure 16.1

Antero-posterior chest x-ray taken in the supine position in a patient in respiratory distress related to acute pulmonary edema. The peri-hilar "bat-wing" appearance, with increased widespread interstitial and alveolar pulmonary markings, is classical for this condition.

the right lower lung field). Similarly, vascular and valvular calcification may provide important clues to the presence of occult cardiovascular disease.

CXR is particularly useful for the identification of pulmonary congestion as a reflection of left ventricular systolic or diastolic dysfunction. Classical findings include upper lobe pulmonary vascular prominence and bilateral pleural effusions. In the acute setting, prominence of the hilar pulmonary vasculature may give rise to a bat's wing or butterfly appearance (Figure 16.1). More commonly, interstitial edema may result in peribronchial cuffing and Kerley B lines, and alveolar edema will give rise to air bronchograms and fluffy opacities within the lung fields bilaterally.

Limitations of Chest X-Ray

CXR however, offers only an insensitive appraisal of underlying cardiac structure and function. The size of the cardiac silhouette on the PA film is commonly cited as an important radiological feature in significant left ventricular impairment; however, the presence of cardiomegaly on CXR is an unreliable determinant of impaired systolic function.[1] Furthermore, the absence of such a finding does not exclude significant systolic or valvular dysfunction.[1] It should be remembered that the majority of patients with clinical features of left ventricular failure will have normal, or near-normal cardiothoracic ratios; however, the presence of an enlarged cardiac silhouette increases in prevalence with increasing chronicity and severity of systolic heart failure.

Echocardiography

Two-dimensional transthoracic echocardiography (TTE) is a readily available, safe, and relatively inexpensive technology able to provide an assessment of cardiac structure, as well as measures of systolic, diastolic, and valvular function. These factors that ensure it remains the initial investigation of choice in the determination of cardiac dyspnea. Cardiac chamber dimensions are commonly performed utilising M-mode echocardiography; however, two-dimensional area and biplane volume calculations are increasingly being performed clinically and results may have significant prognostic implications in the management of heart failure and certain arrhythmias (e.g., atrial fibrillation).

Systolic Function

Left ventricular ejection fraction (LVEF) is the most common parameter utilized for the assessment of global systolic function (Figure 16.2) and provides important information regarding the underlying etiology of clinical heart failure.[2] Although load dependent, LVEF is frequently relied upon to determine the appropriateness and therapeutic response to pharmacologic therapies such as ACE-inhibitor and beta-blocker therapy. Furthermore, this routine left ventricular systolic assessment is widely used to evaluate patient suitability for advanced heart failure therapies such as prophylactic automated implantable cardio-defibrillators (AICD) or biventricular resynchronization pacemakers. In addition to a global systolic assessment, TTE is also useful for identifying regional wall motion

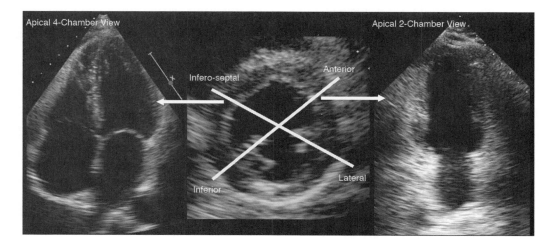

Figure 16.2

The apical 4- and 2-chamber views used to calculate LVEF by TTE. Although widely utilized as a measurement of global LV function, large areas of myocardium are not assessed by this method, as illustrated on the ventricular short-axis image (center).

abnormalities (RWMA) consistent with previous myocardial infarction or other myopathic processes that may benefit from therapeutic intervention.

The development of left ventricular dyssynchrony in the presence of systolic dysfunction is widely acknowledged as a potent contributor to disease and symptom severity in heart failure. Randomized trial evidence currently supports the insertion of a biventricular resynchronization pacemaker for patients with LVEF 35% in conjunction with the presence of ECG evidence of QRS prolongation (bundle-branch block; frequently induced by apical right ventricular cardiac pacing). Not all recipients respond favorably to the insertion of such a device, with up to a third of patients having no benefit, or experiencing a clinical deterioration, following insertion. Accordingly, considerable literature has been focused on better predicting which patients will respond.

Numerous methods currently exist for the detection and assessment of severity of LV dyssynchrony, however no single method has provided sufficiently high, prospective sensitivity and specificity for the identification of biventricular pacemaker responders to allow routine clinical application. Thus, such measures are not included in most current guidelines and currently have only limited utility in borderline cases, or in the optimization of device settings following implantation.

Diastolic Function

It is conservatively estimated that between one-third and one-half of hospitalized patients who were admitted for decompensated heart failure have heart failure with preserved systolic function (HF-PSF).[3,4] Equally, diastolic left ventricular dysfunction (impaired ventricular relaxation/filling) is a common cause of chronic heart failure and exercise-induced dyspnea, particularly in the elderly. As such, a comprehensive assessment of diastolic function is essential in the investigation of acute and chronic dyspnea.

TTE provides a variety of methods for the assessment of diastolic function, however mitral inflow patterns and measurements (such as isovolumic relaxation time) poorly distinguish the presence of diastolic impairment on their own. Spectral Doppler assessments of mitral annulus motion during ventricular diastole (Tissue Doppler) complement the traditional ratio of early (E): atrial (A) mitral inflow in the determination of diastolic cardiac function (Figures 15.3 and 15.4).[5] Such measurements are highly reproducible and have significant prognostic value.[6] The peak early-diastolic mitral annular velocity (E') and the ratio of traditional early mitral inflow, to early mitral annular motion (E/E') are particularly useful measures of diastolic function in various disease states and may be further complemented by the assessment of pulmonary vein inflow characteristics into the left atrium. An elevated E/E' (> 15) is indicative of elevated left ventricular end-diastolic pressure (LVEDP) in HF-PSF, with E/E' < 8 effectively excluding significant diastolic impariment.[7] Equally, Doppler diastolic assessments can assist in the discrimination of myocardial restriction from pericardial constriction, which may both present with exertional dyspnea and features of congestion.

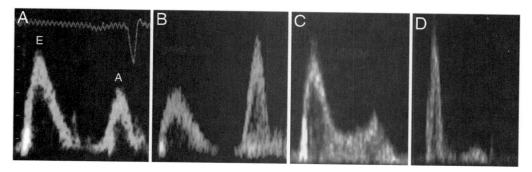

Figure 16.3

Representative patterns of early (E) and atrial (A) mitral inflow—normal (Panel A), abnormal relaxation (Panel B), pseudonormal (Panel C), and restrictive (Panel D).

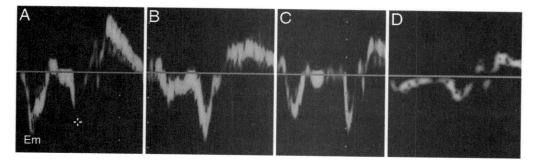

Figure 16.4

Representative tissue Doppler patterns of mitral annular motion—normal (Panel A), abnormal relaxation (Panel B), pseudonormal (Panel C), and the low-velocity restrictive pattern (Panel D). Although the patterns are useful in distinguishing normal mitral inflow from pseudonormal, the comparison of early mitral inflow (E) and early mitral annular velocity (Em) is particularly useful in the estimation of LVEDP.

Although a structural rather than functional parameter, left atrial size/volume should also be considered in the assessment of diastolic function. Impairment in left ventricular relaxation leads to increased LVEDP, necessitating a corresponding increase in left atrial pressure to maintain diastolic ventricular filling. This elevated pressure leads to increased LA wall tension and subsequent dilatation (over time), reflecting elevated LV filling pressures (in the presence of normal mitral valvular function).[8-10] Additionally, increased LA volume is a potent predictor of adverse events such as atrial fibrillation, ischemic stroke, left ventricular failure and heart failure survival.[11-13]

Valvular Function

Although increasing dyspnea is generally a reliable indicator of worsening disease severity, the presence and severity of valvular heart disease may be routinely estimated by a variety of increasingly sophisticated Doppler means. Reliance solely on visual appearance of regurgitant severity on 2D-color images has been demonstrated to be highly unreliable. As such, regurgitant fractions/volumes are increasingly used to provide more clinically relevant results.

In stenotic lesions, stenotic severity is usually accurately assessed utilizing Doppler methods, allowing reproducible calculation of stenotic valvular gradients. Because such measures are flow-dependent, the presence of significant systolic dysfunction, hypotension, or complex valvular disease may lead to substantial underestimation of valvular stenosis severity by Doppler velocity alone. As such, it is appropriate to routinely utilize the more robust assessment of valvular area for stenotic valves, just as regurgitant area/volume are more reliable measures of disease severity for incompetent valves.

Right Ventricular Function

Although echocardiography is the dominant imaging modality utilized for the assessment of the right ventricle in clinical practice, the assessment of right ventricular size and function is relatively insensitive using traditional two-dimensional echocardiography. Assessing RV function is important in patients with dyspnea as changes on this chamber largely reflect increased pulmonary pressures (in the presence of normal pulmonic valve function). The RV therefore can be acutely affected by pulmonary embolism, but more chronically affected in patients suffering from dyspnea secondary to impaired LV function or chronic pulmonary disease. Planimetered RV area (in the apical 4-chamber view) and single-plane short-axis dimensions are commonly used, but correlate poorly with cardiac MRI methodologies, predominantly due to the limitation of echocardiography in accurately visualizing the anterior right ventricular wall and infundibulum, regions which may be responsible for up to 30% of RV volume. Three-dimensional echocardiography may be able to better represent the complex structure of the right ventricle, however these regional imaging limitations persist (see below).

Right ventricular cardiac output may be accurately assessed by Doppler methods (in the absence of significant tricuspid regurgitation), but right ventricular contractility and ejection fraction are not well assessed by standard TTE. Other Doppler and tissue strain methodologies developed for the assessment of right ventricular function (such as myocardial performance index and measures of tricuspid annulus excursion) show promise, but require further clinical validation.

Echocardiography, however, is the preferred noninvasive technique for the evaluation of pulmonary arterial pressure (PAP) through the assessment of peak tricuspid regurgitant jet velocity. This technique provides important diagnostic and prognostic information in the assessment of pulmonary arterial hypertension (PAH) due to a wide variety of etiologies. Moreover, this method for assessing PAP allows for the serial assessment of therapeutic efficacy in the treatment of PAH syndromes. The accuracy of this method is, however, markedly reduced in the presence of eccentric tricuspid regurgitation. As Doppler methods are most accurate when data acquisition parallel to the direction of flow, eccentric tricuspid regurgitation may lead to substantial underestimation of PAP, potentially delaying diagnosis of this significant etiological differential in the assessment of breathlessness.

Limitations of Two-Dimensional Transthoracic Echocardiography

It is important to acknowledge that echocardiography is highly dependent on adequate image quality—frequently impaired in routine clinical practice. Chronic obstructive pulmonary disease, artificial ventilation, obesity, and even cachexia may impair the sonographer's ability to adequately image all regions of the heart (e.g., the anterior left ventricular wall is often difficult to image, as it is most likely to be obscured by overlying lung). Additionally, the presence of arrhythmia (e.g., rapid AF) may also give a false impression of baseline cardiac function. Furthermore, cardiac preload, afterload, and contractile state at the time of the examination may significantly affect assessment of LVEF and chamber dimensions (e.g., hypovolemia may falsely elevate LVEF), and such factors should be considered by the clinician in the interpretation of echocardiographic and other non-invasive imaging findings.

Advanced Echocardiography

Stress Echocardiography

Useful for the exclusion of significant coronary artery disease and for the detection of myocardial viability (see Chapter 14), dobutamine, or exercise stress, echocardiography may also be useful in the assessment of valvular disease severity in the breathless patient, particularly in the presence of significant resting left ventricular systolic dysfunction. Moreover, the assessment of myocardial contractile reserve with dobutamine in the presence of advanced aortic stenosis and low resting LVEF may have significant prognostic benefit in determining which patients will derive greatest benefit from valve replacement, and hence warrant the not-insubstantial procedural risks in this cohort.

Additionally, exercise stress echocardiography is increasingly recognized as an important tool in the diagnosis of subclinical primary pulmonary arterial hypertension (PPAH). The evaluation of changes in RV cardiac output and PAP with exercise may provide substantial clues to the presence of PAH as a cause or contributor to exercise limitation due to symptomatic dyspnea.

Transesophageal Echocardiography

Due to its higher image resolution, transesophageal echocardiography (TEE) is most useful in the evaluation of dyspnea for the assessment of valvular heart disease severity prior to possible therapeutic intervention (particularly mitral valve disease) and in the assessment of intracardiac tumors. LVEF is poorly assessed by this method, although an indicative cardiac assessment is usually possible, and TEE remains widely used in intubated patients for this purpose, particularly by anesthetists and intensive care physicians.

Contrast Echocardiography

The addition of intravenous contrast has markedly improved endocardial border definition in patients with poor baseline echocardiographic images. Not available in all centers, this simple advance has significantly improved evaluation of regional cardiac function, at rest and during stress echocardiographic studies. Moreover, this technique may even allow for the demonstration of regional myocardial hypoperfusion during pharmacological stress.

Unfortunately, however, echocontrast is not without controversy, having been associated with a small number of fatalities leading to a formal U.S. FDA warning. Patients at particular risk from adverse cardiopulmonary reactions include those with known cardiac shunts, clinically unstable or recent worsening of congestive heart failure, symptomatic arrhythmias, QT prolongation, or significant pulmonary disease, including emphysema and pulmonary emboli. Thus, this advance has not been the panacea for poor echocardiographic image quality that had been desired.

Real-Time Three-Dimensional Echocardiography (RT3DE)

Three-dimensional echocardiography now provides an exciting advance in the assessment of myocardial and valvular function and provides new insights in the evaluation of breathlessness in complicated or congenital heart disease cases. Although still reliant on adequate echocardiographic windows, RT3DE LVEF appears to provide a more accurate assessment of global systolic function than traditional 2D echo.[15] Valvular and congenital lesions in particular, may now be appreciated with greater clarity prior to surgical or percutaneous intervention. Moreover, RT3DE is enormously promising in the evaluation of right ventricular function. Able to reduce the need for some of the geometric assumptions inherent in Simpson's rule calculations of RVEF, even RT3DE has difficulty imaging the whole RV in all patients.

NUCLEAR CARDIOLOGY

Nuclear scintigraphic techniques have advanced significantly since their clinical emergence in the 1970s. Since the 1980s in particular, nuclear cardiac imaging has become a widely utilized and trusted noninvasive methodology for the assessment of cardiovascular disease. Single-photon emission computed tomographic (SPECT) and positron emission tomography (PET) techniques assessing coronary perfusion and left ventricular systolic function are widely used in clinical practice. The recent emergence of newer technologies such as cardiac MRI and coronary CT angiography represents a significant challenge to the dominance of nuclear imaging techniques in the routine assessment of cardiovascular disease in clinical practice.

Assessment of Left Ventricular Function

ECG-gated SPECT allows for the assessment of spatial changes in myocardial activity across the cardiac cycle, hence, determination of regional and global myocardial contraction. This technique, routinely using ^{99m}Technetium-labeled tracers, allows for the reproducible quantification of left ventricular volumes, hence, ejection fraction. Such information may be valuable in the serial assessment of systolic function in various cardiomyopathies, particularly those associated with the use of potentially cardiotoxic chemotherapeutic agents. Unlike echocardiography, such techniques are unable to assess diastolic cardiac function, potentially preventing the detection of cardiac injury at an earlier stage.

Myocardial Perfusion Imaging

The exclusion of significant coronary artery disease (CAD) remains a critical consideration in the evaluation of dyspnea, with or without chest pain. As mentioned previously, silent myocardial ischemia is increasingly prevalent in diabetic and elderly patients, but appears to portend a negative prognostic impact similar to symptomatic CAD. Myocardial perfusion imaging (MPI), whether utilizing SPECT or PET techniques, confers a quantitative evaluation of regional myocardial blood flow that has significant therapeutic and prognostic utility. CAD should always be considered in the investigation of dyspnea, particularly where pulmonary function is normal and left ventricular imaging is also normal, particularly if imaging reveals regional wall motion abnormalities indicative of previous ischemic insult. The recent incorporation of coronary CT angiography into the SPECT assessment of myocardial perfusion using combined scanners has added substantially to the utility of this technology, although the clinical role and broader radiation safety of such an approach remains to be determined.

Myocardial Viability

The comparison of regional myocardial perfusion and contractility with SPECT and PET allows identification of dysfunctional, but viable myocardium. Of particular relevance, in the context of chronic coronary ischemia, the historical presumption that "akinetic equals dead" has been dispelled by substantial nuclear and cardiac magnetic resonance (CMR) research. Techniques for the detection of hibernating myocardium may play a crucial role in optimizing therapy in the breathless patient with left ventricular dysfunction. Such technology assists in the prediction of likely clinical benefit from coronary revascularization—whether percutaneous or operative. As such, the evaluation of myocardial viability should become a standard component of the clinical assessment of ischemic cardiomyopathy, particularly where the risks of surgical revascularization are increased—e.g., elderly, renal impairment, or coexistent pulmonary disease.

SPECT techniques for the detection of myocardial viability are well established. Late redistribution images using thallium-201 and technetium-99m analogs allows identification of persistent tracer within viable myocardial cells, with relative signal paucity in nonviable tissue. More sensitive than Dobutamine stress echocardiography, SPECT suffers from relatively low spatial resolution, leading to lower specificity than most other techniques.[16] Of note, SPECT has been demonstrated to be relatively insensitive for the detection of prior sub-endocardial infarction in comparison to CMR.[17] Moreover, tissue attenuation artifacts and radiation exposure remain significant limitations for this technique.

PET appears particularly robust for the detection of both myocardial hypoperfusion and cellular viability, with superior spatial resolution and reduced attenuation artefact in comparison to SPECT. Previously regarded as the gold standard technique for this indication, PET remains limited by scanner and imaging tracer availability. Diagnostic accuracy is comparable to CMR techniques, with PET results identified to have significant prognostic import in the management of patients with ischemic left ventricular dysfunction.

Both SPECT and PET techniques have also been used to identify cardiac sarcoidosis with high clinical accuracy.[18] As such, nuclear imaging techniques may play an important role in the extended evaluation of nonischemic cardiomyopathy, or in the exclusion of cardiac involvement in this condition.

Thromboembolic Pulmonary Vascular Disease

Pulmonary embolus is a common cause of dyspnea in the hospital setting, but may also be seen in ambulatory patients, with or without clinical features of deep venous thrombosis. In recent years, ventilation/perfusion scintigraphy (V/Q) has been largely superseded by the emergence of CT-pulmonary angiography (CTPA) as the preferred method for the exclusion of acute pulmonary embolus. The higher sensitivity and specificity of CTPA, and the reduction in nondiagnostic results has ensured a wane in the popularity of pulmonary scintigraphy. Recent evidence has confirmed V/Q as a viable alternative to CTPA, particularly where renal dysfunction or allergy to iodinated contrast may make CTPA disadvantageous.[19]

Of note, V/Q scanning appears to have a particularly useful place in the exclusion of *chronic* pulmonary thromboembolic disease in the context of chronic pulmonary hypertension, or chronic thromboembolic pulmonary hypertension (CTEPH). With substantially greater sensitivity (97% vs 51%) and comparable specificity (90–95% vs 99%) to CTPA,[20] current pulmonary hypertension guidelines recommend V/Q scintigraphy as the initial test for the differentiation of CTEPH and idiopathic pulmonary arterial hypertension (Figure 16.5).[21] False positive V/Q results may, however, be seen in pulmonary veno-occlusive disease, so HRCT may then be utilized as a secondary investigation to exclude other pathological processes.

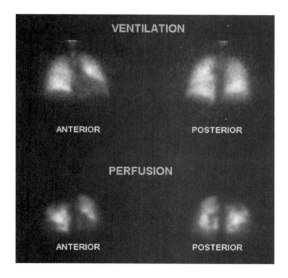

Figure 16.5

V/Q scintigraphy revealing homogenous pulmonary ventilation, but focal, patchy defects in pulmonary perfusion—so called V/Q mismatch. Such findings are highly suggestive of multiple, bilateral pulmonary emboli.

Shunt Quantification

Nuclear scintigraphy with ^{99m}Tc-labeled macro-aggregated albumin may be used in dyspneic patients to detect and quantify right to left shunts where other imaging modalities have suggested such pathology is possible. Although passage of these particles is precluded through the normal pulmonary circulation, arteriovenous malformations, and anatomic communications allowing right to left shunting will allow passage of the labeled albumin into the systemic circulation, where it may be detected and quantified. Although invasive investigation is preferred in the exclusion of pulmonary to systemic shunting, this technique may be of use in selected cases.

Limitations

Nuclear cardiology, like most noninvasive technologies, is widely acknowledged to suffer from potential diagnostic inaccuracy, particularly with respect to myocardial perfusion imaging. Regardless of such concerns, a negative MPI study portends a very low rate of death or non-fatal myocardial infarction—approximately 1% per year.[22] Tissue attenuation is also widely acknowledged as a common cause of false positive results (e.g., due to abdominal obesity or breast tissue). Although methods exist to compensate for this phenomenon, it remains a significant clinical issue in many centers.

CARDIAC MAGNETIC RESONANCE IMAGING

Cardiac magnetic resonance is an exciting, emerging technology able to provide high-resolution cardiac and vascular imaging, overcoming many of the limitations of routine echocardiography and other available imaging modalities. Indeed, CMR is now widely acknowledged as the noninvasive gold standard for the assessment of cardiac systolic function. CMR is particularly suited to the reproducible assessment of systolic ventricular function, identification of RWMAs and quantification of myocardial mass. Congenital defects, cardiac tumors, and pericardial disease are also well assessed by this technique. Additionally, dedicated CMR imaging sequences can be used to accurately quantify flow, enabling reproducible assessment of cardiac output, intracardiac shunts, and valvular function.

The addition of gadolinium-based contrast agents further enhances this technology, improving detection and identification of cardiac masses and intra-cardiac thrombus, as well as allowing quantitative assessment of regional myocardial perfusion in combination with pharmacologic cardiac stressors such as adenosine. Gadolinium-based CMR angiography is particularly useful in the identification and characterization of vascular abnormalities—whether congenital or acquired.

Perhaps the greatest development offered by gadolinium-enhanced CMR imaging is in the identification and quantification of myocardial fibrosis. Delayed-contrast-enhanced imaging takes advantage of the differential in gadolinium contrast wash-out between viable and nonviable myocardial tissue, allowing near-pathology-quality delineation of myocardial fibrosis and prior infarction. Such information is of great utility in the assessment of dyspnea and cardiomyopathies, particularly where disease is subclinical, but of significant prognostic importance (e.g., the detection of arrhythmogenic right ventricular cardiomyopathy in a deceased proband's siblings).

Left Ventricular Structure and Function

CMR's greatest strength in the assessment of cardiac structure is in its excellent contrast between blood pool and myocardium. Where poor endocardial border definition is often a significant factor in the interpretation of echocardiographic images, both black and bright blood CMR sequences allow for the accurate and reproducible assessment of cardiac structure. Although predominantly performed during breath-holding, respiratory gating/averaging can be utilized to acquire images in free-breathing patients, although image quality may be less robust.

Measures of systolic function including stroke volume, LVEF, and cardiac output are reproducibly determined by ECG-gated cine CMR sequences (Figure 16.6). Moreover, because of the systematic assessment of the entire heart, areas of regional hypokinesis can often be detected with greater clarity than by trans-thoracic echocardiography. In particular, the left ventricular apex is more reliably assessed by CMR, allowing for greater sensitivity in the detection of apical intracardiac thrombus that may be missed by other imaging modalities.

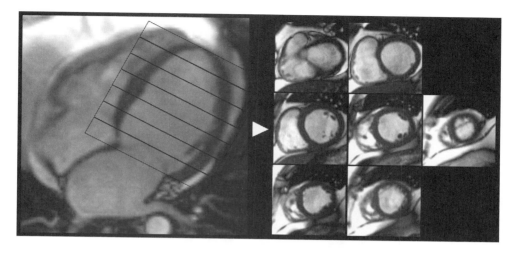

Figure 16.6

CMR assessment of LVEF. The ventricle is divided into evenly spaced short-axis slices, with endocardial and epicardial borders traced (manually or semiautomated) at end-diastole and end-systole to derive myocardial mass, end-diastolic and end-systolic volumes, and hence stroke volume and ejection fraction.

Assessment of Valvular Function and Intracardiac Shunts

CMR is emerging as a robust technology for the assessment of valvular heart disease, but echocardiography remains the preferred method in most patients. Dyspnea caused by valvular dysfunction may be detected by cine CMR as a disruption of normal laminar flow at the level of the dysfunctional valve. Moreover, cine CMR may be used for the high-resolution planimetry of stenotic and regurgitation valves to determine orifice dimensions. Of greatest interest in the determination of valvular disease severity by CMR is the emergence of velocity-encoded sequences to quantitatively assess blood flow. Such sequences allow for the accurate determination of peak stenotic valve flow velocity and valvular regurgitant volumes in the evaluation of valvular heart disease severity. CMR, however, even more so than echo, is significantly disadvantaged by the presence of multi-valve disease.

In addition to the sensitive identification of intracardiac shunting through high-resolution cine imaging, velocity-encoded CMR allows for the accurate quantification of intracardiac shunt severity through the quantification of left and right ventricular outputs (Qp:Qs). CMR has particular utility in the assessment of dyspnea caused by an atrial or ventricular septal defect, able not only to quantify shunt direction and severity, but also provide high-quality structural information regarding septal defect margins useful in guiding potential percutaneous or operative closure. As mentioned previously, significant

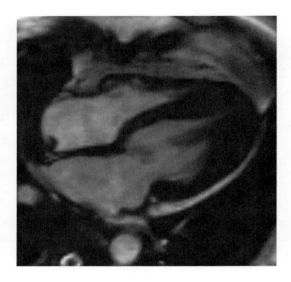

Figure 16.7

Apical HCM demonstrated by CMR. The spade-shaped ventricle and apical myocardial hypertrophy are classical features easily identifiable by CMR.

regurgitant valvular disease, however, limits the accuracy of this, and other, CMR flow techniques.

Right Ventricular Structure and Function

Right ventricular function may be adversely affected by a variety of cardiovascular conditions. Impairment of right ventricular function may have significant prognostic implications in the presence of pulmonary arterial hypertension (both acute and chronic) and cardiomyopathy of ischemic, valvular, and congenital etiology. Frequently considered the forgotten ventricle, right ventricular function can now be accurately assessed by CMR, overcoming many of the previous limitations caused by the asymmetric geometry of this chamber.

Although highly preload dependent, right ventricular volumes and ejection fraction may be reproducibly assessed by cine CMR sequences. Larger than the left ventricle, the normal RV ejection fraction ranges from 47–76% by CMR, with normal volumes varying with gender. Additionally, right ventricular myocardial mass may be quantified by cine CMR for the serial measurement in right ventricular pressure-overload states with dedicated flow sequences used to accurately quantify valvular regurgitation and/or stenosis severity.

Cardiac Ischemia

Adenosine (vasodilator) stress perfusion CMR (with gadolinium) and dobutamine (wall-motion) stress CMR have emerged as new, highly accurate methods for the noninvasive functional assessment of cardiac ischemia. With image quality superior to dobutamine stress echocardiography and markedly improved spatial resolution in comparison to stress SPECT methodologies, these techniques continue to gain increasing favor worldwide for their high diagnostic accuracy.[23,24] Importantly, a negative CMR stress test has highly favorable prognostic implications, with very low rates of cardiac death or nonfatal MI (< 1% at 3 years follow-up).[25] Not only useful for the assessment of regional myocardial ischemia, the viability of regions of previous myocardial infarction can be accurately determined through the addition of delayed-contrast enhanced imaging sequences following gadolinium administration. While cost-effective analyses and longer-term clinical end-point data continue to emerge, these two CMR methodologies offer great promise in the evaluation of regional myocardial ischemia and viability.

Myocardial Inflammation, Infiltration, Fibrosis, and Viability

Myocarditis is associated with myocardial inflammation, hence increased interstitial edema, which is readily detected by T2-weighted CMR sequences.[26] Moreover, inflamed myocardium clears gadolinium slower than noninflamed myocardium, allowing for detection of delayed-enhancement imaging. Focal or patchy hyperenhancement is common in myocarditis, usually in a midwall or subepicardial distribution—as distinct from the subendocardial or transmural distribution of cardiac ischemia.

Hypertrophic and infiltrative/restrictive cardiomyopathies are readily characterized by a combination of cine and contrast-enhanced CMR sequences. Detection of classical hypertrophic cardiomyopathy (HCM) is usually possible by echocardiography, however CMR offers the capacity for serial monitoring of myocardial mass and for the demonstration of myocardial fibrosis, features that have been associated with increased risk for disease progression and sudden cardiac death.[27] Moreover, the detection and characterization of obesity and diabetes-related cardiac dysfunction due to cardiac steatosis has also emerged as a strength of CMR in recent years.

Amyloidosis, sarcoidosis, and rarer forms of myocardial infiltration can be readily detected by delayed contrast-enhanced CMR imaging, in addition to the identification of indirect features of myocardial restriction by cine sequences (such as biatrial enlargement and reduced atrial flow velocity). Gadolinium enhancement is generally globally subendocardial or diffuse in amyloidosis, with a patchy mid-wall and subepicardial distribution in sarcoidosis. Other infiltrative cardiomyopathies have similarly suggestive delayed-enhancement patterns, with CMR potentially contributing substantially to a definitive, etiological diagnosis in breathless patients with evidence of diastolic dysfunction on echocardiography.

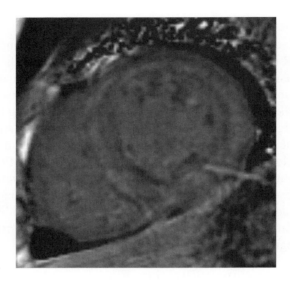

Figure 16.8

Image of advanced myocardial amyloid infiltration. The impaired "nulling" of the blood-pool (gray rather than bright) and "washed out" myocardium are highly suggestive of amyloid infiltration. Additionally, the diffuse myocardial enhancement and "zebra" appearance (best seen over the anterior and lateral walls) are also pathognomonic of amyloid infiltration.

An important use of CMR is the differentiation of ischemic and nonischemic processes in patients with systolic left ventricular impairment. Specifically, nonischemic dilated cardiomyopathy (DCM) may be differentiated from ischemic cardiomyopathy by the absence of subendocardial enhancement following gadolinium administration. A small percentage of idiopathic DCM patients may, demonstrate patchy mid-wall or subepicardial fibrosis by CMR instead,[28] with some recent evidence suggesting such fibrotic changes may portend a poorer prognosis. The addition of low-dose dobutamine stress further enhances the accuracy of CMR viability studies, with a failure of hyperkinesis with dobutamine associated with poorer regional functional recovery in the context of moderate local delayed contrast enhancement.

Pericardial Disease

CMR has emerged as a highly useful technology for the differentiation of myocardial restriction from pericardial constriction in the breathless/congested patient. Although both conditions may cause symptoms of diastolic cardiac impairment, accurate diagnosis is critical to the targeted treatment of symptomatic patients. CMR is a robust method for the evaluation of pericardial thickness and regional fibrosis with pericardial thickness > 4mm associated with > 90% accuracy in the diagnosis of chronic pericarditis.[29] More robust is the real-time, dynamic assessment of right and left ventricular chamber dimensions during free-breathing CMR. Not only is CMR useful in the demonstration of respiratory variation in ventricular volumes, but constriction is often associated with a classical pattern of abnormal septal motion in early diastole that is helpful in distinguishing constriction from restriction.[30]

Pulmonary Vascular Disease

Contrast-enhanced pulmonary MRA currently has an emerging but limited role in the evaluation of acute pulmonary embolus,[31] particularly the acutely dyspneic patient where breath-hold imaging is impractical. In the evaluation of chronic pulmonary hypertension, CMR continues to show promise however. Importantly, CMR remains the method of choice for the serial assessment of right ventricular size and function, factors that have significant prognostic implications. Pulmonary artery compliance and other novel indices of pulmonary vascular reactivity continue to emerge but remain experimental. Moreover, advances in MR imaging, including the development of ventilation/perfusion scanning using contrast-enhanced MR sequences in combination with inhalation of hyper-polarised noble gases, promises a substantially increased future role for MRI in the evaluation of pulmonary hypertension secondary to chronic thromboembolic disease.[32]

CMR Conclusion

Whether in the detection of cardiac structural or functional derangement, or the exclusion of silent myocardial ischemia or previous myocardial infarction, CMR offers substantial clinical utility in the extended assessment of the dyspneic patient.

Limitations of CMR

Diastolic Cardiac Function

Although imaging sequences to duplicate the echocardiographic assessments of mitral valve inflow are relatively robust, sequences evaluating mitral annulus motion in the evaluation of diastolic cardiac impairment remain experimental at this time. Thus, diastolic left ventricular impairment is not well-assessed utilizing current clinical CMR sequences.

Metallic Implants

Implanted or embedded ferromagnetic material is a potential contraindication to CMR. Coronary stents, ASD/PFO closure devices, and most mechanical valves have been safely imaged at 1.5 Tesla, although debate persists regarding the MR safety of some such devices immediately postimplantation and with greater-strength clinical magnets (e.g., 3 Tesla). Magnetic resonance imaging may have significant effects on the electronic function of pacemakers and AICD or may induce an electromagnetic current along the device leads, potentially impairing accurate device sensing, or causing local tissue heating and injury that may impair subsequent device function. Although patients with these devices have been safely scanned under controlled circumstances, such imaging is best performed in experienced centers and only with robust clinical indication. Although safety is paramount, image quality may be significantly impaired by the presence of intrathoracic metallic implants, although sternotomy wires rarely cause clinically meaningful image artifact.

Patient Factors

CMR assessment of cardiac function is highly patient-dependent. Ideally, patients need to be able to understand and comply with simple breathing instructions, with most cardiac sequences assessing dynamic function requiring a 5–15 second expiratory breath-hold (depending on heart rate, patient size, and imaging sequence). Although advances in CMR imaging have markedly improved the temporal resolution of cine studies such that many sequences can now be modified to accommodate free breathing, image quality is generally less robust.

Furthermore, the presence of frequent ventricular ectopy may dramatically reduce image quality, potentially leading to nondiagnostic images. The variable R-R intervals associated with atrial fibrillation also represents a significant obstacle to the use of CMR in the evaluation of breathlessness; however, this issue can often be overcome if the heart rate is well controlled. Claustrophobia is an impediment to imaging in some patients, with approximately 2% of patients unable to tolerate the CMR environment for this reason. Additionally, acutely dyspneic patients are poorly suited to the CMR environment, for many of the reasons stated above. As such, this investigation complements, rather than replaces, echocardiography in the assessment of the underlying etiology of acute and chronic dyspnea.

Nephrogenic Systemic Fibrosis

Although gadolinium-based contrast agents have previously been preferred over potentially nephrotoxic iodine-based agents in patients with renal impairment, gadolinium chelates have recently been associated with a potentially fatal fibrotic condition called Nephrogenic Systemic Fibrosis (NSF). Although still controversial, this condition is believed to occur because of impaired renal clearance of gadolinium-chelate, intravascular dissociation of free gadolinium (a heavy metal) and subsequent deposition in systemic tissues, most notably skin.[33] The FDA and other regulatory bodies have recommended against gadolinium-based contrast administration in patients with glomerular filtration rates (GFR) less than $30mL/min/1.73m^2$, or in the presence of acute renal failure and acute inflammatory states.[2,34] Incidence is estimated at 2.4–3.0% per gadolinium exposure, although severity of underlying renal dysfunction, concurrent inflammatory illness, and gadolinium-dose and -agent are significant contributing factors.[34,35]

COMPUTED TOMOGRAPHY

Computed tomography is used extensively for the high-resolution diagnostic evaluation of pulmonary parenchymal pathology in dyspneic patients. In addition, the field of cardiovascular CT has advanced significantly, related to progressive improvements in image acquisition. Reduced imaging time has resulted in markedly improved image resolution when assessing cardiac structures, despite continuous cardiac motion. Coronary imaging, in particular, has become commonplace, and offers an exciting noninvasive alternative to traditional invasive coronary angiography in the assessment of low- to intermediate-risk chest pain. Radiation dose remains a significant concern in younger patients, and women in particular, because of concerns regarding increased lifetime cancer risk.[36] Despite this, CT provides high-resolution imaging of coronary, systemic, and pulmonary vascular beds and is able to diagnose, or exclude, numerous causes of dyspnea and chest pain.

Coronary Artery Disease

Coronary artery disease should be considered a potential contributor to, or cause of, breathlessness. Myocardial ischemia secondary to significant coronary stenoses is a common, potent cause of myocardial systolic and diastolic dysfunction. Moreover, silent myocardial ischemia presenting as breathlessness is common in diabetic, hypertensive and elderly patients, with evidence indicating a poorer prognosis in such patients. Coronary CT angiography may provide useful noninvasive information regarding coronary anatomy; however, functional imaging of ischemic territories using CT perfusion sequences remains largely experimental. CT imaging of coronary artery bypass grafts (saphenous vein grafts in particular) is often useful in the breathless patient following previous cardiac surgery.

Coronary CTA has also been advocated in the exclusion of congenital coronary abnormalities that may be associated with chest pain, breathlessness, or syncope. The radiation associated with CT lends support to the use of coronary imaging by CMR for this purpose instead (where available), given the usually young age of such patients.

Cardiac Structure and Function

Cardiac CT is able to provide excellent tissue definition in the identification of abnormalities of cardiac anatomy. Left ventricular size and mass, valvular and atrial anatomy, and pulmonary arteries and veins are all reproducibly assessed by CT. The aorta, in particular, is usually very well visualized by CT, with aortic dissection, intramural hematoma, or aortic perforation accurately excluded by CT angiographic techniques.

By extension, cardiac structure can be assessed repeatedly across the cardiac cycle to derive an accurate assessment of cardiac function. Such an approach is comparable in accuracy to CMR; however, radiation dose rises significantly with this approach. As such, CT should not be considered a first-line investigation for the assessment of cardiac anatomy and function.

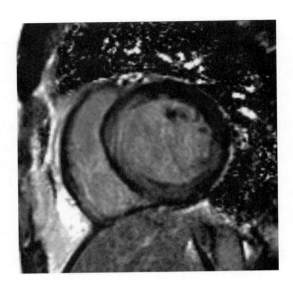

Figure 16.9

Sarcoid cardiomyopathy indicated by extensive, patchy subendocardial and transmural myocardial hyperenhancement in a noncoronary distribution in a patient with hilar lymphadenopathy and pulmonary nodules.

Pericardial Disease

CT is particularly useful in the assessment of pericardial disease in the investigation of the dyspneic patient. The pericardium is usually evident as a thin (1–2mm) structure of soft-tissue density overlying the heart from the insertion of the great vessels to the diaphragm (where it normally thickens to 3–4mm). Epicardial adiposity and pericardial effusions may accentuate the usually thin space separating parietal and visceral pericardial layers; however, CT is particularly useful in the assessment of parietal pericardial anatomy. Focal or more generalized thickening (with or without pericardial calcification) may be a particularly useful finding in a breathless patient with otherwise apparently normal cardiac structure and function by echocardiography. Moreover, cardiac CT (or CMR) should be considered in all cases of presumed pericardial constriction—particularly where echocardiographic Doppler indices are inconclusive. The presence of pericardial thickening (> 4mm) alone is insufficient for the diagnosis of pericardial constriction and must be supported by real-time functional assessment during respiration—an area where CMR has markedly greater utility than CT—or by invasive cardiac hemodynamics.

CT (like CMR) may also demonstrate abnormalities of mediastinal or pulmonary parenchymal anatomy that may infiltrate the pericardium—including neoplasms or infections (e.g., tuberculosis) that are usually not evident on routine transthoracic echocardiography.

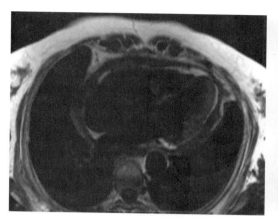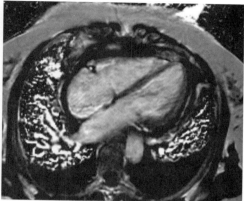

Figure 16.10

Black-blood and post-contrast phase-encoded CMR images indicating the grossly thickened pericardium, right atrial enlargement, and bilateral pleural effusions of pericardial constriction.

Pulmonary Arterial Disease

It is clear that chest CT is the investigation of choice in the exclusion of significant pulmonary parenchymal abnormalities that may contribute to acute or chronic breathlessness. The exclusion of pulmonary thromboemboli should be considered in all acutely, and chronically, breathless patients—particularly where an alternative diagnosis is elusive.

Substantial literature has been devoted to the comparison of CTPA and V/Q SPECT with regard to the most accurate method for detecting PE, with CTPA generally preferred.[37] The diagnostic accuracy of each technology is tied to the pretest probability of PE based on patient clinical factors and biomarkers such as D-dimer results. Numerous scoring systems have been developed to assist clinicians in choosing the most appropriate diagnostic and therapeutic course.[38] Sensitivity for CTPA and V/Q is comparable in patients with normal lung fields on chest x-ray; however, nondiagnostic findings are more common in V/Q scans, particularly in the presence of coexisting cardiopulmonary disease.

CT pulmonary angiography (with contrast) provides high diagnostic accuracy in the assessment of pulmonary emboli, particularly where there is a high pretest clinical suspicion. It has been acknowledged that smaller PE in the more distal, subsegmental pulmonary arteries may be missed by CTPA, though these are less common entities. In PIOPED-II[39], the addition of venous phase CT of the proximal leg veins (CTV) to exclude deep venous thrombosis improved the sensitivity of PE detection (90% vs 83% for CTPA alone), with similar specificity (95% vs 96%). Although still imperfect, a negative CTPA portends a very favorable prognosis, regardless of therapy.[40,41] Additional investigation should always be considered in cases where the level of clinical suspicion is inconsistent with the findings of diagnostic imaging.

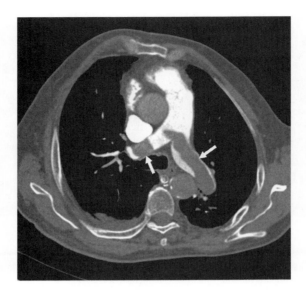

Figure 16.11

CTPA demonstrating two large thromboemboli (represented by contrast filling defects—arrows) within the right and left pulmonary arteries, with an associated small right pleural effusion.

Hemodynamic instability is widely acknowledged as a poor prognostic indicator in the presence of acute PE. Cardiac biomarker data (BNP, cardiac troponin) provide further utility in clinical risk prediction, with elevations of BNP (odds ratio [OR] 9.5), pro-BNP (OR 5.7), and troponin (OR 8.3) associated with substantially increased risk of premature death.[42] Significantly, evidence of asymptomatic right ventricular dysfunction on CT (or echocardiography) is also associated with significantly increased patient mortality, even in hemodynamically stable patients (OR 2.4)[42] and as such, RV dimensions should be assessed in all cases of large pulmonary emboli.

Triple Rule-Out

Much fanfare has been associated with CT in the investigation of chest pain and breathlessness due to the ability of CT to image multiple vascular beds in one sitting. The triple rule-out—exclusion of pulmonary embolus, significant coronary artery disease, and aortic dissection—has been advocated by CT proponents as a noninvasive holy grail for the evaluation of acute chest pain and breathlessness. Associated with increased imaging radiation exposure (to adequately image each of the relevant vascular beds), this investigation has been considered a groper-gram by detractors. On balance, such an approach should only be considered in patients with truly nonspecific clinical features and intermediate to high clinical suspicion, rather than as a routine investigation in all-comers.[43]

Limitations

Radiation

Medical radiation doses have become increasingly scrutinized in recent years, particularly in the context of the burgeoning of CT imaging indications. A not-insignificant lifetime risk of secondary malignancy has been predicted related to diagnostic radiation—particularly in women and younger individuals and for combined cardiac and aortic scans.[36] Improved clinician awareness will play a critical role in minimizing harm from diagnostic studies, and alternative-imaging methodologies such as MRI should be considered (if appropriate), particularly where serial imaging is required.

Contrast Nephropathy

Most cardiovascular CT sequences require the administration of intravenous iodinated contrast. Depending on clinical risk factors (baseline creatinine clearance, presence of diabetes, dehydration, acute illness, etc.), such exposure may have an attendant risk of contrast nephropathy. Although generally self-limited, often this process may go unnoticed, particularly in the outpatient setting where monitoring of renal function is less likely. Coadministration of metformin and other such agents is associated with a markedly increased risk of morbidity in the presence of contrast nephropathy, so care should be taken to consider this possibility in at-risk individuals, and an alternative methodology be considered where appropriate.

Arrhythmia

Although advances have been made in ECG-triggering and off-line reconstruction of CT images, elevated heart rates (> 70 beats per minute), and arrhythmias such as atrial fibrillation and frequent ventricular ectopy often lead to inferior image quality for many cardiac indications. Coronary imaging, in particular, is prone to nondiagnostic imaging in the context of short or irregular R-R intervals. The use of intravenous beta-blockers to slow heart rates and the increasing scan speeds associated with newer CT models (e.g., coronary CTA by 320-slice scanners can now image the whole heart in a single gantry revolution) are expected to lessen this issue substantially in the future.

Incidentalomas

Cardiac CT is becomingly increasingly prevalent in the evaluation of chest pain and breathlessness, in outpatient and emergency department settings. Due to the nature of the investigation, generally a much larger region of anatomy is imaged than is specifically intended. This frequently results in the identification of incidental findings, particularly in elderly patients (up to 40% of cases).[44] Although more than 50% of acute chest pain presentations have a noncardiac source, such incidental findings are often asymptomatic. Identification may trigger substantial patient anxiety and additional investigation, however. Care should be taken to consider this in the choice of imaging investigation—don't look if you don't want to find.

CONCLUSION

Dyspnea, whether acute or chronic, often poses a difficult diagnostic quandary for the clinician. This is particularly true in elderly, comorbid patients where multiple factors may contribute to symptom severity. Meticulous history taking and clinical examination remain at the heart of a successful clinical assessment of the dyspneic patient. That said, imaging plays a crucial role in the determination of organ involvement and disease severity, with results guiding appropriate therapeutic advice and management. Although routine investigations such as the CXR and echocardiography will remain highly valuable components of this assessment, continued advances in noninvasive imaging will ensure CT, MRI, and nuclear techniques will continue to evolve as the new standard of care.

◇◇◇◇◇◇◇◇◇◇◇◇◇

REFERENCES

1. Petrie MC. It cannot be cardiac failure because the heart is not enlarged on the chest X-ray. *Eur J Heart Fail* 2003;5:117-9.
2. Swedberg K, Cleland J, Dargie H, Drexler H, Follath F, Komajda M, Tavazzi L, Smiseth OA, Gavazzi A, Haverich A, Hoes A, Jaarsma T, Korewicki J, Levy S, Linde C, Lopez-Sendon JL, Nieminen MS, Pierard L, Remme WJ. Guidelines for the diagnosis and treatment of chronic heart failure: executive summary (update 2005): The Task Force for the Diagnosis and Treatment of Chronic Heart Failure of the European Society of Cardiology. *Eur Heart J* 2005;26:1115-40.
3. Nieminen MS, Brutsaert D, Dickstein K, Drexler H, Follath F, Harjola VP, Hochadel M, Komajda M, Lassus J, Lopez-Sendon JL, Ponikowski P, Tavazzi L. EuroHeart Failure Survey II (EHFS II): a survey on hospitalized acute heart failure patients: description of population. *Eur Heart J* 2006;27:2725-36.
4. Owan TE, Hodge DO, Herges RM, Jacobsen SJ, Roger VL, Redfield MM. Trends in prevalence and outcome of heart failure with preserved ejection fraction. *N Engl J Med* 2006;355:251-9.
5. Sohn DW, Chai IH, Lee DJ, Kim HC, Kim HS, Oh BH, Lee MM, Park YB, Choi YS, Seo JD, Lee YW. Assessment of mitral annulus velocity by Doppler tissue imaging in the evaluation of left ventricular diastolic function. *J Am Coll Cardiol* 1997;30:474-80.
6. Yu CM, Sanderson JE, Marwick TH, Oh JK. Tissue Doppler imaging a new prognosticator for cardiovascular diseases. *J Am Coll Cardiol* 2007;49:1903-14.
7. Paulus WJ, Tschope C, Sanderson JE, Rusconi C, Flachskampf FA, Rademakers FE, Marino P, Smiseth OA, De Keulenaer G, Leite-Moreira AF, Borbely A, Edes I, Handoko ML, Heymans S, Pezzali N, Pieske B, Dickstein K, Fraser AG, Brutsaert DL. How to diagnose diastolic heart failure: a consensus statement on the diagnosis of heart failure with normal left ventricular ejection fraction by the Heart Failure and Echocardiography Associations of the European Society of Cardiology. *Eur Heart J* 2007;28:2539-50.
8. Appleton CP, Galloway JM, Gonzalez MS, Gaballa M, Basnight MA. Estimation of left ventricular filling pressures using two-dimensional and Doppler echocardiography in adult patients with cardiac disease. Additional value of analyzing left atrial size, left atrial ejection fraction and the difference in duration of pulmonary venous and mitral flow velocity at atrial contraction. *J Am Coll Cardiol* 1993;22:1972-82.
9. Basnight MA, Gonzalez MS, Kershenovich SC, Appleton CP. Pulmonary venous flow velocity: relation to hemodynamics, mitral flow velocity and left atrial volume, and ejection fraction. *J Am Soc Echocardiogr* 1991;4:547-58.
10. Sousa AC. Left atrial volume as an index of diastolic function. *Arq Bras Cardiol* 2006;87:e27-33.
11. Benjamin EJ, D'Agostino RB, Belanger AJ, Wolf PA, Levy D. Left atrial size and the risk of stroke and death. The Framingham Heart Study. *Circulation* 1995;92:835-41.
12. Modena MG, Muia N, Sgura FA, Molinari R, Castella A, Rossi R. Left atrial size is the major predictor of

cardiac death and overall clinical outcome in patients with dilated cardiomyopathy: a long-term follow-up study. *Clin Cardiol* 1997;20:553-60.

13. Vaziri SM, Larson MG, Benjamin EJ, Levy D. Echocardiographic predictors of nonrheumatic atrial fibrillation. The Framingham Heart Study. *Circulation* 1994;89:724-30.

14. Bonow RO, Carabello BA, Kanu C, de Leon AC, Jr., Faxon DP, Freed MD, Gaasch WH, Lytle BW, Nishimura RA, O'Gara PT, O'Rourke RA, Otto CM, Shah PM, Shanewise JS, Smith SC, Jr., Jacobs AK, Adams CD, Anderson JL, Antman EM, Faxon DP, Fuster V, Halperin JL, Hiratzka LF, Hunt SA, Lytle BW, Nishimura R, Page RL, Riegel B. ACC/AHA 2006 guidelines for the management of patients with valvular heart disease: a report of the American College of Cardiology/American Heart Association Task Force on Practice Guidelines (writing committee to revise the 1998 Guidelines for the Management of Patients With Valvular Heart Disease): developed in collaboration with the Society of Cardiovascular Anesthesiologists: endorsed by the Society for Cardiovascular Angiography and Interventions and the Society of Thoracic Surgeons. *Circulation* 2006;114:e84-231.

15. Jenkins C, Bricknell K, Hanekom L, Marwick TH. Reproducibility and accuracy of echocardiographic measurements of left ventricular parameters using real-time three-dimensional echocardiography. *J Am Coll Cardiol* 2004;44:878-86.

16. Camici PG, Prasad SK, Rimoldi OE. Stunning, hibernation, and assessment of myocardial viability. *Circulation* 2008;117:103-14.

17. Wagner A, Mahrholdt H, Holly TA, Elliott MD, Regenfus M, Parker M, Klocke FJ, Bonow RO, Kim RJ, Judd RM. Contrast-enhanced MRI and routine single photon emission computed tomography (SPECT) perfusion imaging for detection of subendocardial myocardial infarcts: an imaging study. *Lancet* 2003;361:374-9.

18. Nishiyama Y, Yamamoto Y, Fukunaga K, Takinami H, Iwado Y, Satoh K, Ohkawa M. Comparative evaluation of 18F-FDG PET and 67Ga scintigraphy in patients with sarcoidosis. *J Nucl Med* 2006;47:1571-6.

19. Sostman HD, Stein PD, Gottschalk A, Matta F, Hull R, Goodman L. Acute pulmonary embolism: sensitivity and specificity of ventilation-perfusion scintigraphy in PIOPED II study. *Radiology* 2008;246:941-6.

20. Tunariu N, Gibbs SJ, Win Z, Gin-Sing W, Graham A, Gishen P, Al-Nahhas A. Ventilation-perfusion scintigraphy is more sensitive than multidetector CTPA in detecting chronic thromboembolic pulmonary disease

as a treatable cause of pulmonary hypertension. *J Nucl Med* 2007;48:680-4.

21. Galie N, Torbicki A, Barst R, Dartevelle P, Haworth S, Higenbottam T, Olschewski H, Peacock A, Pietra G, Rubin LJ, Simonneau G, Priori SG, Garcia MA, Blanc JJ, Budaj A, Cowie M, Dean V, Deckers J, Burgos EF, Lekakis J, Lindahl B, Mazzotta G, McGregor K, Morais J, Oto A, Smiseth OA, Barbera JA, Gibbs S, Hoeper M, Humbert M, Naeije R, Pepke-Zaba J. Guidelines on diagnosis and treatment of pulmonary arterial hypertension. The Task Force on Diagnosis and Treatment of Pulmonary Arterial Hypertension of the European Society of Cardiology. *Eur Heart J* 2004;25:2243-78.

22. Iskander S, Iskandrian AE. Risk assessment using single-photon emission computed tomographic technetium-99m sestamibi imaging. *J Am Coll Cardiol* 1998;32:57-62.

23. Nagel E, Lehmkuhl HB, Bocksch W, Klein C, Vogel U, Frantz E, Ellmer A, Dreysse S, Fleck E. Noninvasive diagnosis of ischemia-induced wall motion abnormalities with the use of high-dose dobutamine stress MRI: comparison with dobutamine stress echocardiography. *Circulation* 1999;99:763-70.

24. Watkins S, Oldroyd KG, Frohwein S. Magnetic resonance myocardial perfusion imaging: a new era in the detection of reversible myocardial ischemia. *Heart* 2007;93:7-10.

25. Jahnke C, Nagel E, Gebker R, Kokocinski T, Kelle S, Manka R, Fleck E, Paetsch I. Prognostic value of cardiac magnetic resonance stress tests: adenosine stress perfusion and dobutamine stress wall motion imaging. *Circulation* 2007;115:1769-76.

26. Ordovas KG, Reddy GP, Higgins CB. MRI in nonischemic acquired heart disease. *J Magn Reson Imaging* 2008;27:1195-1213.

27. Moon JC, McKenna WJ, McCrohon JA, Elliott PM, Smith GC, Pennell DJ. Toward clinical risk assessment in hypertrophic cardiomyopathy with gadolinium cardiovascular magnetic resonance. *J Am Coll Cardiol* 2003;41:1561-7.

28. McCrohon JA, Moon JC, Prasad SK, McKenna WJ, Lorenz CH, Coats AJ, Pennell DJ. Differentiation of heart failure related to dilated cardiomyopathy and coronary artery disease using gadolinium-enhanced cardiovascular magnetic resonance. *Circulation* 2003;108:54-9.

29. Masui T, Finck S, Higgins CB. Constrictive pericarditis and restrictive cardiomyopathy: evaluation with MR imaging. *Radiology* 1992;182:369-73.

30. Giorgi B, Mollet NR, Dymarkowski S, Rademakers FE, Bogaert J. Clinically suspected constrictive pericarditis:

MR imaging assessment of ventricular septal motion and configuration in patients and healthy subjects. *Radiology* 2003;228:417-24.

31. Fink C, Ley S, Schoenberg SO, Reiser MF, Kauczor HU. Magnetic resonance imaging of acute pulmonary embolism. *Eur Radiol* 2007;17:2546-53.

32. Kreitner KF, Kunz RP, Ley S, Oberholzer K, Neeb D, Gast KK, Heussel CP, Eberle B, Mayer E, Kauczor HU, Duber C. Chronic thromboembolic pulmonary hypertension - assessment by magnetic resonance imaging. *Eur Radiol* 2007;17:11-21.

33. Boyd AS, Zic JA, Abraham JL. Gadolinium deposition in nephrogenic fibrosing dermopathy. *J Am Acad Dermatol* 2007;56:27-30.

34. Sadowski EA, Bennett LK, Chan MR, Wentland AL, Garrett AL, Garrett RW, Djamali A. Nephrogenic systemic fibrosis: risk factors and incidence estimation. *Radiology* 2007;243:148-57.

35. Deo A, Fogel M, Cowper SE. Nephrogenic systemic fibrosis: a population study examining the relationship of disease development to gadolinium exposure. *Clin J Am Soc Nephrol* 2007;2:264-7.

36. Einstein AJ, Henzlova MJ, Rajagopalan S. Estimating risk of cancer associated with radiation exposure from 64-slice computed tomography coronary angiography. *Jama* 2007;298:317-23.

37. Stein PD, Woodard PK, Weg JG, Wakefield TW, Tapson VF, Sostman HD, Sos TA, Quinn DA, Leeper KV, Jr., Hull RD, Hales CA, Gottschalk A, Goodman LR, Fowler SE, Buckley JD. Diagnostic pathways in acute pulmonary embolism: recommendations of the PIOPED II Investigators. *Radiology* 2007;242:15-21.

38. Tapson VF. Acute pulmonary embolism. *N Engl J Med* 2008;358:1037-52.

39. Stein PD, Fowler SE, Goodman LR, Gottschalk A, Hales CA, Hull RD, Leeper KV, Jr., Popovich J, Jr., Quinn DA, Sos TA, Sostman HD, Tapson VF, Wakefield TW, Weg JG, Woodard PK. Multidetector computed tomography for acute pulmonary embolism. *N Engl J Med* 2006;354:2317-27.

40. van Belle A, Buller HR, Huisman MV, Huisman PM, Kaasjager K, Kamphuisen PW, Kramer MH, Kruip MJ, Kwakkel-van Erp JM, Leebeek FW, Nijkeuter M, Prins MH, Sohne M, Tick LW. Effectiveness of managing suspected pulmonary embolism using an algorithm combining clinical probability, D-dimer testing, and computed tomography. *Jama* 2006;295:172-9.

41. Quiroz R, Kucher N, Zou KH, Kipfmueller F, Costello P, Goldhaber SZ, Schoepf UJ. Clinical validity of a negative computed tomography scan in patients with suspected pulmonary embolism: a systematic review. *Jama* 2005;293:2012-7.

42. Sanchez O, Trinquart L, Colombet I, Durieux P, Huisman MV, Chatellier G, Meyer G. Prognostic value of right ventricular dysfunction in patients with haemodynamically stable pulmonary embolism: a systematic review. *Eur Heart J* 2008;29:1569-77.

43. Gallagher MJ, Raff GL. Use of multislice CT for the evaluation of emergency room patients with chest pain: the so-called "triple rule-out". *Catheter Cardiovasc Interv* 2008;71:92-9.

44. Burt JR, Iribarren C, Fair JM, Norton LC, Mahbouba M, Rubin GD, Hlatky MA, Go AS, Fortmann SP. Incidental findings on cardiac multidetector row computed tomography among healthy older adults: prevalence and clinical correlates. *Arch Intern Med* 2008;168:756-61.

CHAPTER 17

Congenital Heart Disease Assessment

Karen S.L. Teo, MBBS, PhD, FRACP
Philip J. Kilner, MBBS

INTRODUCTION

Improvements in medical and surgical approaches over the past few decades have allowed for correction of major congenital cardiac defects and the survival of many pediatric patients with congenital heart disease (CHD) into adulthood.[1] It is also important to recognize in adult patients the features of the more common congenital defects that have not been previously diagnosed.[2] In the adult patient without previously known congenital heart disease or surgery, defects that are encountered include: (1) valvular abnormalities such as bicuspid aortic valve, pulmonary stenosis, mitral and tricuspid valve anomalies, (2) left ventricular outflow tract and aorta abnormalities such as subaortic stenosis, supravalvular aortic stenosis, sinus of Valsalva aneuryms, aortic coarctation, (3) septal defects and shunt lesions such as atrial septal defects, ventricular septal defects and patent ductus arteriosus, (4) coronary anomalies and fistulas, and (5) complex congenital heart disease.

The care of the adult patient with congenital heart disease will require the initial assessment of suspected or known CHD, continuing care of patients and in many patients, surgical or nonsurgical intervention. The imaging of congenital heart disease plays a crucial role in both the initial as well as follow-up assessment and management. This has traditionally been with echocardiography, although cardiovascular magnetic resonance (CMR) is playing an increasing role in the assessment of CHD to guide management as it is able to provide functional and morphological information even in complex anatomy.[3] CMR is the gold standard imaging for the assessment of ventricular volumes and function.[4] The use of diagnostic catheterization may also potentially be reduced if information can be obtained with noninvasive imaging such as CMR, which provides information about function and physiology in addition to anatomy.[5]

ECHOCARDIOGRAPHY

Transthoracic echocardiography remains the primary imaging technique for the assessment of simple and complex congenital malformations, particularly in the younger patient or infant. The echocardiographic approach to the assessment of complex congenital heart disease involves the segmental analysis of the heart.[6-8] This approach assesses (1) apex position (2) situs of the atria, (3) atrioventricular relationship, and (4) ventriculoarterial relationship. In valvular abnormalities, echocardiography allows assessment of valvular morphology as well as stenosis and regurgitation severity by echo-Doppler determination of velocity. [9] However, it may be difficult to obtain sufficient information with transthoracic echocardiography in the adolescent and adult population after surgery because the interposition of scar tissue and lungs.[10] Transesphageal echocardiography (TEE), a semi-invasive technique, provides additional diagnostic information that transthoracic echocardiography doesn't including valvular function and shunt assessment.[10] Three-dimensional echocardiography is a new technology that is not widely available, but has the potential to provide unique imaging planes and projections of the septae, atrioventricular, and semilunar valves.[11] Three-dimensional echoacardiography, like CMR, also permits volumetric analyses independent of geometric assumptions.[12]

CARDIOVASCULAR MAGNETIC RESONANCE

The value of CMR in the assessment of congenital heart disease was first recognized in the 1980s.[13, 14] It is free of ionizing radiation and therefore is acceptable for lifelong follow-up. It is uniquely versatile in terms of tissue characterization and measurements of myocardial function and flow.[15] The ability of CMR to image in arbitrary planes complemented by three-dimensional angiography allows it to obtain superior anatomic and functional data, including the right ventricle and pulmonary arteries. CMR is replacing car diac catheterization as the modality of choice for anatomic and functional characterization of congenital heart disease when echocardiographic imaging is inadequate.[16]

ANATOMY ASSESSMENT IN CONGENITAL HEART DISEASE

The anatomy in congenital heart disease can range from simple to complex and may be preoperative or postoperative. In complex congenital heart disease, defining morphology of the atria and ventricles is crucial and requires a systematic examination of the atria, atrioventricular connections, ventricles, and ventriculoarterial connections, as well as conduits and baffles. Although echocardiography may provide this information, in the adult population in particular, poor acoustic windows because of body habitus or interposition of scar or lung tissue may limit adequate images.[5, 10] CMR can acquire images in multiple and complex planes and is not affected by artifacts from calcification or surgical patch materials in the postoperative patient.

A CMR study in a patient with CHD includes contiguous axial images (in horizontal, coronal and sagittal views) that provide initial information about morphology and allows further detailed images in regions of interest to be acquired. In addition, serial cine images are acquired to provide comprehensive information about congenital anatomy. Currently, CMR already has clinical applications in the assessment of great artery anatomy (aorta and pulmonary arteries), venous connections (systemic and pulmonary veins), extracardiac conduits and baffles, intracardiac shunts (atrial and ventricular septal defects), and in the assessment of complex congenital heart disease.

FUNCTION AND PHYSIOLOGY ASSESSMENT IN CONGENITAL HEART DISEASE

CMR can provide information on the ventricle such as ventricular volumes, ventricular mass, stroke volume, and ejection fraction and is now established as the gold standard technique for the assessment of RV volume, mass, and function.[17, 18] Other imaging modalities such as echocardiography and angiography are able to provide this information; however, as CMR does not rely on geometric assumptions, even abnormally shaped ventricles can be assessed for volume and function. In particular, the assessment of the right ventricle is important in congenital heart disease, where it may be a subpulmonary RV and support the pulmonary circulation or may be a systemic RV and support the systemic circulation.[19]

CMR FLOW ASSESSMENT IN CONGENITAL HEART DISEASE

A CMR technique that is used to assess flow is based on the principle that the phase of flowing spins relative to stationary spins along a magnetic gradient changes in direct proportion to the velocity of flow.[20] This allows the quantification of blood flow velocity and volume flow in cardiac chambers and great vessels.[15, 21] Two sets of images are usually acquired simultaneously and then reconstructed in magnitude, providing anatomic information and in phase, providing velocity information.[20] This technique has been validated for the measurement of aortic and pulmonary flow representing left and right ventricular stroke volumes,[15, 22] thus allowing quantification of left-to-right shunts,[23] quantitative assessment of valvular regurgitation, and the peak flow velocity in valvular stenosis.[21, 24]

GADOLINIUM-ENHANCED MR ANGIOGRAPHY

The accurate diagnosis of vascular anomalies in congenital heart disease is important for both prognosis and management.[25] Contrast-enhanced MR angiography is noninvasive and provides information about vascular anatomy of the aorta, pulmonary vessels, and collateral vessels, including major aortopulmonary collaterals.[26, 27] Multiple cross-sectional images can be obtained with a single breath-hold and the images can be reconstructed offline to obtain images similar to conventional angiography, which can be viewed in multiple planes.

EVALUATION OF SPECIFIC CONGENITAL HEART LESIONS

Shunt Lesions

Atrial Septal Defects

Atrial septal defects are the most common congenital cardiac malformation diagnosed in adults and account for approximately 10% of all congenital heart lesions.[28] Many adult patients with secundum-type atrial septal defects (ASDs) are able to have these defects fixed percutaneously. Accurate delineation of not only the defect size in an atrial septal defect, but also its geometry and margins are important for the assessment of suitability for percutaneous device closure of the defect.[29] Transesophageal echocardiography has traditionally been used to assess this information, however it is semi-invasive.[30, 31] CMR (see Figure 17.1) is not only able to provide this information,[32] but provides additional information, including the amount of shunting determined from pulmonary to systemic flow (Qp:Qs) using velocity encoded cine (VEC) sequences[33, 34] and stroke volume differences. Associated anomalies including the pulmonary venous drainage can also be assessed with gadolinium-enhanced magnetic resonance angiography.[35]

Ventricular Septal Defects

Ventricular septal defects (VSD) may be an isolated finding or may be in association with complex congenital heart disease. The clinical significance of VSDs depends on the defect location, size, and magnitude of the shunt. The long-term outcome in small

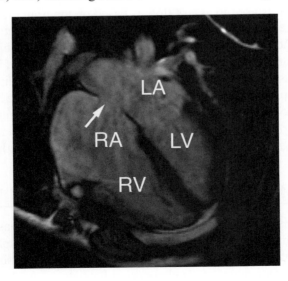

Figure 17.1

Steady state free precession CMR image in horizontal long axis view showing a secundum atrial septal defect (arrowed). Defect margins can also be clearly seen (RA, LA = right and left atria; RV, LV=right and left ventricles).

restrictive VSD is excellent.[36] VSDs associated with other cardiac anomalies or a large shunt are generally corrected in childhood. If uncorrected, these are associated with a large left-to-right shunt with progressive pulmonary and left heart dilatation.[37] Associated defects should also be assessed such as tricuspid regurgitation and regurgitation.

Conotruncal Defects

Tetralogy of Fallot

In Tetralogy of Fallot (TOF), the primary morphologic abnormality is anterocephalad deviation of the outlet septum resulting in varying degrees of right ventricular outflow tract obstruction, ventricular septal defect, an overriding aorta, and right ventricular hypertrophy. Surgical repair involves patch closure of the ventricular septal defect and an infundibular or transannular right ventricular outflow patch to relieve the obstruction.[38] The overall survival of patients who have had operative repair is excellent, reported to be 85% at 32 years.[39] However, adult patients may present with complications such as pulmonary regurgitation, residual right ventricular outflow tract (RVOT) obstruction, RV and LV dysfunction, and aortic regurgitation with or without aortic dilation.[40] Follow-up imaging thus requires assessment of right and left ventricular volumes and function, residual RVOT obstruction, VSDs, aortic root dilation, RVOT aneurysms or akinetic regions, and to quantify pulmonary regurgitation.[40-43] The timing of pulmonary valve replacement in repaired TOF remains controversial. There is however a considerable amount of research that has been published using CMR to assess repaired TOF in adults,[41, 42, 44-46] and in particular, the impact of pulmonary regurgitation on RV function and indications for pulmonary valve replacement.[43, 47-49] Detection of fibrosis with delayed gadolinium CMR after TOF repair has also been shown to have potential for arrhythmic risk stratification.[50]

Transposition of the Great Arteries

In transposition of the great arteries (TGA), the aorta arises from the right ventricle and the pulmonary artery from the left ventricle. Associated abnormalities include ventricular septal defects, left ventricular outflow tract obstruction, and coarctation of the aorta. Surgical management options include atrial switch (Mustard or Senning operations), arterial switch and the Rastelli operation.

TGA Treated by Atrial Switch Operation (Mustard and Senning Operations)

Atrial switch operations involve the removal of the atrial septum and creation of a baffle from right atrial wall and atrial septal tissue (Senning operation) or insertion of a baffle from pericardium and synthetic tissue (Mustard operation). Late survival data show the most frequent cause of death being sudden cardiac death and systemic right ventricular failure .[51] Imaging of patients after Mustard or Senning requires assessment of pulmonary venous flow path, superior and inferior vena cava limbs of the systemic venous flow paths, and systemic right ventricular function (see Figure 17.2).

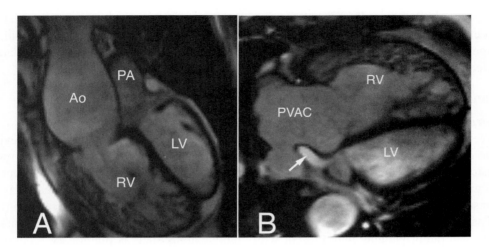

Figure 17.2

(A) CMR images after the Mustard operation showing the parallel relationship of the great vessels in a long-axis image, and (B) the baffle (arrowed) as well as the pulmonary venous atrial compartment (PVAC).

TGA Treated by Arterial Switch

The arterial switch operation involves the transection of the aorta and pulmonary artery at a level above the valve sinuses and the coronary arteries are detached from the aorta and sutured in place to the neoaorta.[52] Imaging postarterial switch requires assessment for RVOT stenosis, pulmonary artery branch stenoses, the neoaortic valve and biventricular function. The patency of the reimplanted coronaries and LV perfusion may also need assessment.

TGA Treated by Rastelli Operation

The Rastelli operation is performed in patients with TGA who also have a VSD and pulmonary or subpulmonary artery stenosis. Blood is redirected so that the systemic ventricle supports the circulation. A valved conduit is placed from the right ventricle to the pulmonary artery and left ventricular outflow is via the VSD and a patch to the aortic root. [53] Imaging requires assessment of the reconstructed flow path, RVOT, RV to pulmonary artery stenosis, LVOT, biventricular function, and possible residual shunt.

SINGLE VENTRICLE

Fontan Operations for Functionally Single Ventricle

The Fontan operation for patients born with a single effective ventricle reroutes systemic venous return to pulmonary arteries, without passage through an intervening ventricle.

Modifications to the original procedure have resulted in total cavopulmonary connection by either an intra-atrial tunnel or an extracardiac conduit.[54] Imaging following the Fontan operation requires thorough assessment of the cavopulmonary connections, the ventricle, the atrioventricular valve, the ventricular outflow tract, and any residual leaks or collaterals development. It is crucial to assess the cavopulmonary paths for obstruction and this can be done with cine CMR imaging as velocity mapping. Contrast-enhanced 3D angiography is an alternative to imaging the cavopulmonary paths.

AORTA

Aortic Coarctation

CMR allows the assessment of native coarctation diagnosed beyond childhood with a view to percutaneous intervention with stenting or surgery, to assess recoarctation or aneurysm formation in repaired coarctation, and any associated pathology such as stenosis or regurgitation of a bicuspid aortic valve, or LV hypertrophy. The nature and severity of coarctation can be obtained with cine imaging using steady-state free precession sequences and measurement of velocity across the coarctation with velocity mapping[21, 55] (see Figure 17.3).

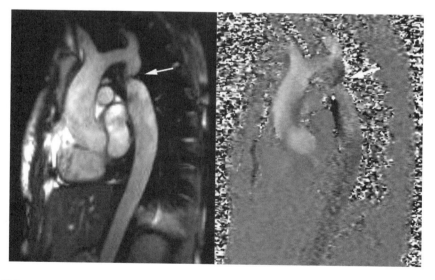

Figure 17.3

Aortic coarctation assessed with CMR using steady-state free precession cine imaging (coarctation site arrowed, beyond subclavian artery) and with "in-plane" velocity mapping.

CONCLUSION

The imaging of congenital heart disease plays a crucial role in both the initial as well as follow-up assessment and management. While echocardiography is the primary investigation of congenital heart disease, cardiovascular magnetic resonance (CMR) with its ability to give unrestricted access to cardiac structures will continue to play an increasing role in the diagnosis and follow-up of adults with congenital heart disease.

◇◇◇◇◇◇◇◇◇◇◇◇◇

REFERENCES

1. Garson A, Jr., Allen HD, Gersony WM, Gillette PC, Hohn AR, Pinsky WW, Mikhail O. The cost of congenital heart disease in children and adults. A model for multicenter assessment of price and practice variation. *Arch Pediatr Adolesc Med.* Oct 1994;148(10):1039-1045.

2. Brickner ME, Hillis LD, Lange RA. Congenital heart disease in adults. Second of two parts. *N Engl J Med.* Feb 3 2000;342(5):334-342.

3. Babu-Narayan SV, Gatzoulis MA, Kilner PJ. Non-invasive imaging in adult congenital heart disease using cardiovascular magnetic resonance. *J Cardiovasc Med (Hagerstown).* Jan 2007;8(1):23-29.

4. Weber OM, Higgins CB. MR evaluation of cardiovascular physiology in congenital heart disease: flow and function. *J Cardiovasc Magn Reson.* 2006;8(4):607-617.

5. Hirsch R, Kilner PJ, Connelly MS, Redington AN, St John Sutton MG, Somerville J. Diagnosis in adolescents and adults with congenital heart disease. Prospective assessment of individual and combined roles of magnetic resonance imaging and transesophageal echocardiography. *Circulation.* Dec 1994;90(6):2937-2951.

6. Van Praagh R. The segmental approach to diagnosis in congenital heart disease. In: Bergsma D, ed. *Birth Defects: Original Artical Series.* Baltimore: Williams & Wilkins; 1972.

7. Therrien J. Echocardiography. In: Gatzoulis MA, Webb, G.D. and Daubeney, P.E.F., ed. *Diagnosis and Management of Adult Congenital Heart Disease.* Edinburgh: Churchill Livingstone; 2003:35-47.

8. Shinebourne EA, Macartney FJ, Anderson RH. Sequential chamber localization—logical approach to diagnosis in congenital heart disease. *Br Heart J.* Apr 1976;38(4):327-340.

9. Li W, Davlouros PA, Kilner PJ, Pennell DJ, Gibson D, Henein MY, Gatzoulis MA. Doppler-echocardiographic assessment of pulmonary regurgitation in adults with repaired tetralogy of Fallot: comparison with cardiovascular magnetic resonance imaging. *Am Heart J.* Jan 2004;147(1):165-172.

10. Hoppe UC, Dederichs B, Deutsch HJ, Theissen P, Schicha H, Sechtem U. Congenital heart disease in adults and adolescents: comparative value of transthoracic and transesophageal echocardiography and MR imaging. *Radiology.* Jun 1996;199(3):669-677.

11. Marx GR, Su X. Three-dimensional echocardiography in congenital heart disease. *Cardiol Clin.* May 2007;25(2):357-365.

12. Heusch A, Rubo J, Krogmann ON, Bourgeois M. Volumetric analysis of the right ventricle in children with congenital heart defects: comparison of biplane angiography and transthoracic 3-dimensional echocardiography. *Cardiol Young.* Nov 1999;9(6):577-584.

13. Higgins CB, Byrd BF, 3rd, Farmer DW, Osaki L, Silverman NH, Cheitlin MD. Magnetic resonance imaging in patients with congenital heart disease. *Circulation.* Nov 1984;70(5):851-860.

14. Didier D, Higgins CB, Fisher MR, Osaki L, Silverman NH, Cheitlin MD. Congenital heart disease: gated MR imaging in 72 patients. *Radiology.* Jan 1986;158(1):227-235.

15. Kilner PJ, Gatehouse PD, Firmin DN. Flow measurement by magnetic resonance: a unique asset worth optimising. *J Cardiovasc Magn Reson.* 2007;9(4):723-728.

16. Wood JC. Anatomical assessment of congenital heart disease. *J Cardiovasc Magn Reson.* 2006;8(4):595-606.

17. Katz J, Whang J, Boxt LM, Barst RJ. Estimation of right ventricular mass in normal subjects and in patients with primary pulmonary hypertension by

nuclear magnetic resonance imaging. *J Am Coll Cardiol.* May 1993;21(6):1475-1481.

18. Longmore DB, Klipstein RH, Underwood SR, Firmin DN, Hounsfield GN, Watanabe M, Bland C, Fox K, Poole-Wilson PA, Rees RS, et al. Dimensional accuracy of magnetic resonance in studies of the heart. *Lancet.* Jun 15 1985;1(8442):1360-1362.

19. Davlouros PA, Niwa K, Webb G, Gatzoulis MA. The right ventricle in congenital heart disease. *Heart.* Apr 2006;92 Suppl 1:i27-38.

20. Didier D, Ratib O, Beghetti M, Oberhaensli I, Friedli B. Morphologic and functional evaluation of congenital heart disease by magnetic resonance imaging. *J Magn Reson Imaging.* Nov 1999;10(5):639-655.

21. Kilner PJ, Firmin DN, Rees RS, Martinez J, Pennell DJ, Mohiaddin RH, Underwood SR, Longmore DB. Valve and great vessel stenosis: assessment with MR jet velocity mapping. *Radiology.* Jan 1991;178(1):229-235.

22. Kondo C, Caputo GR, Semelka R, Foster E, Shimakawa A, Higgins CB. Right and left ventricular stroke volume measurements with velocity-encoded cine MR imaging: in vitro and in vivo validation. *AJR Am J Roentgenol.* Jul 1991;157(1):9-16.

23. Hundley WG, Li HF, Lange RA, Pfeifer DP, Meshack BM, Willard JE, Landau C, Willett D, Hillis LD, Peshock RM. Assessment of left-to-right intracardiac shunting by velocity-encoded, phase-difference magnetic resonance imaging. A comparison with oximetric and indicator dilution techniques. *Circulation.* Jun 15 1995;91(12):2955-2960.

24. Kilner PJ, Manzara CC, Mohiaddin RH, Pennell DJ, Sutton MG, Firmin DN, Underwood SR, Longmore DB. Magnetic resonance jet velocity mapping in mitral and aortic valve stenosis. *Circulation.* Apr 1993;87(4):1239-1248.

25. Herlong JR, Jaggers JJ, Ungerleider RM. Congenital Heart Surgery Nomenclature and Database Project: pulmonary venous anomalies. *Ann Thorac Surg.* Apr 2000;69(4 Suppl):S56-69.

26. Ferrari VA, Scott CH, Holland GA, Axel L, Sutton MS. Ultrafast three-dimensional contrast-enhanced magnetic resonance angiography and imaging in the diagnosis of partial anomalous pulmonary venous drainage. *J Am Coll Cardiol.* Mar 15 2001;37(4):1120-1128.

27. Prasad SK, Soukias N, Hornung T, Khan M, Pennell DJ, Gatzoulis MA, Mohiaddin RH. Role of magnetic resonance angiography in the diagnosis of major aortopulmonary collateral arteries and partial anomalous pulmonary venous drainage. *Circulation.* Jan 20 2004;109(2):207-214.

28. Hoffman JI, Kaplan S, Liberthson RR. Prevalence of congenital heart disease. *Am Heart J.* Mar 2004;147(3):425-439.

29. Harper RW, Mottram PM, McGaw DJ. Closure of secundum atrial septal defects with the Amplatzer septal occluder device: techniques and problems. *Catheter Cardiovasc Interv.* Dec 2002;57(4):508-524.

30. Cao Q, Radtke W, Berger F, Zhu W, Hijazi ZM. Transcatheter closure of multiple atrial septal defects. Initial results and value of two- and three-dimensional transoesophageal echocardiography. *Eur Heart J.* Jun 2000;21(11):941-947.

31. Cooke JC, Gelman JS, Harper RW. Echocardiologists' role in the deployment of the Amplatzer atrial septal occluder device in adults. *J Am Soc Echocardiogr.* Jun 2001;14(6):588-594.

32. Durongpisitkul K, Tang NL, Soongswang J, Laohaprasitiporn D, Nana A, Kangkagate C. Cardiac magnetic resonance imaging of atrial septal defect for transcatheter closure. *J Med Assoc Thai.* Aug 2002;85 Suppl 2:S658-666.

33. Beerbaum P, Korperich H, Barth P, Esdorn H, Gieseke J, Meyer H. Noninvasive quantification of left-to-right shunt in pediatric patients: phase-contrast cine magnetic resonance imaging compared with invasive oximetry. *Circulation.* May 22 2001;103(20):2476-2482.

34. Piaw CS, Kiam OT, Rapaee A, Khoon LC, Bang LH, Ling CW, Samion H, Hian SK. Use of non-invasive phase contrast magnetic resonance imaging for estimation of atrial septal defect size and morphology: a comparison with transesophageal echo. *Cardiovasc Intervent Radiol.* Mar-Apr 2006;29(2):230-234.

35. Geva T, Greil GF, Marshall AC, Landzberg M, Powell AJ. Gadolinium-enhanced 3-dimensional magnetic resonance angiography of pulmonary blood supply in patients with complex pulmonary stenosis or atresia: comparison with x-ray angiography. *Circulation.* Jul 23 2002;106(4):473-478.

36. Gabriel HM, Heger M, Innerhofer P, Zehetgruber M, Mundigler G, Wimmer M, Maurer G, Baumgartner H. Long-term outcome of patients with ventricular septal defect considered not to require surgical closure during childhood. *J Am Coll Cardiol.* Mar 20 2002;39(6):1066-1071.

37. Valente AM, Powell AJ. Clinical applications of cardiovascular magnetic resonance in congenital heart disease. *Cardiol Clin.* Feb 2007;25(1):97-110, vi.

38. Kawashima Y, Kitamura S, Nakano S, Yagihara T. Corrective surgery for tetralogy of Fallot without or with minimal right ventriculotomy and with repair of the pulmonary valve. *Circulation.* Aug 1981;64(2 Pt 2):II147-153.

39. Murphy JG, Gersh BJ, Mair DD, Fuster V, McGoon MD, Ilstrup DM, McGoon DC, Kirklin JW, Danielson GK. Long-term outcome in patients undergoing surgical repair of tetralogy of Fallot. *N Engl J Med.* Aug 26 1993;329(9):593-599.

40. Gatzoulis MA. Tetralogy of Fallot. In: Gatzoulis MA, Webb, G.D. and Daubeney, P.E.F., ed. *Diagnosis and Management of Adult Congenital Heart Disease.* Edinburgh: Churchill Livingstone; 2003:315-326.

41. Davlouros PA, Kilner PJ, Hornung TS, Li W, Francis JM, Moon JC, Smith GC, Tat T, Pennell DJ, Gatzoulis MA. Right ventricular function in adults with repaired tetralogy of Fallot assessed with cardiovascular magnetic resonance imaging: detrimental role of right ventricular outflow aneurysms or akinesia and adverse right-to-left ventricular interaction. *J Am Coll Cardiol.* Dec 4 2002;40(11):2044-2052.

42. Geva T, Sandweiss BM, Gauvreau K, Lock JE, Powell AJ. Factors associated with impaired clinical status in long-term survivors of tetralogy of Fallot repair evaluated by magnetic resonance imaging. *J Am Coll Cardiol.* Mar 17 2004;43(6):1068-1074.

43. Therrien J, Provost Y, Merchant N, Williams W, Colman J, Webb G. Optimal timing for pulmonary valve replacement in adults after tetralogy of Fallot repair. *Am J Cardiol.* Mar 15 2005;95(6):779-782.

44. Oosterhof T, Mulder BJ, Vliegen HW, de Roos A. Cardiovascular magnetic resonance in the follow-up of patients with corrected tetralogy of Fallot: a review. *Am Heart J.* Feb 2006;151(2):265-272.

45. Samyn MM, Powell AJ, Garg R, Sena L, Geva T. Range of ventricular dimensions and function by steady-state free precession cine MRI in repaired tetralogy of Fallot: right ventricular outflow tract patch vs. conduit repair. *J Magn Reson Imaging.* Oct 2007;26(4):934-940.

46. Meadows J, Powell AJ, Geva T, Dorfman A, Gauvreau K, Rhodes J. Cardiac magnetic resonance imaging correlates of exercise capacity in patients with surgically repaired tetralogy of Fallot. *Am J Cardiol.* Nov 1 2007;100(9):1446-1450.

47. Henkens IR, van Straten A, Schalij MJ, Hazekamp MG, de Roos A, van der Wall EE, Vliegen HW. Predicting outcome of pulmonary valve replacement in adult tetralogy of Fallot patients. *Ann Thorac Surg.* Mar 2007;83(3):907-911.

48. Oosterhof T, van Straten A, Vliegen HW, Meijboom FJ, van Dijk AP, Spijkerboer AM, Bouma BJ, Zwinderman AH, Hazekamp MG, de Roos A, Mulder BJ. Preoperative thresholds for pulmonary valve replacement in patients with corrected tetralogy of Fallot using cardiovascular magnetic resonance. *Circulation.* Jul 31 2007;116(5):545-551.

49. Knauth AL, Gauvreau K, Powell AJ, Landzberg MJ, Walsh EP, Lock JE, del Nido PJ, Geva T. Ventricular size and function assessed by cardiac MRI predict major adverse clinical outcomes late after tetralogy of Fallot repair. *Heart.* Feb 2008;94(2):211-216.

50. Babu-Narayan SV, Kilner PJ, Li W, Moon JC, Goktekin O, Davlouros PA, Khan M, Ho SY, Pennell DJ, Gatzoulis MA. Ventricular fibrosis suggested by cardiovascular magnetic resonance in adults with repaired tetralogy of fallot and its relationship to adverse markers of clinical outcome. *Circulation.* Jan 24 2006;113(3):405-413.

51. Gelatt M, Hamilton RM, McCrindle BW, Connelly M, Davis A, Harris L, Gow RM, Williams WG, Trusler GA, Freedom RM. Arrhythmia and mortality after the Mustard procedure: a 30-year single-center experience. *J Am Coll Cardiol.* Jan 1997;29(1):194-201.

52. Jatene AD, Fontes VF, Paulista PP, Souza LC, Neger F, Galantier M, Sousa JE. Anatomic correction of transposition of the great vessels. *J Thorac Cardiovasc Surg.* Sep 1976;72(3):364-370.

53. Rastelli GC, McGoon DC, Wallace RB. Anatomic correction of transposition of the great arteries with ventricular septal defect and subpulmonary stenosis. *J Thorac Cardiovasc Surg.* Oct 1969;58(4):545-552.

54. de Leval MR, Kilner P, Gewillig M, Bull C. Total cavopulmonary connection: a logical alternative to atriopulmonary connection for complex Fontan operations. Experimental studies and early clinical experience. *J Thorac Cardiovasc Surg.* Nov 1988;96(5):682-695.

55. Mohiaddin RH, Kilner PJ, Rees S, Longmore DB. Magnetic resonance volume flow and jet velocity mapping in aortic coarctation. *J Am Coll Cardiol.* Nov 1 1993;22(5):1515-1521.

Index

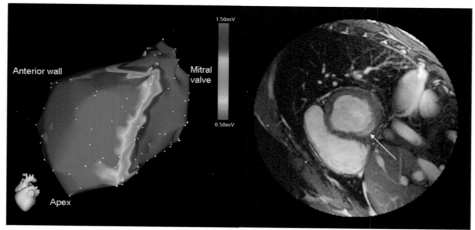

Color Plate 1

Left Panel: A voltage map of the left ventricle in a patient with a prior anterior wall infarction. The map was created by sampling electrograms point by point with a catheter maneuvered around the ventricular endocardium. The electrogram voltage is color coded and plotted in the three-dimensional structure created by this electroanatomic mapping system (CARTO™). The red area represents low voltage regions or scar with purple representing myocardium with normal voltage. The infarct borderzone is represented by the intermediate colors. The VT substrate is often contained within the scar or its border region, which can then be identified with further mapping and potentially targeted for catheter ablation. Right Panel: Cardiac MRI in a different patient. This demonstrates delayed hyperenhancement (arrow) in the subendocardium of the anterior wall of the left ventricle, consistent with scar from a prior infarct.

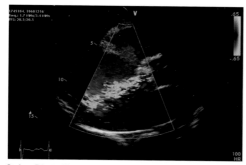

Color Plate 2

Severe aortic regurgitation directed over the anterior mitral valve leaflet. The left ventricle is moderately enlarged.

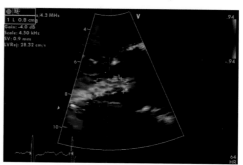

Color Plate 3

Zoomed view of the vena contracta (arrows) in severe aortic regurgitation.

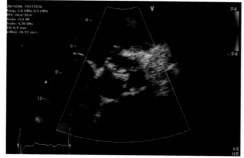

Color Plate 4

Central jet of aortic regurgitation seen from the short-axis view.

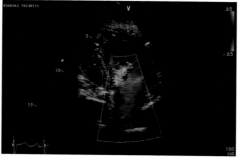

Color Plate 5

Apical 4-chamber view of aortic regurgitation mixing with mitral inflow.

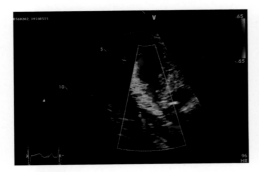

Color Plate 6

Apical long-axis view of severe aortic regurgitation during diastasis.

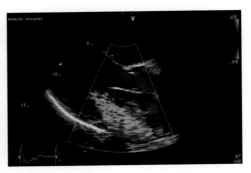

Color Plate 7

Long-axis view of severe mitral regurgitation. The jet occupies most of the atrium, has a wide vena contracta, and has proximal flow acceleration.

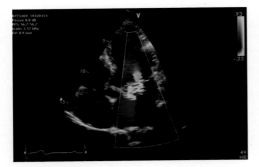

Color Plate 8

Apical 4-chamber view of severe mitral regurgitation due to posterior leaflet pathology.

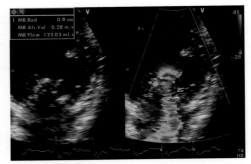

Color Plate 9

Zoomed 4-chamber view of severe mitral regurgitation showing a wide vena contracta and a pronounced PISA.

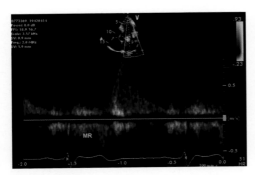

Color Plate 10

Systolic flow reversal in the pulmonary veins as recorded by pulse wave Doppler is a sign of moderate to severe mitral regurgitation.

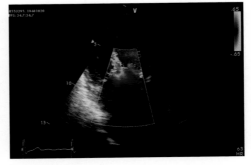

Color Plate 11

Apical 3-chamber view showing flow acceleration/aliasing as blood crosses the stenosed mitral valve.

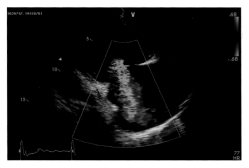

Color Plate 12

Parasternal right ventricular inflow view of severe tricuspid regurgitation.

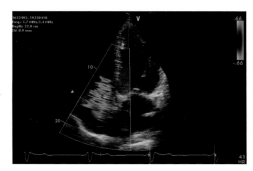

Color Plate 13

4-Chamber view of severe tricuspid regurgitation.

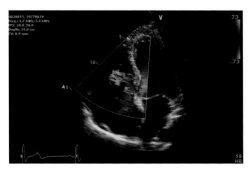

Color Plate 14

Severe tricuspid regurgitation in Ebstein's anomaly with jet directed behind the relatively immobile septal leaflet.

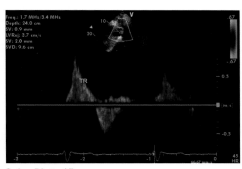

Color Plate 15

Reversal of hepatic vein flow in severe tricuspid regurgitation.

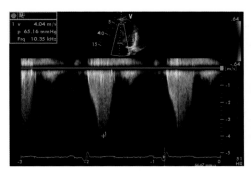

Color Plate 16

Dagger-shaped continuous wave Doppler indicating dynamic LV outflow obstruction.

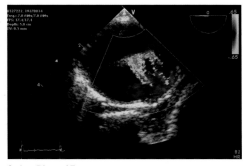

Color Plate 17

Surgically constructed fenestrations ensure equalization of pressure between the lumens.

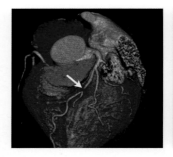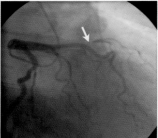

Color Plate 18

With coronary CTA, tight stenosis without calcifications can well be visualized. However, retrograde filling of distal coronary segments remain a pitfall in CTA.

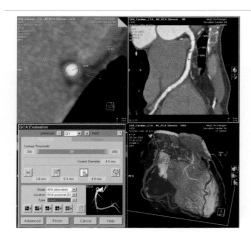

Color Plate 19

Postprocessing software may help in the reporting of a coronary CTA dataset by quantifying the degree of stenosis.

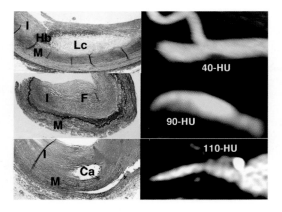

Color Plate 20

The difference in density might give an idea of the component of atherosclerotic plaques in the coronary arteries. Low dense plaques more likely contain lipid or thrombus material, intermediate dense plaques commonly consist of fibrous tissue and calcium.

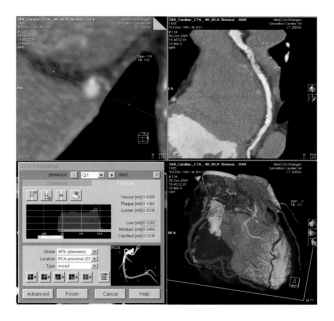

Color Plate 21

Postprocessing software may support in the assessment of atherosclerotic coronary plaques. However, the measurement is often difficult to reproduce.

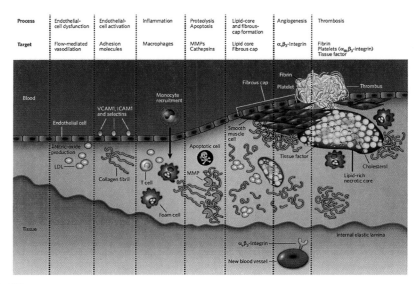

Color Plate 22

Simplified representation of the development and progression of an atherosclerotic lesion. Pathophysiological processes and associated potential targets for molecular imaging of atherothrombosis are indicated. ICAM: intercellular adhesion molecule; LDL: low-density lipoprotein; MMP: matrix metalloproteinase; NO: nitric oxide; VCAM1, vascular cell adhesion molecule-1.

Modified from Sanz & Fayad 2008.

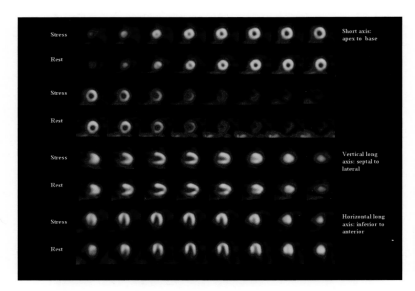

Color Plate 23

Normal stress rest perfusion images in a patient who had Tc-99m Sestamibi for rest and stress imaging.

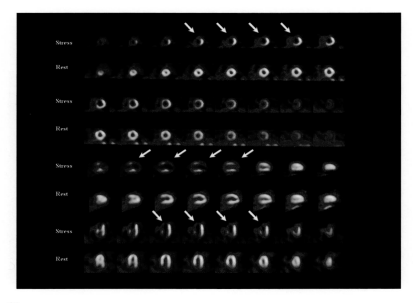

Color Plate 24

Abnormal stress perfusion and normal rest perfusion in a patient who had Tc-99m Sestamibi for rest and stress imaging. The perfusion defect is in the vascular territory of the left anterior descending coronary artery. Additionally, there is a visual impression of dilation of the left ventricular cavity on stress images compared to the rest images. This suggests transient ischemic dilation of the ventricle, and occurs with severe and extensive myocardial ischemia.

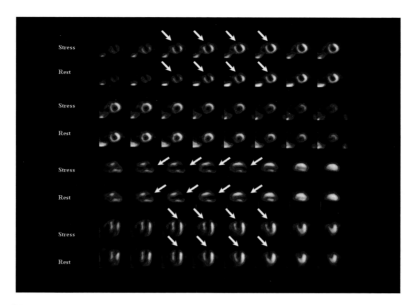

Color Plate 25

Abnormal stress and rest perfusion imaging in a patient with prior left anterior descending coronary artery infarction. The ventricular cavity shape is abnormal, consistent with presence of remodeling of the ventricle, associated with apical thinning and aneurysm.

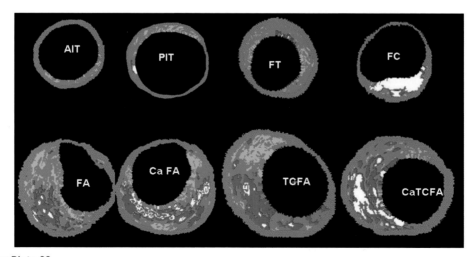

Color Plate 26

IVUS-Virtual Histology proposed lesion types. AIT: adaptative intimal thickening; PIT: pathological intimal thickening; FT: fibrotic plaque; FC: fibrocalcific; FA: fibroatheroma; CaFA: calcified fibroatheroma; TCFA: thin-capped fibroatheroma.

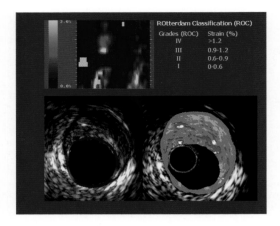

Color Plate 27

IVUS-palpography. In the upper left side, the palpography strain map is opened up. The local strain is calculated from the gated radiofrequency traces using cross-correlation analysis and displayed, color-coded, from blue (for 0% strain) to red to yellow (for 2% strain). Plaque strain values are assigned a Rotterdam Classification (ROC) score ranging from 1 to 4 (ROC I = 0—< 0.6%; ROC II = 0.6—< 0.9%; ROC III = 0.9—< 1.2%; ROC IV = >1.2 %). At the bottom, in the same cross-sectional area a high-strain spot (ROC III) is shown (left); in the Virtual Histology (VH) image (right) a confluent necrotic core area in contact with the lumen is seen, suggesting an IVUS-derived thin capped fibroatheroma. The IVUS-VH color-code is fibrous tissue (green), fibro-fatty tissue (light green), necrotic core (red) and dense calcium (white).

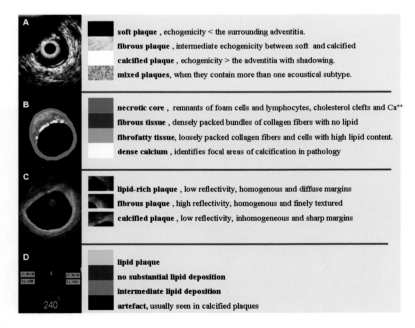

Color Plate 28

Multi-imaging in the coronary arteries. The same coronary segment (represented by one frame) has been imaged by 4 different imaging techniques: grayscale IVUS (panel A), IVUS-virtual histology (panel B), optical coherence tomography (panel C) and intravascular magnetic resonance spectroscopy (IVMR). Of note, in the upper left quadrant of the plaque, a calcified area is seen in three imaging modalities, but not in IVMR where an artifact is observed. On the right hand side, the different plaque and tissues types across the coronary imaging techniques is shown.

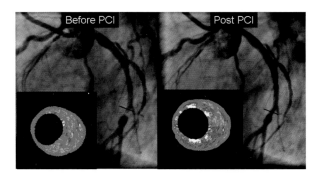

Color Plate 29

IVUS-virtual histology in stented segments. In the left hand side, a coronary angiogram of the left coronary system shows on the distal segment of the left circumflex artery an eccentric lesion. A prestenting Virtual Histology (VH) frame showed a fibrotic type of plaque (location of VH frame is indicated by a black line). On the right hand side, the post-stenting VH frame is depicted. Of note, at the lumen and surrounding areas an increase in the amount of "dense calcium" and "necrotic core" is observed. This is due to the presence of stent struts that are misclassified by VH. PCI, percutaneous coronary intervention.

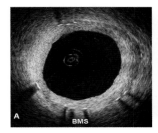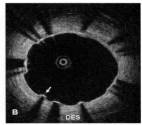

Color Plate 30

OCT and stent. Panel A: Demonstrates the optical coherence tomography (OCT) imaging of a bare metal stent 4 months following implantation. The circumferential tissue struts are visible with shadowing induced by the metal. The neointimal tissue measured between 140 and 220 microns in thickness. Panel B: OCT imaging of a drug-eluting stent (DES) at 4 months follow-up showing the circumferential struts with a very thin neointimal layer (10–40 microns thick). The arrow indicates a strut with no visible tissue coverage.

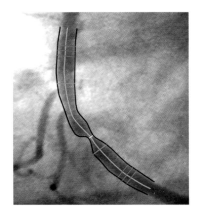

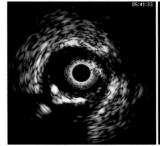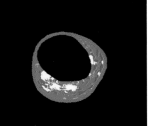

Color Plate 31

Illustrative example of measurements obtained during quantitative coronary angiography.

Color Plate 32

Illustrative example of plaque composition derived from radiofrequency analysis of intravascular ultrasound imaging.

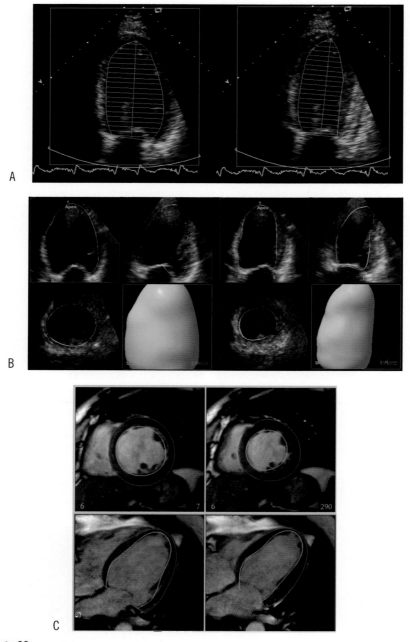

Color Plate 33

Comparison of end-systolic and end-diastolic LV volumes with 2D and 3D echocardiography against the reference standard of cardiac magnetic resonance. Analysis of LV volume using 2DE Simpson's method of discs (A) shows an EDV of 204 mls and ESV of 141 mls. Analysis of LV volume using 3DE (B) shows an EDV of 262 mls and ESV of 165 mls. The use of cardiac magnetic resonance (CMR) (C) shows EDV of 272 mls and ESV of 174 mls. The use of this guide-point CMR approach requires long-axis images for orientation of the apex and base, with measurements performed in the short-axis views.

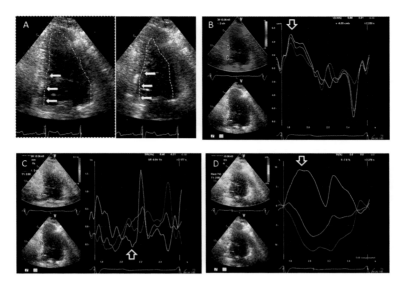

Color Plate 34

Application of quantitative techniques to evaluate regional function after myocardial infarction. Standard 2D echocardiography (A) shows akinesis of the basal and mid inferior walls (arrows). Tissue velocities (B) show a minor gradation of systolic velocity (open arrow) from base to apex, but reduced basal function is not appreciated due to tethering. Strain rate imaging (C) shows reduced and delayed basal inferior systolic strain rate (yellow line, marked with open arrow), with minor delay of the midwall segment (turquoise). Tissue velocity-based strain (D) shows lengthening of the basal septal segment (open arrow) and reduction of the midwall segment (turquoise).

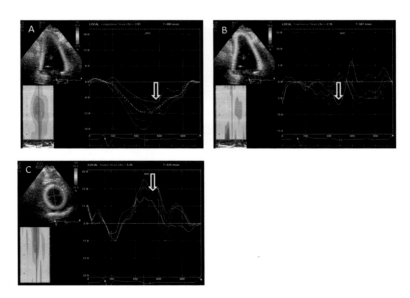

Color Plate 35

Longitudinal (A) and radial (B) assessments of 2D strain from the apical view show delay of the basal inferior systolic strain (yellow line, marked with open arrow). The mid-inferior wall dysfunction is more readily appreciated on radial strain (blue and purple curves) in the mid-LV short axis (C).

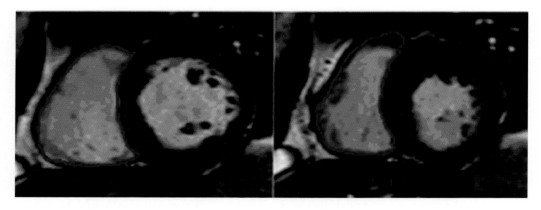

Color Plate 36

Assessment of RV volumes and EF using CMR. The left panel shows EDV, with ESV on the right panel.

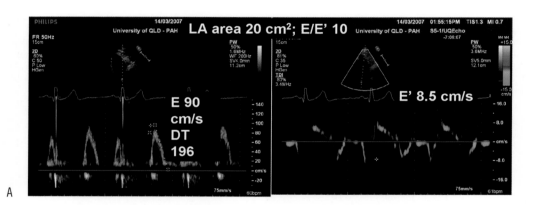

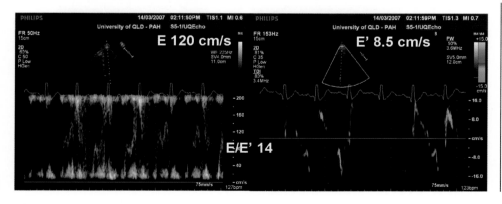

Color Plate 37

Assessment of LV filling pressure using the E/E' ratio at rest (A) and after exercise (B).

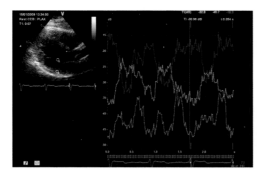

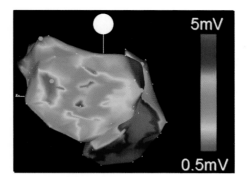

Color Plate 38

Measurement of integrated backscatter (IB) from an image in raw data format. Myocardium (in yellow) shows cyclic variation of IB. Calibrated IB is based on comparison of reflectivity relative to pericardium (red) or blood-pool (blue).

Color Plate 39

Voltage map created with the CARTO mapping system. Using a Navistar™ mapping/ablation catheter, which has a location sensor in its tip; contact with the myocardial wall allows the recording of a local bipolar electrogram. The maximum amplitude of the voltage may be represented on the constructed anatomy as a continuum of color from low voltage (0.5mV) to high voltage (5mV).

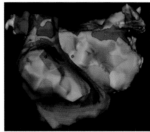
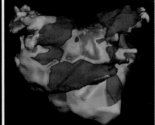

Color Plate 40

Automated comflex fractionated electrogram mapping with NavX Fusion™.

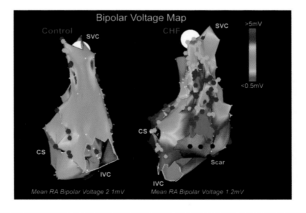

Color Plate 41

Bipolar right atrial voltage mapping using the CARTO mapping system in congestive cardiac failure. Voltage is color-coded on the right hand scale (red areas are low voltage, blue areas are the highest voltage). Areas of gray indicate scar (voltage ≤ 0.05mV). In congestive cardiac failure, the mapping defined areas of low atrial voltage, electrical silence, and widespread fractionated signals.

Printed with permission from Sanders et al.[1]

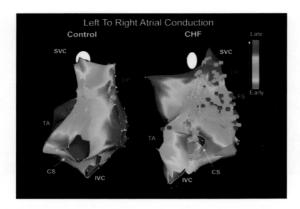

Color Plate 42

Left to right atrial conduction in patients with congestive cardiac failure.

Printed with permission from Sanders et al.[1]

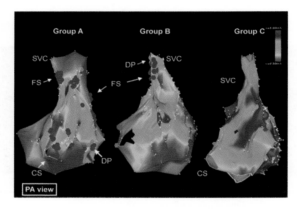

Color Plate 43

Electroanatomical bipolar voltage mapping in three age groups. (Group A ≥ 60, Group B 31–59, Group C ≤ 30). Voltage is color-coded on the right hand scale (red areas are low voltage, blue areas are the highest voltage). The mapped bipolar voltage was significantly lower at all right atrial sites in the older age groups. Notice the clustering of fractionated signals and double potentials on the right atrial posterior wall.

Printed with permission from Kistler et al.[2]

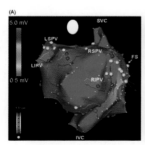 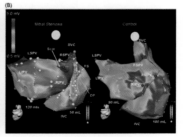

Color Plate 44

Electroanatomical map of a patient with mitral stenosis (A) Voltage is color-coded on the left-hand scale (red areas are low voltage, blue areas are the highest voltage) Gray areas denote scar with recorded voltages 0.05 mS. (B) Note the markedly enlarged LA (100ml) resulted in significant deformation and compression of the RA (58ml). In this extreme example observed, both atria demonstrate extensive regions of low voltage associated with regions of scar and fractionated signals (FS, pink tags).

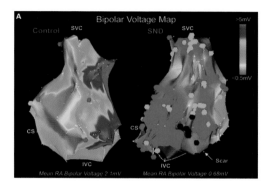
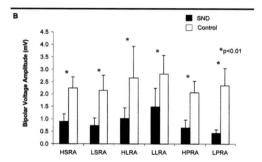

Color Plate 45

(A) Bipolar voltage mapping in a patient with sinus node disease (right) and an age-matched control (left). Areas of electrical silence (voltages ≤ 0.05 mV) are demonstrated in gray. The patient with sinus node disease demonstrates significantly greater number of double potentials (blue dots) and fractionated signals (brown dots). (B) Regional bipolar voltage showing a reduction in average voltage in each atrial site analyzed.

Printed with permission from Sanders et al.[3]

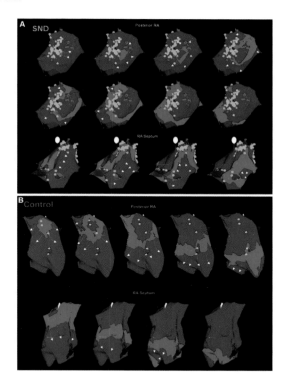

Color Plate 46

Propagation map across the right atrium in sinus node disease (SND) compared to controls. In sinus node disease (A), there are numerous sites of slowed conduction (brown dots—fractionated signals) and conduction block (blue dots—double potentials) with marked heterogeneity in depolarization septally and anteriorly. In controls (B), there is simultaneous activation of the crista terminalis (yellow dots) with rapid depolarization septally and anteriorly.

Printed with permission from Sanders et al.[3]

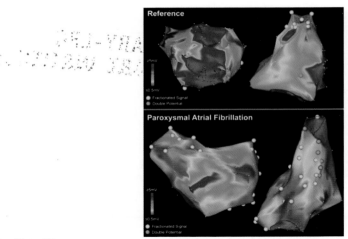

Color Plate 47

Electroanatomical mapping in paroxysmal atrial fibrillation. Representative CARTO maps of a patient with atrial fibrillation (bottom) and a reference patient (top). In addition to having greater regions of low voltage (red), the patient with atrial fibrillation has more evidence of conduction abnormalities in the form of fractionated signals (pink tags) and double potentials (blue tags). They were mainly found clustered at the high-posterior and high-septal right atrial regions and the left atrial septum and roof.

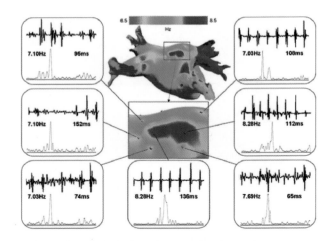

Color Plate 48

Relationship between dominant frequency and complex fractionated electrograms in drug-refractory atrial fibrillation. Anterosuperior view of the left atrium with the roof en face displaying dominant frequency (DF) data on a color spectrum. High DF areas (blue-purple) are seen in the pulmonary veins, basal left atrial appendage, and the left atrial roof. A zoomed view of the area of high DF at the roof is shown with the corresponding points (inset). One second electrograms, frequency spectra (3–15Hz), and corresponding DF and complex fractionated electrogram-mean (CFE-mean) values for each of the local seven points contributing to the color map are shown in linked boxes. The central point of highest DF is fast and regular, with surrounding points showing either increased CFE-mean suggesting increased fractionation of electrograms in that area, lower DF, or both.

1. Sanders P, Morton JB, Davidson NC, Spence SJ, Vohra JK, Sparks PB, Kalman JM. Electrical remodeling of the atria in congestive heart failure: electrophysiological and electroanatomic mapping in humans. *Circulation* 2003;108(12):1461-1468.

2. Kistler PM, Sanders P, Fynn SP, Stevenson IH, Spence SJ, Vohra JK, Sparks PB, Kalman JM. Electrophysiologic and electroanatomic changes in the human atrium associated with age. *J Am Coll Cardiol* 2004;44(1):109-116.

3. Sanders P, Kistler PM, Morton JB, Spence SJ, Kalman JM. Remodeling of sinus node function in patients with congestive heart failure: reduction in sinus node reserve. *Circulation* 2004;110(8):897-903.